Best Wishes,

'L.A. 2000:'

Sex Asylum

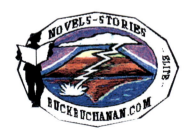

'L.A. 2000:'
Sex Asylum

A Contemporary Novel

By

Buck Buchanan

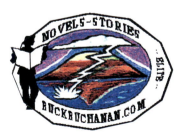

Editorial & Graphics work by ~
Sandy St. Pierre

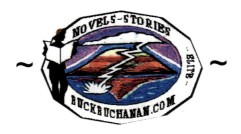

Copyright © 2000, 2001 by Buck Buchanan
All rights reserved. No part of this book may be reproduced, stored in a retrieval system, or transmitted by any means, electronic, mechanical, photocopying, recording or otherwise, without written permission from the author.

ISBN 0-75960-975-6

This book is printed on acid free paper.

1stBooks - rev. 3/19/01

Special thanks to Kevin Kearney
For his 5' X 6' original oil painting
'Elysian Fields,'
Used for the cover layout
~ View Kearney paintings at BUCKBUCHANAN.COM ~

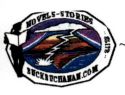 ~ **READER COMMENTS ON THE NOVEL** ~

From: Dr. David Simon: davidraphaelsimon@compuserve.com
Clearwater Medical Center, Clearwater, FL
To: Buck Buchanan: BUCKBUCHANAN.COM
Subject: *'L.A. 2000:' Sex Asylum*

Hello Buck!!

I wanted to let you know that I just finished ***'L.A. 2000:' Sex Asylum***, and thoroughly enjoyed it! In fact, I couldn't put it down. I don't know if you wanted feedback or not, Buck, but I thought I'd offer you my two cents.

I really like the way you write. In particular I enjoyed the seamless way in which you conveyed your philosophical ideas about love, religion, and psychology through the characters in **Sex Asylum** without seeming preachy and without interrupting the flow of the story and the integrity of the characters. I also really enjoyed the richness of your metaphors and your use of language. What was it you said about the smog laying over L.A. "like plastic wrap over a chocolate cake," or something like that. The characters were all very 'real,' believable, and alive to me, and the story itself was extremely engrossing. As I said, it was difficult for me to put it down once I got into it.

So that's my 2 cents, Buck. I thoroughly enjoyed reading ***'L.A. 2000:' Sex Asylum***. You've made me a fiction reader once again!

All the best,
Dr. David Simon

* * *

From: Barbara Lee, Ph.D.: lee@hal.fmhi.usf.edu
Louis de la Parte Florida Mental Health Institute
University of South Florida, Tampa, FL 33612
To: Buck Buchanan: BUCKBUCHANAN.COM
Subject: *'L.A. 2000:' Sex Asylum*

Hi, Buck!

Hope the new century is looking optimistic.

How's your new book of short stories coming along? My own writing is going way slow.... chapter due Dec 31 isn't done yet. Curses.

Since I haven't gotten to the comment that I promised you, let me try an off-the-cuff one...

I was a little skeptical of the setting for *'L.A. 2000:' Sex Asylum*, because I have worked, as well as been a patient in, those kinds of mental health programs. At first, it annoyed me a little that it seemed like a therapist was getting away with behavior that would never be tolerated...or would it?! While written a little large (murder is, after all, kind of uncommon in any work setting,) the effect of power -- or the lack of it -- on the characters rang true as the Liberty Bell before it cracked.

I quickly came to a point where I could not put it down, caring about and *needing* to know what would happen to the characters, and even the "bad guys." The sexuality/sensuality scenes were wonderful, explicit without being pornographic. No one who has not been in a mental hospital against their will, in restraints, could appreciate fully the portrayal of the patients and their experiences.

I was one of the lucky ones who does have this special appreciation, and the plot and characters unfolded for me smoothly, not giving away the end until the end, and then doing so in a most satisfactory way!

I hope to see more of this kind of writing from you, Buck!

Best regards,
Barbara Lee, Ph.D.

* * *

Chapter 1

Morton Allison eased to a stop in front of his small apartment just south of the Santa Monica Freeway, a little north of View Park. It was 3:00 a.m., that eerie, incomprehensible moment in Los Angeles when all became silent for ten breathless minutes before resuming its frenzy of sirens and faraway bursts of gunfire.

Morton sighed and glanced into the bed of the old half-ton pickup at his camping gear, all covered over with highway dust. It had been a long drive in from the mountains. His left arm was in a cast up to the elbow. He had to reach across with his right to shoulder the door open. That's what you got when you mixed it up too close in other people's lives, broken bones.

The place seemed different somehow. Smaller maybe? Or was it regret he was feeling for turning in his resignation and bolting the Fraction House without a decent goodbye to his friends? He'd become lonely in his heart, and he wanted out of schizophrenia. For that matter, he'd been talking about leaving California altogether. He'd done all he could at Dar/Neese, he felt. Getting sucked deeper into the lives of the insane wouldn't do anybody any good.

As he walked across the worn spot in the grass Morton heard a tiny rattle. The next door neighbors were peering at him from behind their louvered glass windows. They wouldn't speak, he'd come to expect that, yet through the moonlight he could make out their chilling scowls, the old L.A. anonymity weighing them down.

Before he left Dar/Neese Morton tried to get this idea through to the hot new blonde, Annise Chastain, in their training sessions. The bottom line was that the *clients* were besieged by this schizophrenic anonymity of the heart. Maybe he should have sensed something off-kilter, what with her quick-draw defenses of things Morton considered pretty frivolous. About her name, for instance. "It's not *Anise*, Morton. Please, that's a cocktail. Try to say it right, will you? It sounds exactly like 'Denise' only with a kind of cool European accent, if you know what I mean." He didn't know, of course. And as far as weirdo psychological concepts regarding L.A.'s Collective Unconscious insanity—alas, with Annise so many of Morton's ideas just wouldn't seem to take. Well, so be it. Accept what you couldn't change in a woman, that was his motto, but for Godsake don't let a fluke of nature, like her stunning looks for instance, cause you to seek haven in passion too early.

The neighbors continued to glare as Morton approached with his nylon traveling bag. Something was up.

He paused under the awning's tattered moon shadow to fish for his key. He glanced down. A stain of blood as big as a person's liver was pooled on the landing. It was fresh and shiny, just beginning to gel in the thick night air. The door, he noticed, was ajar.

Morton stepped off the landing and edged alongside the building. He stretched to his tiptoes and was able to see through the front window.

On the small oriental rug in front of his recliner, slashed over with bars of moonlight, lay the body of a woman. She was bent into the self-protective fetal curl Morton had become familiar with as a Psychiatric Counselor at the Dar/Neese Fraction House. Dr. Harvey Mueller, the Freudian, had labeled this posture 'Fear Factor A' in his scholarly papers, and for once Morton hadn't disagreed.

He reached into his rear pocket and withdrew the cellophane packet containing his ever present pair of latex gloves. In the asylum or in the street he was never without these, precaution against those messy eventualities that tended to crop up with the more radical clients. He snapped one over his good hand with a second nature so ingrained he hardly associated it with crisis. Yes, he was still in the contact mode.

Morton hurried inside. He knelt and carefully turned the woman by her shoulders.

"Muriel! My God, what's happened to you?" he exclaimed.

A puddle of vomit was seeping into the rug under her chin. Her eyes were dark and sunken, her lips ballooned like two sausages. She was wearing a frock dress, oddly one Morton hadn't seen before. He could see day old scabs where it had slipped off her shoulders and ridden up over her knees. Splotches of red showed through the fabric at her crotch. He leapt to the phone and started to dial 911. But no, it was dead. The utilities had lapsed weeks ago when he first decided to leave L.A.

Muriel coughed and began to spit blood. Morton saw then how she had her hand wedged in that stylized way across her face. One finger was jammed into her ear, one covered her eye, another pushed closed the nostril. Her thumb pressed hard across her lips. He recognized this as one of her old defense mechanisms, a self-distortion of the senses designed to block out events she didn't feel strong enough to handle. This fingers to the face business had always preceded a full-fledged breakdown.

Morton pried her hands from her face. Her pupils were shrunken to pinpoints, indicative of narcotic use. This was strange. She'd always been limited to antidepressants and mood elevators. Occasionally Harvey tossed in a tranquilizer to keep her leveled off, but never narcotics.

"Muriel, how did you get here? Did you take street drugs? Were you raped?" He thought a moment. "Did that goddamn Joseph have anything to do with this?"

Joseph Schopen was the rakish Clinical Supervisor at the Fraction House, one of your Italian looking ladies' man types who used a dandyish approach to disarm his prey. Joseph was Harvey's strong arm man in the trenches. The Gestapo, Morton called him, though for legal reasons you had to be careful about your accusations these days.

Muriel gave a tense shake of her head. "No, Joseph didn't have anything to do with it."

Morton lit a candle. He eased Muriel against the base of the recliner. Then he jerked off his T-shirt, wet it from the dusty, half full fifth of vodka he'd left on the coffee table, and began wiping at the blood and spittle around her mouth. Some of her teeth were loose and oozing out a weird yellowish fluid. She was worn out and ravaged, but underneath all the dirt and bruises as beautiful and unpretentious as ever.

"I'm going next door to call an ambulance," said Morton.

He started away, but Muriel clutched herself low where the blood stain was and gave a violent dry heave.

"Jesus Christ! Were you stabbed? Look, we've got to get these clothes off you!" cried the counselor.

Morton grabbed the steak knife he used to open mail and started hacking at the flimsy cotton dress. He ripped a jagged line from hem to neck, then peeled it slowly apart. She had no panties on, no bra. Bloody smears streaked like willow branches over her thighs. Morton doused again with the vodka and wiped frantically at the stains.

"I know this stings. I'll be gentle," he said.

Though traumatized, Muriel became immediately aware of the rough plastic cast as he tended to her. Her eyes grew big.

"Oh, no, I really did break it," she said beginning to stroke his arm. "I'm so sorry, Morton. I was trying to *stop* you from falling down those steps. You know that, don't you?"

On top of all the swelling he saw tears beginning.

"I know," soothed the counselor.

"Morton—" All at once she gasped, "I love you. I love you so much!"

The words came in a raspy whisper. They were barely audible through the bubbles of blood and gleaming saliva. This was Muriel Gonska for you, enthusiastic to the very end.

Her hand quivered as she touched the blondish two weeks' growth on Morton's face. Her eyes were blue glaciers with small, conic volcanoes flaming inside, quite striking even for a schizophrenic. In terms of mental health she'd come a long way from those early days two years ago when she was first discharged from Roselawn, the state mental institution.

"Your hair is so yellow. You've been in the sun," said Muriel. She drooled a bit of saliva. "Your jaws look hollow.

You're handsomer. But you haven't been eating right, have you?"

Morton peeled off the rubber glove. He cupped her face.

"How did you get in here, Muriel? Can you please tell me what's going on?"

"I used your spare key," she said.

"My spare key?"

"I knew where it was from when we came here with Joseph that time. You were so proud of your new apartment. But you'd locked yourself out. You'd hidden a key under the bush. Remember?"

"But Muriel, look at you. I mean—"

She laid her arms heavily over Morton's shoulders. In her exhaustion she began to draw him toward her. The cut away pieces of the dress flopped off her hips exposing her youthful nakedness to the soft, flickering light of the candle.

"Help me, Morton," she uttered low. "Please help me."

The counselor shook his head. "What am I going to do with you, Muriel?" he muttered. "What in the world am I going to do with you?"

She looked longingly at him. "What do you *want* to do with me?" she said.

* * *

Chapter 2

Suddenly a powerful white light flooded the room. Morton raised the cast to shield his eyes. People gathering on the landing. Vehicles were screeching to a halt out front. One was an ambulance, for he could see the red strobe flashing erratically across the ceiling.

"Good Lord! He's raped her!" someone cried.

The counselor knew the voice. It was Joseph Schopen, the Gestapo.

"Don't move, Allison. Just don't make any moves," hissed Joseph. "Goddamn, Harvey, look what he's done to her!"

Morton felt the floors creak as all three hundred pounds of Dr. Harvey Mueller lumbered into the room.

The fierce beam of Joseph's five-cell flashlight skidded wildly over Muriel's flesh. He pointed at the steak knife, which rested cockeyed on her bare stomach.

"He's stabbed her," declared Joseph.

There was a jittery, hair on end tremor in Joseph's words that didn't mix well with his square jaw and steel arm tactics. The Gestapo stared Muriel up and down the way he did those girls in the boob bars he frequented. One thing about Joseph Schopen—he'd always been blatant regarding his lechery, which *was* a kind of honesty, wasn't it?

"Joseph, I'm glad you're here," began Morton.

In the confusion the counselor accidentally bumped Muriel's legs farther apart. The moment turned strangely sordid. Morton was still clutching the half empty fifth of Sopov vodka he'd been using to treat Muriel's wounds.

Joseph shot forward and snatched the bottle. He caught Morton's cast with his jodhpur style boot and wedged it against the base of the recliner. Harvey shook his great head at the sad spectacle.

The paramedics stormed in with stainless steel suitcases and giant flood lights. In the hubbub Morton and Joseph were shoved aside. The Gestapo swaggered to the door and angled his muscular, weightlifter's physique as if to bar Morton's exit.

"I just got home. She was here when I—" began the counselor.

"Shut up," said Joseph. He turned to Harvey. "I've suspected something like this out of him all along."

Beads of perspiration sprouted on the doctor's cheeks and forehead. He began to frantically pat his pockets. The psychiatrist wasn't fast at many things, but in a blink he found his thumb-size nitroglycerin vial and slipped one of the tablets under his tongue.

Through the screen door Morton could see another vehicle pulling up. It was a van. Even from a distance the bold printing on the side was clearly visible. ROSELAWN STATE MENTAL INSTITUTION, it said.

"Damn, it's Priscilla," whispered Harvey. He checked his watch. "And our Second isn't here yet."

~~~

Priscilla. That would be Priscilla Daddio, Ph.D., Roselawn's own infamous Clinical Supervisor. Two years ago Priscilla had let Muriel and her enormous funding block slip through Roselawn's greedy hands. She wasn't about to have it happen again. Her pitch black hair was up, but as usual the pins weren't holding and long tails bounced over her ears as she hustled across the street.

Joseph said, "I'll handle this. She's got no right busting in here."

Morton noticed for the first time the compact Sharp camcorder slung over Joseph's shoulder. This was used to update the documentary he'd been keeping of Muriel's progress. She'd become their showcase client, and if things went right she would soon be living on her own in the frightening outside world. This would give Dar/Neese a sort of super accreditation and thereby bring in the hefty state funds.

Morton took a swift step and jerked the camcorder, lanyard and all, right off Joseph's arm. Quickly he swung it toward Muriel and the paramedics and pulled the trigger. He was able to spin a full 360 degrees before the Gestapo got a chokehold on the counselor.

"What's the matter?" grunted Morton tugging at Joseph's forearm. "Don't want to document a regression in your prize pupil? It'd look awfully bad for the Fraction House." Joseph tightened his grip. "Priscilla could swipe Muriel and her money right from under your nose. Not to mention the fifty thousand her old man slips you under the table each year."

The broken wrist made Morton an inept fighter. Joseph's gold chains jingled in the counselor's ear. The Gestapo's irritating *Paca Roma* cologne mixed with the odor of his last smoked cigarette. Morton's eyes watered.

Joseph regained control of his camcorder. He stepped back and aimed it flush at the counselor, moving it side to side across his bare chest. Morton tried to stop him, but the supervisor kneed him aside with one of his homespun martial arts moves. The videotape hummed as Joseph scanned Muriel's exposed body and zoomed in on her private parts.

"Priscilla's here!" called Priscilla Daddio from the doorway. She pushed up her hair and squeezed past Harvey.

"What is Joseph Schopen doing to Morton? And why is Muriel Gonska naked?" she asked.

Priscilla had the curious habit of addressing everyone, including herself, by their given name. This was due to her belief that mental illness was brought on, more or less, by the use of personal pronouns. You. I. Her. Me. These words, she believed, splintered a patient's understanding as to exactly whose identity was being discussed. According to Priscilla, if you didn't know yourself by your rightful name then who the hell were you? This kind of confusion, to Priscilla Daddio's mind, could drive a person plumb crazy in short order.

A police car pulled up. Harvey tugged Joseph aside.

"Get that Priscilla out of here," he said to Joseph. "And make sure the cops stay outside. If they arrest Allison Roselawn will get Muriel for sure."

Joseph gripped Priscilla's arm and hustled her into the courtyard. They made a good looking couple until you realized how much they hated each other. Both harbored aspirations for the Dar/Neese Directorship, Harvey's position, but neither had the class to be very secretive about it.

Harvey positioned himself in the doorway. He was a doctor, yes, but he was a soft, approachable guy nonetheless. Morton eased over.

"How you doing, Harvey?"

"Not bad," he said affably.

They looked on as the paramedics attended to Muriel. After a little first aid she didn't seem as bad off as Morton originally feared. She was haggard and ashen, but not verging on death by a long shot.

"I didn't do anything to her, Harvey. You know that, don't you?" said Morton.

Harvey shrugged his mammoth shoulders. He wore a dark brown beard threaded with bright strands of gray, very attractive, really.

"Probably you didn't. But we've got to document it anyway," said the Freudian.

"How did you know she was here? I didn't even know until an hour ago," said Morton.

Harvey reached into his suit coat for his pipe.

"Well, we made Muriel her own Guardian. You know, to get her ready for the apartment. I guess she took advantage of us. She bolted the day after you quit."

"She's been out two weeks?" said the counselor, shocked.

Harvey stroked his beard thoughtfully. "That's right. There were only a few places she could run to. Her parents, which wasn't likely. Roselawn. Or, well, here. We all know how close you two were."

"You do?"

"We're not as blind as you make us out, Allison. We told the police to contact Dar/Neese if there was an alert from any of those places. I guess your neighbors called. Frankly, we'd about given up hope."

"I see," said Morton.

"I'm not sure how Roselawn knew," continued the psychiatrist. "I wouldn't put it past Priscilla to be monitoring the police shortwave. She's shrewd, you know."

"I know," agreed Morton.

A red sports car zoomed up, jumped the low curb and came to a halt in the middle of the courtyard. Morton peered through the screen door.

"Ahhh, here comes our Second," said Harvey.

"Annise? *She's* your Second!" exclaimed Morton.

"Why not? You trained her for your position, didn't you?"

"Uh, yeah. But she's not skilled enough yet. I mean, she *admits* she's not skilled enough."

~~~

A 'Legal Second' was the formal term for a person brought in to witness some bizarre incident with one of the clients. In fact, Morton himself, knowing the value of affidavits when it came to discrepancies of opinion, had been the innovator of this procedure. Such advice to Harvey and Joseph in those early days got him quickly up the Fraction House ladder. Later though his ideas were seen as a little too perceptive, a little threatening to the higher ups.

Ideally the Second would be one of the direct-contact counselors. This person was charged with writing up an eye witness account meant to put into perspective the biases of the police, Roselawn, the Fraction House Administration, and so on. Seconds got to use a lot of fancy psychological jargon in their reports. Morton found this could pull serious weight with big wheels like the State Arbitrators, who decided where the high-end funding went. Official looking documents and scrawled signatures, that's what made the modern psychiatric world go round.

"Annise! Over here!" called Harvey.

Annise waved, then emerged from her low slung Mazda Miata. Even through the dimness of the L.A. night you could see her over-grateful smile at Harvey's correct pronunciation of her name. She wore tight fitting western-style Levi's and a pair of tall cowboy boots. *Very* stylish.

As was typical of her, she didn't do exactly what her boss requested. Instead she strolled up to Joseph and Priscilla, who were standing with two police officers by the Roselawn van. Morton detected an extra wiggle in her stride—a hint perhaps of those late night hot toddies she was so fond of?

Harvey continued to motion with his pipe, and finally she came. Her gleaming mass of blonde hair swung silkily behind like a white cape in the florescent glow of the streetlights. She had a small pad and pencil. Already she was taking notes.

"Joseph gave me the run down," said Annise. "He's calling it date rape. Priscilla's going with simple abduction. Oh, and assault and battery too, I think she said."

Annise shot a quick glance at Morton. As a psychiatric counselor she was the jump in with both feet type.

"I'm sure it was none of that," said Harvey evenly.

"Well, Joseph didn't say that to the police, of course," she whispered.

As Morton had learned, Annise tended to pause halfway through doorways. Like a cat you never knew which way she would go when it began closing. Quirky? Maybe. On the other hand, considered the counselor, one could envision plenty of raw material to work with later.

Harvey put his hand in the small of Annise's back and nudged her inside. She surveyed the scene: the open vodka bottle, Morton's bloody T-shirt, the gaunt, shivering client.

The paramedics assisted Muriel to her feet. They'd replaced her damaged dress with a green hospital gown. The flood lights clicked off. Suddenly the pouty oval of Muriel's lips was put in sharp relief under the flickering candlelight.

Annise turned to Morton with a slitting of her eyes. "You and your women," she said. "Christ, even two weeks on the lam couldn't make *that* chick look bad."

Annise touched self-consciously at her makeup, then whipped out her pad and started to write.

* * *

Chapter 3

Morton went to Muriel. He wanted to be certain she was OK in the head before they whisked her off to some high pressure Emergency Room. He knew they'd have to test for semen. Hell, before it was over they might even be calling *him* in for a specimen. Any way you looked at it it wouldn't be pretty.

Morton whispered something into Muriel's ear. She listened, then whispered back. Although eye contact had traditionally been her weak point she gazed solidly at Morton as he guided her toward the door.

Harvey broke in. "Just a moment people," he said, and everyone stopped in their tracks. "Allison, I'd like to ask you to come back to Dar/Neese. We want to stabilize Muriel at any cost, you know that. Our new blonde—or, rather, Annise needs you too. We have to get her completely grounded if she's going to be Muriel's primary caseworker."

The paramedics waited. Muriel was all ears. Morton shuffled his feet nervously.

"A minute ago I was a rapist," noted the counselor. "And now you're trying to rehire me? I don't get it, Harvey."

"We're all anxious to get Muriel into her apartment. It does none of us any good if she falls apart at the last minute. It's no secret you're the one who pulled her up by the bootstraps. Right now Dar/Neese is still in a supervisory position. We can allocate the funds to give her her freedom, but if she all of a sudden crumbles—Anyway, you know as well as I do that if Priscilla gets hold of her she'll stay locked up for the next twenty years."

Harvey frowned and snapped the bowl of his pipe against his palm.

"We're aware you're on the, uh, unorthodox side," continued the psychiatrist. "But we need you, Allison. If you're back on our payroll this incident will go under the rug. Otherwise—"

Joseph appeared at the screen door. "Otherwise very ugly charges might be filed against you," snorted the Gestapo. "The cops are waiting for the go ahead. By the way, Priscilla's got this down as a kidnapping. That's fifteen to life," he added.

Morton scratched his stubble. Mental illness. Damn if it didn't run deeper than just the ones they locked away. A long moment passed.

"Muriel, do you want me back?" asked Morton.

Muriel looked at Annise, then back to Morton.

"Yes," she peeped.

Morton turned to Annise. "Do *you* want me back?" he asked.

Annise glanced at Muriel, then back to Morton. "Yes. Yes, I do want you back," she said.

"Settled!" confirmed Harvey. "We'll see you first thing in the morning."

Morton said, "Uh, that's a bit soon, Harvey. How about Monday? That way I could have the weekend."

"Monday it is," boomed the doctor of psychiatry. "Let's make it for noon with Joseph. He'll handle all the paperwork."

The neighbors, shack-ups Morton suspected, had edged over to the landing. They were exactly thirty years old, terrified, possibly on drugs. Joseph poked his head out the screen door and had a few covert words with them. Since when was the Gestapo buddies with the neighbors?

In Joseph's moment of inattention Priscilla Daddio jogged across the lawn and took hold of Muriel's arm.

"Priscilla still cares for Muriel," said Priscilla guiding Muriel away. "And Muriel's friends at Roselawn miss Muriel very badly." They stopped at the curb.

The paramedics opened the back of the ambulance and helped the fragile patient inside. Like in a Halloween movie Joseph magically appeared behind the vehicle. The engine roared to life. Then, in a split second lunge, the Gestapo swooped through the double doors and snapped them shut.

"What the—" Morton started toward the ambulance, but it was too late.

The overhead flasher went on, and the ambulance surged into the distance.

Back-lit by the high-tech halogen lamps the counselor could see Muriel's swollen face flattened anxiously against the window. Over her shoulder Joseph's steel-wool five o'clock shadow crowded alongside.

* * *

Chapter 4

Morton and Annise lingered in the yard as the vehicles pulled away. In the east the sun was rising. A pale lemon-yellow halo illuminated the tops of the houses. Under the slow bloom of morning Annise looked even fresher. In a matter of minutes the two were completely alone.

Without turning her head Annise said, "I know you've been running away from the Fraction House. I'd like to ask you something. Was any of it because of me?"

That Annise Chastain. She had a unique way of seeking out where you were vulnerable, then showering you with an extra degree of affection as a reward.

In her eyes Morton could see a faraway sense of guilt. Her pupils had compressed into black dots in the morning sun. In a curious way her gaze struck him as similar to the lost, narcotic-blown eyes of Muriel. Why was that?

"No, it didn't have anything to do with you," he said.

"By the way, I like the shirtless look," she whispered.

They were close there on the grass. The giant L.A. sun was up now and warming their faces. Morton could see the tiny blonde hairs on Annise's arms fanning in the breeze. There'd been opportunities before, but the timing never seemed quite right. He leaned and kissed her.

To his surprise she kissed back. He grasped her waist and drew her to him. She allowed her body to form up against his, the body of a starlet with all the race track curves and high, firm embankments you might someday navigate.

"I saw the bottle of vodka you and Muriel were sharing," said Annise.

Morton tensed. He was irritated with defending himself. But she gripped his hand and said, "Maybe you could pour us one."

"You want me to pour you one? At seven in the morning?"

"Why not? I'm off today," she said.

Coyishly she dipped her head. A small clattering sound came from behind. Those snoopy neighbors again.

Annise slipped a hand under her hair, and in that sultry, acidic way intrinsic to your sexy L.A. blondes lifted it far out to the side, as if thinking. When she let go it all poured uniformly into place, a great platinum waterfall raining over her breasts and reaching southward to her hips. A hot chill raced down Morton's spine.

"Do you like it with ice? I don't have any ice in there," he said.

"Oh no, a shot glass is fine with me," said Annise.

They looked carefully at one another, then pivoted and headed back to the duplex.

* * *

Chapter 5

On Monday Morton arrived at the Fraction House at 11:30 a.m. He made his way up the three flights of stairs and down the long hallway of Administrative Offices. He knew Joseph took an early lunch, and sure enough he was already gone.

In the past Joseph's door was kept tightly locked. Lately however Morton had found it propped conspicuously open. This was due to one of Joseph's so called 'Dictums,' which, like Martin Luther's *95 Theses*, were a list of regulations tacked onto the cafeteria door. The most recent of these invited clients to enter his office for a talk at any time, day or night. One of the Joseph's earliest Dictums however, stated that except for pre-scheduled Therapy Sessions no patients were allowed on the third floor. Interesting approach to the open-door policy, thought the counselor.

Morton looked both ways, then stepped into the Gestapo's fastidiously neat office. Several rows of prescription pill bottles were lined on the coarse, oak-grained desk next to the octagonal Specter computer. It was odd, the medicines not being under lock and key like everything else.

Joseph was a chemistry aficionado. He had a home lab kit where he played scientist, testing this and that drug concoction, then trying them out on— Who? Himself? The clients? Well, maybe his potions just changed colors in the vials and he left it at that.

The Gestapo's own prescription Dexedrine Spansules were there, which suppressed his appetite and kept him trim. Next came the confusing array of newer psychotropic drugs used by Gordon Theodoricus, the so called 'Synthetic Paranoid,' and numerous other clients down on C-Wing.

Nearby were Harvey's cardiac meds. Cardizem. Lasix. Potassium. Nitroglycerin. Lately the Freudian had been so sickly he couldn't be counted on to remember the times and dosages, so the task fell to Joseph. This seemed unusual, but pills were the name of the game at the Fraction House. Someone had to take charge, and Joseph was the one.

The barbells he used during his free time were by the window, the iron discs stacked compulsively from large to small. A pill popping, weightlifting chain smoker, reflected the counselor? Well, at least he didn't jog, which combined with his other habits might be dangerous to his health.

The thick handwritten log books, Anecdotals, they were called, lay open across his three foot square scratch pad. This was where the staff charted what happened with the clients each day.

Morton glanced cautiously into the corridor, then leafed through the log books until he came to the current sections on Muriel.

There did seem to be problems. Harvey had her back on the Tofranil in doses more than twice as high as in the early days. New spells of depression were leaving Muriel so washed out Stacy Lung, who'd once worked in tandem with Morton, described her as "a living mummy."

All this occurring in a mere two weeks? Hard to believe. Joseph was her psychotherapist. His notes would be in the imposing metal file cabinet in the corner marked 'Strictly Confidential.' Morton jerked the handle, but it was locked. No big deal. He'd see Muriel later in the day and get the story directly from her.

The counselor sighed and flopped into the same comfy leather chair he'd been interrogated—ummm, interviewed in, rather—that fateful day two years ago. He remembered admiring Joseph's slight lisp as the Gestapo congratulated him for entering the great field of psychiatric counseling.

"As supervisor over the forty some patients we house here," Joseph told Morton, "I feel I've developed a certain, oh, call it insight into these things. Which is why we're teaming you with two of our most challenging clients." He shook his fingers for emphasis. "I'm sure you and Gordon Theodoricus will do wonderfully together. He's our famous Synthetic Paranoid.

Harvey's written him up in the journals a hundred times. And Muriel too, of course. She's our resident 'Incested Schizophrenic.' Here in L.A. they're psychiatric celebrities. You're smiling," noted the supervisor. "That's good, Allison. That's a very good sign."

A lot had changed since then. Particularly with Muriel. These weren't the old days anymore. For one thing, Joseph was driving that alien looking early 90's Jaguar that only the uninitiated thought looked sporty. Where he found the money was anybody's guess.

Morton leaned back now and rested his feet on Joseph's desk. In so doing he happened to nudge a stack of green 'Mental Adequacy' forms the Gestapo used to evaluate suspicious staff members. Underneath was a manila envelope with the words: EMERGENCY DEPARTMENT, CEDARS-SINAI MEDICAL CENTER, stamped across the top.

Cedars-Sinai? That's where they took Muriel! He checked his watch. Five of twelve. And Joseph was a punctilious son of a—

Morton rifled the envelope. He found photocopies of Muriel's ER evaluation. Quickly he read through the data. 'Facial contusions. Severe dehydration. Acute anxiety reaction during examination.' Well, what'd they expect?

He continued down the page. They'd performed a pelvic exam. He could barely make out the physician's handwriting. 'Evidence of vaginal trauma. Specimen taken.'

Hurriedly Morton ran his finger down the margin. Under lab results he found, 'Spermatozoa verified.'

～～

Suddenly he heard the clatter of the Handicap Access Elevator Joseph and Harvey used. The counselor thrust the folder into place, then pulled one of the fat Anecdotals open across his lap. Joseph rounded the corner.

"You weren't reading those, were you, Allison? They're highly confidential. Besides, you're not officially on the payroll," he said placing a hand on his hip.

"I was just going to lock them up in case someone unauthorized came nosing in."

Joseph frumped his lips. He eyed the layout of his desk. Satisfied, he plucked the Anecdotal from Morton's lap, stacked it with the others and walked to the file cabinet.

"You won't be working your three day round-the-clock stint anymore, Allison," said the supervisor. "We want you as a payrolled nine-to-fiver. In terms of documentation it'd look best that way to the Arbitrators."

"And my duties?" Morton asked.

Joseph slung his kid leather satchel—Morton called it a purse—over the back of his chair. Nervously he tidied the Mental Adequacy forms. Nervous? This wasn't like Joseph. In fact, he needed those Dexie uppers to boost to the warp speeds required for success at the Fraction House.

"Awful lot of drugs you got there." Morton nodded toward the prescription vials. "Ever think that might be an artificial answer to getting these people into the mainstream?"

"Get off your high horse, Allison. Nowadays drugs *are* mainstream," countered the Gestapo.

Now there was a point hard to argue with.

"We're primarily interested in Annise," continued Joseph. "Not *interested*. You know what I'm saying. To keep her training going forward like before is all."

Morton gave a small smile. Regarding Annise Chastain, both knew what the supervisor was interested in.

"Great. I'll be able to concentrate fully on Muriel," returned Morton.

"Ummm, there's something we should clarify. We need you here. On the premises, I mean. We have to insure that you and Muriel achieve full closure on your Freudian bonding and your nutty relationship and all."

"Closure?"

"What I'm saying, Allison, is it's important for you to be nearby. We can't have Muriel bouncing off the walls at the very moment she's supposed to be moving into her own apartment. But we can't exactly have you hanging out with her either, if you get what I'm saying."

"I can't be hanging out with her?"

"No. We need you to be here *for* her, but not *with* her. Understand?"

Morton shook his head.

"Don't look so sour. It's only politics for Christsake. You and I both know how these bureaucratic things go. We're making a special exception and giving you Temporary Custody of her. Mind you, it's not to be used. It's only for the paperwork, in case she happens to bolt over to your place again. Think of it as a formality rather than a reality. We kept her original pairing with Gordon Theodoricus, so you should like that."

Joseph reached for a batch of forms. "Sign these and we're ready to rock and roll," he said.

Morton looked over the papers. He jutted his jaw in a way that made his lower teeth extend over his uppers. It was a trait he exhibited when he questioned authority.

"This Temporary Custody form. It's blue, not pink like the old ones," said Morton. "The wording looks different too. Harvey make a change?"

"Not Harvey. I made the change. And yes, it's new," huffed the Gestapo.

"What's this at the bottom? It says, 'Custody Repeal.'" Morton pointed at the fine print.

Joseph reached into his pocket for his razor knife, the one he used to slit open the heavy boxes of drugs from Carney Apothecary. He began obsessively sliding the blade in and out of the aluminum handle.

"Oh, that means you had Custody at one time and you're *re*-appealing now to get it back. It's typical protocol, Allison. There's a lot of changes shaking around here."

The Gestapo pushed over the usual Confidentiality Statement.

"Sign this too," he said. "And this one here is your new Dar/Neese Employment Agreement. Lay down your John Hancock for Christsake and let's get on with things."

The stack of papers was intimidating. Each form needed to be signed in triplicate. Morton penned his name in the appropriate columns, then passed the papers back to Joseph.

"The way the funding is these days everybody wants a piece of Muriel's pie. Priscilla. Her goofy parents. Even Dar/Neese. We're all after a good healthy bite. The State Arbitrators are mighty picky. Frankly, there's a humongous mess here, Allison. Especially since she ran off and got herself raped over at your place."

"Now hold on!" Morton came to his feet.

Joseph threw up his hands. "Forget I said that. Please, Morton, can't you work with us? It's all for Muriel's good."

The supervisor kept declaring how open he was being, but somehow the counselor felt nasty secrets stacking up across the wide oak desk.

"You may not be aware of how bad this is, Allison. But Muriel has really gone to the dogs these last weeks."

Joseph rambled on about 'Crisis Overloads' and 'Autosuggestive Impulses,' concepts he'd swiped from Harvey. But with all the fancy lingo it was hard to put a finger on exactly what he was getting at.

"Muriel's escape was quite out of character," explained the supervisor. "It wasn't much more than her hiding out in your apartment. You know, sleeping in your bed, nibbling at your leftovers."

This seemed strange. A few cans of Spaghetti O's had been opened. The bedclothes were rumpled, yes. But two weeks? Couldn't be.

"What about her bloody teeth? What about the blood at her crotch?" questioned Morton.

"You know these schizos. They admit nothing. I got it on good authority she snuck over to her parents' place in Burbank and had an ugly run-in with her father. You know Wojeck."

Morton's jaw began to jut.

"It's very common for an incest victim to return to her first molester, Allison. It's in all the literature. They're looking for the abuse in adulthood they think they deserve for giving in to the son of a bitch in childhood."

Morton shifted in his chair. Knowing Muriel that wasn't likely.

"I've got two years of solid growth down on videotape," proceeded the supervisor. "Shots of her all dressed up and moving into this new apartment could really climax my work."

Morton pursed his lips. "Well, you *are* her therapist. I suppose you deserve to reap the rewards."

"I've got to run," said Joseph.

He shouldered his purse, picked up a batch of papers, and the two men walked down the hallway—the Gestapo wide, stout, ruggedly dark of skin and hair; the counselor tall and thin with a light complexion.

Morton skidded as they reached the top of the steps, the very flight he'd fallen down the day before he turned in his resignation. He'd been planning to leave anyway and that tumble was the last straw, particularly with the wrist broken so badly. They paused.

"By the way, that's a terrific looking cast. Your schizo can really throw a punch," snickered Joseph.

At the time Morton had felt some kind of blow, or a bump maybe, he wasn't sure. Muriel was upset about his departure, true, but had she actually—

"It wasn't a punch," said Morton. "Muriel wouldn't do that. I slipped on your fancy buffing job."

Joseph had dismissed the housekeepers months ago from their third floor duties. "Snoopy maids," he called them. He compulsively waxed the upstairs floors himself, keeping them ice rink slick.

'L.A. 2000:' Sex Asylum

The counselor shuffled his feet. "It doesn't seem as oiled up as in the old days, Joseph. What's the matter, not following up on your fetishes?"

"No need to anymore, Allison," returned the supervisor. "With that busted arm I've got you down to half throttle. I'm not worried."

Morton cradled the newfangled plastic cast with its Velcro attachments and complicated traction devices. Was Joseph being facetious? People often told the truth by accident. You had to keep your eyes open for these things. The Gestapo pointed down the stairwell to the oversized window he'd installed to view the goings on in the Organic Therapy Garden.

"You're lucky you didn't crash right through there," observed Joseph nodding toward the window. "That's half inch glass, Allison. It'd cut you in two like a frankfurter."

"I thought the Joint Commission was making Harvey change it to shatterproof Plexiglas," said Morton. "Too many clients stagger down this way after their Therapy Sessions. It's not safe, Joseph."

"Maybe, but Plexiglas is terribly hazy. You know as well as I do I have to see who's zooming who in the bushes," said the Gestapo.

Morton made a mug.

Joseph turned serious. "Look, here's your paycheck for the upcoming week. I know it's unusual to get your money ahead of time, but Harvey wanted to show how much we think of you."

Morton noticed the figure. It was almost double what he'd earned before he resigned.

Joseph handed him another paper. "And this is a recommendation letter. You can read it later. Harvey really crows about you," said Joseph with obvious distaste.

Hmmm, maybe Dar/Neese *was* changing. Maybe Harvey Mueller did appreciate all the soul and heart Morton had poured into the clients.

Joseph said, "One more thing. God knows why, but Muriel does seem to trust you. And I guess her goof-ball parents think they've got some far out kind of rapport with your unhinged counseling style. Anyway, Harvey felt we had to invite you."

"Invite me to what?"

"Muriel's big Termination Meeting is scheduled for the end of the month. We're hoping to have all the loose cannons muzzled by— Or rather, the loose ends tied up by then."

"So Emily and Wojeck are coming?" asked Morton. Emily was Muriel's brassy, redheaded mother.

"Yes. And Wanda Novice, the Social Worker, will be there," replied Joseph.

"What about the new blonde? I mean, Annise Chastain?" asked Morton.

Joseph narrowed his gaze. He got a cigarette out and wedged it behind his ear for quick access when he cleared the front doors.

"The blonde? Yes, if she ever gets over the flu. Or the hangover, or whatever it is. Can you believe it, the wench called in sick today? She's not even through with her orientation and she calls in sick."

Morton experienced an inner tremor for Annise's well being. He was aware that when the Gestapo was so vocal in his criticism of someone it usually meant he was backhandedly attracted to them. Annise and *Joseph*, pondered the counselor in a dark corner of his mind?

"Now listen, Morton, the Dar/Neese Board of Directors is going to reevaluate Muriel's status. So far nobody from the Arbitrators' office knows she's trying to revert to her old ways. We're counting on you to get her back to normal. Well, normal*ized*, as we say. Our reputation— Let me rephrase that. Muriel's welfare is at stake here. We simply cannot allow Priscilla to steal her back. You agree, don't you?"

"I'll do what I can," said Morton.

"I know you're not in love with the Administration around here, but would you try to be a little bit respectful of Harvey and me this time around? Especially since the family is going to be there?" Joseph gritted his teeth, then stiffly offered his hand. "Can we please agree on that much?"

"Sure, Joseph, we can agree on that much."

Morton extended his left arm and in an awkward fingers-to-fingers clasp the two warily jiggled hands.

* * *

Chapter 6

Morton walked down the block from the Fraction House and ordered lunch at Vera's Russian Diner. He was a regular there, and the place gave him a sense of stability amidst the frantic pursuit of taboo pleasures known as the L.A. lifestyle. He waved to the group of red-faced oldsters who hung out at the counter during the day drinking coffee and bitching about death. They waved back enthusiastically, all eight of them.

As he worked over his BLT Morton remembered that Gordon and Muriel were scheduled for afternoon activities in the Recreation Room.

When he returned along the sidewalk he saw Muriel staring out through the blurry Plexiglas window. The faded aluminum siding of the exterior was in sharp contrast to the snazzy tiling and soundproofing of the inside. He looked closer. A figure was there beside her. Joseph again? Damned if that Gestapo wasn't everywhere these days.

Morton gave a wave and his old-time smile. No response. Her eyes were glazed over like a couple of Vera's twice baked doughnuts. This wasn't good.

~~~

Morton passed through the lobby and negotiated the maze of hallways leading to the Recreation Room. Slowly he opened the door. Inside, the walls were tiled with a bold Aztec mosaic. The psychedelic purples and greens seemed to vibrate free of the mortar as they crossed the retina, causing Morton a kind of vertigo. Concerned for the clients, he'd brought this up to Harvey early on. "It might make *you* queasy, Morton," clarified the Freudian. "But you've got to remember our people are *already* dizzy. To them that mosaic is as still as an island in a sea of utter lunacy."

Morton was relieved to see that it was Gordon Theodoricus, the Synthetic Paranoid, standing beside Muriel at the window, not Joseph after all. He angled to catch Muriel's eye but she wouldn't turn her head.

Gordon and Morton were old buddies. They exchanged a discreet nod, then Gordon headed over to the long Clay-Work table.

Gordon Theodoricus was a very socially aware paranoid. For instance, he'd concluded that life was a horribly unnatural phenomenon. Strange cancers were cropping up everywhere. Unidentified bacteria waited patiently for him on the seat of every toilet. Weirder people with wilder ideas were lurking around each corner. So Gordon set out to build what he called "resistance." To get a resistance, of course, you had to ingest the very things likely to kill you to stay safe. As he'd explained it to Morton, "The more poison gets in me the more protected I am against poison."

This theory governed every phase of Gordon's life. He refused to wash vegetables in order to get pesticides into his liver and thereby resist liver cancer. He went jogging only if the Air Index was rated in the dangerous Triple-X category, which kept his lungs healthy. He scanned the labels of foods to buy items with as many preservatives, artificial colorings, nitrites and nitrates as possible. Although he was right handed he used his left one for awkward sexual practices. Presumably this confused his genes into thinking it wasn't him doing it. Moreover, everyone he instinctively liked he decided to immediately detest. "That way, Morton, I don't have to reverse my opinion later when they turn out to be assholes, like you're doing all the time."

Well, there he had a point. At any rate, Gordon and Morton had always gotten along well. In fact, Gordon was next in line to get his freedom. The same battle taking place with Muriel—the vying for funding between Roselawn and the Fraction House—all this was likely to occur with Gordon. Priscilla's nastiness, Joseph's nastiness—

The paranoid took a seat beside Sally Featherman. Sally was designated an 'Echolalic,' which meant she repeated everything you said. She was also termed 'Echopraxic,' which meant she copied a person's gestures to a T, going as far as sneezing when they sneezed, or burping when they burped.

Wanda Novice, the stocky, tenderhearted Social Worker, was overseeing things from the high-backed chair at the far end of the Clay-Work table. Like many of your California in-crowd Wanda was a health food freak. Her on-the-job lunch lay unraveled on a long strip of wax paper. Today she was having a sandwich of mung bean sprouts and lentil paté lubricated with a small jar of organically grown papaya juice, which she kept uncapping, sipping, recapping, as if it were some holy elixir. Morton tasted it once, but like her bee pollen and her yellow carrot juice he felt it best to stick with Vera's Russian coffee.

"Afternoon, Wanda. Afternoon, Sally," said Morton smiling.

"Afternoon, Wanda. Afternoon, Sally," echoed Sally Featherman mimicking the offbeat way Morton had smiled. Not all, reflected the counselor, had come as far as Muriel.

The snakes and oblong balls Gordon and Sally were fashioning out of Play-Doh—blatant phallic symbols according to Harvey—lay strewn across the grainy, unvarnished wood.

"I guess you're filling in for Annise, eh Wanda?" said Morton walking over and patting her shoulder.

"Yeah. As a matter of fact she just phoned. She's been up all night long, poor thing. She thinks she can make it in around four."

Quietly, to keep it from the clients, Morton said, "By the way, Wanda, what do you think of our new Annise?"

"One of the finest things I've seen around here so far," she said. The Social Worker winked.

Wanda's body unconsciously rippled. Quickly she smoothed her short-cropped hair. Sexual preferences, one couldn't help noticing, ran in diverse directions around the Fraction House.

"That's my opinion too," said Morton giving a secret wink of his own.

Just then the door opened. Stacy Lung, Morton's ex-girlfriend, stuck her head in. "We still on for our Friday clubbing, Wanda?" she called. She spotted Morton and frowned.

Wanda gave one of her militaristic salutes, which meant 'absolutely yes she was.' Stacy nodded and snapped closed the door.

Muriel was leaning against the windowsill, staring out at the heavy Los Angeles traffic. She was wearing her khaki walking shorts and her standby Grateful Dead T-shirt. The teddy bear Morton had given her before he quit, Little Morton, she'd named it, was propped conspicuously nearby. The counselor was touched.

Wanda whispered, "Muriel has missed you terribly. I'm so glad you're back."

Even considering her runaway, Muriel was no longer the skinny, neurotic waif who'd first entered the Fraction House. No, you couldn't mistake her for a teenager anymore, noted Morton observing the womanly S of her body.

The counselor approached her. "Well, Muriel, I'm back, for better or worse!" he said. He wasn't a good one for phrasing complicated emotions.

Muriel rotated toward him. The moment their eyes met she started with the funny sideways grin she used in the old days when Morton became confused about the more delicate aspects of mental illness. She really had come an incredible distance. Much of it, according to Harvey's reports anyway, was due to Dar/Neese's state of the art therapy programs.

Of particular impact was the powerful Regressive Therapy Joseph used on her. Every Wednesday and Friday Muriel climbed into the special gold-trimmed bathtub. She was required to be nude, another of Joseph's Dictums. Patiently, soothed by the tepid water, one assumed, she waited for Joseph to regress her.

The supervisor would loosen his tie, and with his resonant, lady killer voice tell her things her parents or her last therapist had told him. Bit by bit he'd lead her backwards through her life.

First to those nasty teenage indiscretions she likely committed at Roselawn. On into puberty and the insecurities of first menstruation. And then, carefully... ever so carefully, back into infancy. Until finally, yes, he had taken her *into the womb*.

As he did this Muriel was shown infantile drawings of different types of trauma she might have encountered during those formative months. For example, of a pregnant mother falling forward onto her belly; or of Daddy accidentally dropping the newborn baby on its head, of Daddy's hairy sex organs, of daughter's hairless sex organs, and so on. A box of Crayola Crayons was kept nearby in case Muriel got angry and wanted to put a black X over the father's genitals if she felt hatred for her father, or perhaps a red X over the mother's stomach, if, say, Muriel hated herself when she was in the womb.

It was common knowledge that Joseph was beset with a certain degree of OCD, or Obsessive/Compulsive Disorder. For unknown reasons, he peeked from the Therapy Room into the hallway every six minutes. This accounted for his meticulous setting of all Dar/Neese clocks, which had to match to the second the readout on his gold Rolex watch. In the realm of mental health psychological problems among the staff were common. But they had Prozac now. They had Depakote. They had Zoloft and Lithium to control the bad urges. The Gestapo however fancied drugs that fed his obsessions. Like Dexies. Like cocaine.

So it was with Joseph.

And such was one of the drawbacks of mental institutions in general—they attached to themselves, from the Administration on down, the very personalities they were trying to cure.

～～

Morton now reached out with his good hand and began to massage Muriel's neck. As usual, he couldn't stifle his tendency to be overly direct. He didn't mention her recent escape, but came immediately to the goings on in those confidential Therapy Sessions.

Morton said, "I'm trying to find out if Joseph is doing anything weird in there, Muriel."

"Everything Joseph does seems weird to me. He's been doing it a long time, you know."

"Doing what a long time?"

Silence. It was apparent she wasn't going to answer.

"But is it productive? I mean, is anything accomplished?" pursued the counselor.

"Oh, yes. Joseph gets the coloring book filled in just about every time. And he lets me use all those expensive shampoos and creme rinses," said Muriel.

"*Joseph* fills in the book? Makes the X's and all?" Morton was amazed.

"Only if I don't know where to put them. And he always gives me my Tofranil shot before we start so he won't get nervous," explained Muriel.

"But does it help you? That's the important thing," probed the counselor.

She thought it over. Eyes that distinctive lunar blue roaming into the distance. Auburn hair glistening in the afternoon sunlight as it struck in through the west-facing window. Tiny upturned nose, which made her look more youthful than her twenty-five years. Body full-grown, but not quite real somehow, not seeming to fit her yet.

"I'm serious, Muriel. I want to know if all this business in the Therapy Room is of any benefit to you."

"About the same benefit you and Stacy Lung got when you two used to sneak in there," she answered.

Morton was floored. "Me and Stacy! How did you know— I mean, are you trying to say you and Joseph—"

But he caught himself. Experience had taught him it was best to lie low when the first bombshell dropped.

"So, uh, you feel it's of use?"

"In a way I think it is," she returned. "Because I always get twice as clean as I normally would. Joseph says being clean is everything being dirty isn't."

"Well, I suppose there must be something to it," sighed Morton.

"Joseph practices what he preaches too, Morton. Because when I finish he takes off his suit and tie and gets in himself. I can hear him scrubbing from way down the hall."

"In the same water? He actually gets in the same water you were in?" cried the counselor.

A moment passed. Muriel slowly turned her head.

"What are you trying to say, Morton? Wouldn't *you* get in my water?"

* * *

Chapter 7

One way or another Muriel had improved. She'd entered the Fraction House at twenty-three as a 'Delusional Schizophrenic' with no control over her bowels, a tendency toward kicking and scratching attacks on staff, and a phobia to all food smells except spaghetti, which Harvey said she probably wasn't served as a child.

Roselawn, where she'd been housed since age twelve, sent her files along. They were sketchy though on what first landed her there, and her parents offered only enough background information to know that ugly, incestuous traumas had occurred. Muriel, as was typical of your Roselawn graduates, all of whom had at some point been certified as loonies, wasn't talking.

After two years at the Fraction House, the same two Morton was employed there as it happened, Muriel had become a new person. Off the antidepressant drugs. Standing upright instead of her original hunched-over shuffle. Even venturing tenuous eye contact. At last she was prepared to show the skeptical psychiatric world how successful the Dar/Neese Rebonding Program could be.

The bowel problem? Well, that was solved when the Fraction House discovered her allergy to orange juice, which Roselawn served during their famous Vitamin-C Psyco-Reversal Experiment. Now, however, at the critical moment, the old introversion was taking her over, a nervous oblivion, which at times verged on outright catatonia. Morton took his friend by the hands and made her face him.

"Look, Muriel, you've got to quit this staring out the window bullshit. We're going to start a brand new regimen. We're going to get back to paying close attention to your real self," he said.

"My real self?" echoed Muriel.

"Sure. How else are you going to see reality if not through yourself? A person should be aware of what people are thinking about them, else they're liable to step out of line and do something totally off the wall."

Muriel shuddered.

"You've got to look for your inner self, Muriel. I can tell you're ready to find it."

"Yes... I... I do feel I'm finding things. But I'm so weak inside. My knees even wobble."

"The self you find may be weak, but the one that searches is strong. All you need to do is buckle down and take a long hard look," persisted the counselor.

"In the mirror?" she asked.

"Well, that's a start."

"But you always say what other people think is none of my business, don't you?"

Morton paused. "In two years a person says a lot of things, Muriel. It's what I'm saying now that's important."

"Isn't it vanity though to sit around reflecting on yourself? That's what a lot of them at this place do. The nuts *and* the staff."

Morton's brow creased.

"And anyway, none of us can see who we really are, whether we look in the mirror or at the things we do all day. Can we, Morton? I mean, can we?"

One thing about sane people was you could always identify their limits. With people like Gordon and Sally Featherman, with Muriel too for that matter, you couldn't even guess their limits, which was kind of exciting, in its way.

"There's something I have to know, Muriel. It's about your escape," said Morton. "Answer me yes or no. I don't want any of that run-around psycho-babble you're so good at."

"OK," said Muriel humbly.

"Did someone have sex with you when you were out those weeks?"

"Sex?"

"That's right, sex. You know what sex is," waved the counselor.

"Yes," returned Muriel. "It's the dirty stuff in back of the linen closet that leads up to intercourse."

"Right," said Morton. "But the question is, who was it with?"

"My father you mean? Is that what you're asking?" wondered Muriel.

"Did you go to your parents' place? I don't know if you're aware of this, Muriel, but rape is a Capital Offense. Which means even the dopey government thinks it's one of the worst crimes around."

"A Capital Offense?"

"Well, it used to be Capital. Which meant they hung the guy. Or chopped his head off in the guillotine. Or fried him in the electric chair. It might be a felony now, I'm not sure."

A long silence came.

"If I told you I was raped what would you do?" she asked finally.

"I'd make sure I had a good night's sleep. Then I'd get hold of the bastard and have a special Therapy Session up in Joseph's office," said the counselor.

"You mean you'd strangle him?"

"You do know what rape is, don't you?" asked Morton.

"Yeah," muttered Muriel low. "Isn't it when somebody gives you something you didn't really want in the first place?"

"No, it's when somebody *takes* something you didn't *want* to give them in the first place," corrected the counselor. "And then it's gone from you and you feel empty."

A look of confusion came over her.

Muriel said, "Don't people sometimes have to be prostitutes to survive? You hear it all the time in L.A. Most of the counselors here say they have to be prostitutes to make a living. So if you have to be an accountant or something— I mean, if a prostitute has to have sex and can't tell you to keep somebody from being killed—"

"Who are you talking about, Muriel?"

"I'm talking about you and me," she said.

"And Joseph? Are you trying to protect that son of a— I mean, it sounds like you're saying Joseph did it and you don't want me to kill him. Is this what you're saying? Was Joseph the one who took something away you didn't want to give him?"

Muriel hesitated. "Took away?" she replied. "I'm not positive I know what you're saying. But if you want to, Morton, we can check under the hood. I'm pretty sure I have all the parts I started with."

"Well, uh, that won't be necessary," stammered the counselor.

Muriel's skin mottled under the strange mix of sun and florescent light reflected off the screwy Aztec tiles.

"I'm so excited talking to you like this, Morton," she said quickly. "I'm excited and happy in my belly right now at this moment I'm living in. Thank you for coming back and being my counselor all over again."

Never before had Muriel telegraphed her sensuality this graphically. It was as if she'd had a ten year delay in the onset of puberty, and like a lot of your precocious L.A. nymphos was about to come of age in grandstand style.

Once again Morton began to massage her neck. It was one of their little endearments, a kind of psychological safe zone. This time the fine strawberry hairs on her neck radiated a mystical twist of heat. A crimson blitzkrieg of passion welling there, only shrouded, as if under the cloak and dagger of her repression and her shyness.

Muriel shot a look to Gordon, her longtime friend. Muriel and the *paranoid*, wondered the counselor for a bizarre instant? They *were* of age. They'd been paired partners for years. And after all, beginning love was like an electric current. It projected its own trembly light over hard and fast reality. Well, romance had more sides than a seal, especially around the Fraction House. Ignore no clues.

What was it he'd been saying about Muriel seeking her real self? She was right, she wouldn't find it in the looking glass. Hers was a self of flowing mercury, a river balled up until the viscous walls would at last burst and redefine itself as... What? Womanhood maybe? A lover of mankind perhaps, like in the religions? Or possibly, just possibly a lover of one man. Of a good man. Like... Well, like Gordon Theodoricus, for instance. At least, hoped Morton running his forefinger inside his cast to where the stitches were, not some cold-hearted man of the streets like Joseph Schopen, her miserable fucking therapist.

~~~

The door opened and into the Recreation Room stepped Annise Chastain. The ends of her platinum hair met the hem of her short pink skirt at high thigh. Wanda's mouth dropped open. A few steps behind trailed Joseph, and the shift from sensitive inner meditations to hardcore day-in-the-life facts of the matter jerked up their heads like a blast of smelling salts.

Muriel tensed, and Morton watched helplessly as by degrees she retreated into her shell. The blitzkrieg of passion evaporated. The flowing river of mercury froze hard on her magenta cheeks, like evening sun on a cold, white lake. Morton started to speak, but it was no use, for she'd turned again to the window, rigid as bone.

* * *

Chapter 8

Annise Chastain hovered in the center of the room, beaming at them all. A lot of new counselors were like that, operating under the assumption they ought to compensate for a potentially depressive place by injecting a double dose of the upbeat.

"Oh, Wanda, thanks *so* much for picking up the slack," said Annise hurrying past Sally and Gordon.

Annise's cream colored mohair sweater was V'd deep at the neck. Morton could see the contrasting black lace of her bra through the loose knitting. Quite sensual indeed! He watched as she leaned far forward and gave Wanda a grateful buss on the cheek.

Morton strode over to Joseph by the ancient steam radiator.

"Listen, Joseph, there's a—"

"As you can see, I got hold of your blonde," interrupted the supervisor. "I decided to drop by her place and see what was up." Joseph fingered his gold Spanish horn necklace. "I was a little slow getting back here. That idiotic paper lantern over her bed can really get on a guy's nerves."

"You mean you—" Morton's gut wrenched. He took a second to compose himself.

"Muriel never went to her father's," whispered the counselor. "She was raped, Joseph. I know that now."

The Gestapo's eyes generally carried a suave somnolence. At Morton's remark they peeled sharply open.

"Muriel told you this?" he asked.

"You know as well as I do she doesn't talk about anything emotional," said Morton.

"She wasn't raped."

"They found sperm in her."

"She was out there two weeks. She had to make her way somehow," defended Joseph. He shrugged and scratched at his heavy five o'clock shadow. Morton could feel him steeling up.

'L.A. 2000:' Sex Asylum

"Where did you get that information about the sperm, Allison?"

"Is it true?"

"I'll tell you what it is," said the Gestapo showing his teeth. "It's fucking confidential. I'm warning you, Morton, butt out of this. You're interfering with the smooth running of a schizophrenic agency. I mean, an agency with schizophrenics in it. Sandra Dar is aware of everything. Me and Harvey are handling it on the Administrative end. That's all you need to know."

"For your information, the correct wording is Harvey and I," said Morton. "You better get it straight, Joseph, if you're trying to pin this cover-up on her father. He's a big dude, you know. And he'll be there at her Termination Meeting."

Joseph said, "Somebody did it. Why not Wojeck? She doesn't have to remember it. The mentally ill are notorious for blocking out traumatic events."

"So she *was* raped! I thought so!" exclaimed Morton.

Annise looked suddenly up. She'd been making small talk with Gordon and Sally.

"Raped?" gasped the blonde, thrusting her hand to her mouth. She stared over at Morton.

"Raped?" cried Sally Featherman glaring at Joseph and slapping her hand over her mouth the way Annise had done.

With a brusque motion Joseph summoned Annise to the empty end of the Clay-Work table. They engaged in a cozy tête-à-tête. For a cold moment Morton noticed the supervisor's arm disappearing behind one of the heaping mounds of clay. It happened fast, if it happened at all, but Morton could have sworn he saw the lady killer reaching around for a pat on Annise's miniskirted behind.

The Gestapo marched out from behind the table. "I'll be in my office," he announced, heading for the exit. The door closed hard, almost a slam.

* * *

Chapter 9

Annise looked like a million dollars. She came toward Morton, totally unaffected. Such was her way, responding to each new incident as if there were no history, no Joseph Schopen or Wanda Novice, no addled Sally Featherman clogging up her lust for the next event. Her lavender scent with a hint of musk imbedded permeated the sterile air of the Recreation Room. Morton touched her arm. Her skin was milky soft, her cheeks scientifically rouged. It occurred to him in a subliminal way that it might well have taken till four in the afternoon to do it up with such high style.

"Are you feeling all right?" asked Morton.

Annise jabbed playfully at his ribs. "Oh, sure. A couple of hot toddies got me on my feet in short order."

Silence.

"Laugh, will you! I'm kidding for Christsake."

Annise took hold of the fingers protruding from Morton's cast and tugged him into the middle of the room.

"Listen, I've got something important to lay on you." She snuck a peek at Muriel. "I've made a big decision, Morton. It's about, well, you know—" And then she whispered, "*Us*."

"Us?" said Morton.

The counselor intuited an emotional turbulence at the window. He feared Muriel was overhearing. She snatched Little Morton and clutched him to her breast.

"I've thrashed this around all weekend, and I've decided we can—" Annise hesitated. "Well, you know, go ahead and—"

Morton leaned close. "Yes?"

Annise fanned her hair with that patented L.A. flair. "Have sex, Morton," she said self-consciously. "I've finally got all the angles figured out. No kidding, we can have all the sex we want from now on. Do you believe it?"

"Sex?"

"I realize we can't go into it right now, but there's something I need to explain. It has to do with a man very dear to me."

Morton glanced at the radiator where Joseph had stood. "Your father?" he asked hopefully.

She shook her head. By now he'd gathered the weight of her religious leanings.

"*The* Father?" he asked. His brow helplessly furrowed.

"It's a bit complicated," warned Annise. "I promise I'll spell it all out as soon as possible."

Not her father. Not *the* Father. What was left, the ex-boyfriend? Well, that wouldn't be so bad, would it?

Morton watched as web-like strands of Annise's hair twirled tiny circles under the air conditioning vents. What a woman, he reflected. What a curious piece of spark and scent she was.

"Sometimes life can feel so good," observed the counselor nonchalantly. "Hanging out with the clients. Feeling easy. It's almost like it couldn't really exist. Like say purgatory or someplace. Isn't that where you go if you sin just enough to be really happy inside?"

He smiled at his thought. During her training they'd learned how to quibble, and there could have been something here, she being so fiercely Catholic and all, but this time it didn't come.

"In a way I feel wonderfully lucky to be standing here with you, Annise," said Morton gently.

"What'd you say? I'm sorry, Morton. I was checking Muriel out is all. Look, she's crying."

It was true. Muriel's face was buried deep in Little Morton's fuzzy chest.

"Christ, she's weeping like a baby," said Annise. "Damn, it's so sad. Isn't there something you can do?"

Gordon, Sally and Wanda all stared at them.

Annise grasped his elbow. "Hey, let me try something on her," she said. "I know it's early in my training, but it might do the trick."

At the thought of a personalized intervention the blonde's eyes went big and bright. Morton turned away and went to Muriel.

For many seconds they gazed silently at each other, the recovering schizophrenic and the counselor with the unhinged style. But the vibes were clearly wrong, screwy and scrambled and loaded with yesterday's meanings. Why was he feeling so harried these days? California itself dictated an a-priori confusion, true, but this was a fresh level of discomfort, more than simply mismatched ground clutter. Let's see, there was Muriel's self, Annise's self, Joseph's self too, he guessed, but what about *Morton's* self? What about the self you brought to others as if it were the real you? Honesty. Was that what you believed you were, or what you pulled from your back pocket like a pack of cat-eyed marbles to impress the kids down the block? The counselor stole a look at Annise. He thought of the line in the Monkeys' song, 'Then I saw her face/Now I'm a believer!' Ah, her countenance *so* perfect. The hair like dream hair. These days it wasn't so much who you loved, it seemed, it was who you were bent on fuc—

Muriel wiped her eyes. "How's your arm, Morton? I saw the way that blonde jerked it." She lifted the cast and stroked the fingers sticking out.

"It was OK a minute ago, but it seems to be hurting right now," said Morton.

"The head—I mean, the mind tells the body to make it hurt. On days like this I hurt all over."

"You know, Muriel, I've been hurting all over too."

"These last weeks things have felt so far apart, Morton," she continued. "Inside me, I mean. Like if you had a million infinities in your heart, and kept feeling them instead of what's really there."

"What is really there?" he asked carefully.

"I'm not sure. But it's supposed to be reality. Isn't that what you're always telling me?"

Morton tugged at his earlobe.

Muriel said, "I kept thinking and thinking about all the infinities in a person. In everything really. In rocks. In trees. But I got scared because I kept thinking there's gonna be a lot more infinities than realities. If you see it that way you might fall through one of the holes in the world. And in infinity, Morton, you just keep on falling."

This was the way Muriel talked. You never quite took the full meaning, but it always made a kind of lopsided sense.

"Yesterday I took a walk. Joseph let me go alone," she went on. "Annise told me you aren't exactly going to be my counselor anymore, but would you like to know what I was thinking of?"

"Of course I'd like to know."

"You. I thought about you the whole time. Is that bad?" She breathed deep.

Morton took her hands. "I'm sorry, Muriel. I know the timing was off. My quitting, I mean. But sometimes things start changing and—"

Annise rushed over. "I just thought of something really wonderful. Oh, I'm sorry, I'm interrupting you two."

Muriel lowered her eyes.

"I had this idea. Would you mind if I suggested it, Muriel?" said Annise.

"No, I wouldn't mind," answered Muriel slowly. Sweet, sensitive Muriel Gonska, as always.

"I know you've been troubled lately," pampered Annise. "But when you get down and out it's the very best thing there is."

"It is?" said Muriel.

"Absolutely yes it is. I understand this may sound strange at first, but I'm Roman Catholic, and I swear to God it works for me practically every time."

"It does?" said Muriel.

"Uh huh. It's prayer, girl. Prayer to the Almighty." Annise stepped back. "You really ought to give it some thought."

"Prayer?" echoed Muriel.

"Have you tried it?"

"No, but I had a number of friends who tried it."

"Beautiful! So you know what I'm talking about," exulted Annise.

"Sort of. I remember two or three hundred of them doing it all at once."

"What were they praying for?" asked Annise, intrigued.

"Release. They kept praying and praying to be released from their troubles," said Muriel.

"Fabulous! So tell me what happened?"

"I don't know. I haven't talked to them for a couple of years."

Annise frumped her lips. "Good God, sweetheart, why in the world haven't you? I mean, if they were truly your friends? This doesn't sound right at all. Friends are *the* most precious things in the world, Miss Gonska. If they mean something to you you should be visiting them and yapping on the phone as often as you possibly can. That's what I do."

Under the fire of Annise's gaze Muriel dipped her head. "I wanted to talk to them," she replied humbly.

"Why didn't you?"

"Because they never got out of Roselawn," she said.

Silence.

"They never got out of— Ohhh, I seee. I'm sooo sorry." Annise glanced around for her purse. "Well, I didn't say it worked every time," hedged the blonde.

"It's OK," consoled Muriel. "I'm sure they're all still praying, so you can feel good about that."

~~~

Muriel invariably absorbed only the good of people, of Harvey, of Wanda, even of Joseph. Morton wished he could be that way. Then again she *was* considered off her rocker.

Annise, on the other hand, exhibited an approach to psychosis so desirous of the warm and golden-hearted her occasional clumsiness seemed to slip right through the cracks. What was more, she never acted melancholy about it like many of the other caseworkers did. Like Morton himself sometimes did.

Muriel pushed away from the windowsill and walked out of the Recreation Room.

Wanda shot to her feet.

"Shit, she's trying to bolt!" cried Annise starting after her. Morton held her back.

"Muriel's free to go where she wants inside the compound. You have to let her be," he instructed them.

Wanda eased down. Morton stepped into the hallway. A moment later Annise joined him. They began to walk.

"She's so brilliant, and yet so terrified," sighed the blonde. "I know exactly how she feels. Reality can be a bad mother, Morton. But at least there's heaven. What would we do if we didn't have a heaven?"

She slipped her arm into his, ultra-taboo according to Joseph's 13th Dictum, and on they continued down the hallway.

* * *

Chapter 10

Muriel was long gone. Up ahead appeared Stacy Lung and Perry Barwick, the reticent Speech Pathologist, with a group of about ten clients.

During the last year relations had been uncomfortable between Stacy and Morton. As she moved by the counselor noticed her dirty blonde hair had been dyed a bright platinum, and ten inches of it sheared off, leaving a stiff, curled-under pageboy.

Another of Joseph's Dictums was that no verbal banter was to go between staff when passing in the hallways, like in elementary school. For the first time since the rule had been instituted everyone obeyed it. The silence was flat out eerie.

Trina Lopez, the resident RN, followed ten feet behind the queue in her familiar corralling manner, escorting them toward the Nursing Station for afternoon meds.

Trina was a wealth of esoteric medical knowledge. If anything, she was *overly* insightful, one of your myopic anteaters forever nosing around Joseph and Harvey's prescription dosages and meticulously charting how they reacted in the patients. Dangerous work.

Although a uniform wasn't required, Trina sported a starched nurses' cap, a white calf-length lab coat and a physician's strength Littmann stethoscope everywhere she went, including into Vera's Diner where she and Morton conducted their most intriguing discussions. To certain individuals at the Fraction House Trina's crisp attire reflected a cracked, overdone pride in her profession. But Morton had discovered that people who wore thick, coke bottle glasses, like Trina, and didn't have the finest of looks maybe, were able to find the self-assurance they needed through an extra hour or two at the ironing board. He appeared to be the only one who didn't fault her for her dress code.

Morton and Annise stepped aside to let the group pass.

"Qué pasa, chiquita?" called Morton to Trina.

"Mucho. Joseph estrangula a Harvey en el bañyo," returned Trina. "Puedes salvarle?"

Morton laughed.

"What'd you say?" asked Annise quickly.

"I said, 'What's happening, babe?'" replied Morton.

"What'd Trina say?"

"She said Joseph's strangling Harvey upstairs in the bathtub and I better go save him."

Annise narrowed her eyes. "That's ridiculous. Joseph couldn't strangle him. Harvey's so much bigger," she said.

Morton stared at her.

Sam Lorenzo, the 'Inertial Catatonic' who continued to walk when he was walking, and refused to start walking when he was still, spotted Morton and embarked upon a slow reduction of pace. Anything, really, could hang the guy up. It was the nature of the Dar/Neese program that certain patients were close to normal, like Muriel; others only partially mentally ill, like Gordon; while a few, like Sam Lorenzo, were totally gone. This mix was supposed to mimic mainstream L.A. society and thereby act as a proving ground for a kind of cracked social integration. That Joseph, he really knew his nuts, you had to give him that.

Stacy and Perry Barwick continued along, disregarding Sam. This was an aspect of Joseph's Behavior Modification Therapy, which he called the IBB Program, or, Ignore Bad Behaviors. Trina, too, hurried on by.

Sam came to a rare stop, his feet working up and down in place, like a mime.

"Why in the world do you do things so slow, Sam?" asked Annise spontaneously.

"I do everything slooowww. I eat slooowww. I talk slooowww. I tie my shoes slooowww," replied Sam.

"I know, but *why*?"

"I walk slooowww. I sit down—"

"But why for Godsake?" cried Annise throwing up her hands.

"Because... Because I'm slooowww," said Sam.

Joseph had persuaded Harvey to put Sam on drugs that depressed the central nervous system—Thorazine, Mellaril, Trillafon, a couple of the benzodiazepines—under the theory that slowing him down would ultimately speed him up the way listening to sad songs when you were dejected made you more cheerful by keeping you crying and upset. Sam's speeds were slow, slower, and stop. It was hard for Morton to see the underlying success, which Joseph insisted was there.

"Wait! I just remembered, I'm on duty now!" exclaimed Annise. "I bet Wanda thinks I'm a total basket case, walking out on her like I did." The blonde scurried away. A few seconds later she came rushing back and grasped Morton by his newly shaved cheeks.

"I've really got to run. I want to thank you though for coaching me. You're doing a great job, you truly are, Morty."

"It's Morton, Annise. I prefer Morton, if you don't mind."

"So are we still looking at Saturday for the movies?" she asked.

He nodded.

"Super! In the meantime promise you'll have a hot toddy on me down at The Amazon Bar & Grill."

"OK," said Morton.

She smiled, kissed him on the lips and once again trotted off down the dimly lit corridor. Sam continued to march in place as the two males watched Annise's hips work seductively into the distance under her pink miniskirt.

Why was it that in her very walk there resided an exotic psychological meaning? Some value over and above the simple bell curve of mere physical attraction? Was it the smoke screen of her presentation? Was it those high-flown overtures to champagne style that enticed him, he wondered, as she disappeared around the bend with an unconscious bump and grind. That Annise Chastain, a washbasin overfull of coltish L.A. enthusiasm right to the very end!

Morton gave Sam Lorenzo a friendly whap between the shoulder blades. "Nice, eh Sam?" he remarked.

Sam initiated a slow turn of his head in Morton's direction.

"Niiiccce," agreed the Inertial Catatonic, his lips creaking with the beginning of a smile which would take the next half hour to complete.

* * *

Chapter 11

On Saturday morning Morton telephoned Annise. Their intention was to make a deeper probe of the clients Morton was especially familiar with. Neither however seemed sure how to go about this part of the training. Their conversation started well, then stalled. The movies were scheduled for later in the evening, yes, but the rest of the day lay ahead like a large empty room. So when Annise suggested a leisurely drive up to Simi Valley, to the "wine country," as she called it, Morton quickly agreed. An expedition, that was the thing!

After much consideration the counselor donned his gray tweed pants with the red suspenders, and his balloon-sleeved Renaissance shirt.

The drive into the valley was lovely. In and out of the beige, river-washed canyons. Up the impossibly steep grades into the cypress green glory of the Santa Monica mountains.

Once at the vineyards Annise delighted both the polyester clad tourists and the burly grape-stomping workers with her long peasant style dress. Of note too was her revealing plum-colored blouse with the racy leather thongs strapped medieval style down the front.

Annise wasn't your porcelain, china doll type either. She knew how to have fun. This was clear when they grinned at each other, and separated from the tour group long enough to take a whiz between the dusty rows of vines. That was the nice thing about Annise Chastain—you got to do what you wanted without the tedious yards of explanation another woman might ask for, a Stacy Lung, for example. What was more, she had the balls to do it *with* you! She had so many facets, plus a kennel full of fur-lined femininity to boot.

Theirs was a long, soporific afternoon in the California sunshine. They toured three—or was it four of the elegant castle-shaped wineries?—returning at last by way of the rugged Pacific Coast Highway. As they wound their way back toward

L.A. above Malibu their cheeks glowed rosy with the effects of the day.

It was twilight. Annise had her black driving gloves on, and Morton couldn't help but feel a special grace in the way she maneuvered her little Mazda sports car through the hairpin turns.

Off to the right they could see the whitecapped waves of the Pacific rolling gently onto the wide sand beaches. Ahead were the bluish, Tinkertoy skyscrapers and freeway loops of the city.

"I noticed you didn't stop around to see me at the Fraction House this week," said Annise.

"Joseph had me up in Administration. I'm organizing the paperwork for Muriel's Termination Meeting." Morton paused. "I get the feeling they're trying to keep me away from you two."

"But they rehired you to hang out with us, didn't they?"

"Joseph told me I'm supposed to be there for her, but not *with* her. I can't figure it out. Sometimes I think he's a bastard in sheep's clothing."

"Joseph? I can't believe that. He's been sweet as pie to me. And you know he takes Harvey out to those rich dinners all the time."

"What's so good about rich dinners? If I had a dark eye I'd say Joseph's trying to kill him with steak and booze."

Annise and Morton frowned at one another.

"I guess I thought you might sneak down for a visit," she said. "It's fun to do things a little wrong sometimes."

She punched the cigarette lighter. "Gordon Theodoricus loves your ass, Morton. You could at least stop in to see him. In fact, he's actually been endangered lately."

"Endangered?" said Morton.

"He keeps looking backwards out of his bicycle glasses. You know, the ones with the little rearview mirrors on the sides. He wants to see if you're coming and then smashes into walls and things."

Morton held up his bad arm. "This thing's broken in a couple of places. I'm not sure I can risk it with those younger guys on C-Wing. They'll want to give the cast a big hug."

"It's such a shame about your wrist. I feel for you, Morton. But sometimes we don't have any control over these things," said Annise sympathetically.

"That's the truth," agreed the counselor. "Right when you're about to say goodbye to your best friend some goon throws marbles on the floor and you go flying down the steps. And there's not a damn thing you can do about it."

"Who threw marbles on the floor?" said Annise looking out the window.

Several moments passed.

"They tell me Muriel used to be a very deranged—or rather, dynamic client," said Annise. "Joseph showed me footage of her. He's been doing his video, you know, for records and all. I suppose she's kind of cute, if you like those types."

"What types?" wondered Morton.

Annise gave him a sideways stare. "Modeling types you'd probably call it."

"Modeling? Muriel doesn't have the personality for that sort of thing."

"No," agreed Annise. "But a lot of those girls who go around in the buff don't need to worry about their personalities."

"In the buff! Joseph showed you a video of Muriel in the buff?"

"It's not so unusual, Morton. The other videos he had were a lot less artistic than Muriel's."

"The other videos! Jesus Christ, Annise, what's going on over there?"

She wheeled into the next turn.

"I'm not as naïve as you seem to think, Morton," she replied. "I need this kind of thing. I've been sheltered from the nitty-gritty my whole life. If you saw our place in Pasadena you'd know what I mean. It's so goddamned ritzy. Joseph's helping me break free of—how did he put it?—yeah, my 'past bondage,' he calls it."

"That's a pile of bullshit, Annise. Joseph does things for his own gain. If you hang around the Fraction House long enough you'll find that out."

Annise at last came up with her cigarettes. The lighter had popped out a while back. She punched it in again.

* * *

Chapter 12

Back in L.A. they decided to drop in at The Shamrock, the Irish style lounge over on La Brea Annise was partial to. It wasn't quite dark yet. They parked, leaving a short walk to the bar.

Morton took her elbow, and they crossed the street at the pace dictated by the high heels she'd slipped on in the car. It was then Morton began to comprehend the enormity of the woman's appeal. Her shape, her stride, every detail of movement and gesture was a piece of patented ultra-femininity. He tried to ignore the beeping horns and neck craning. It was as if the public took her for common property in an instantly astounded way.

How much the counselor was influenced by this he didn't know. It was to her credit, probably, that Annise didn't notice these goings on around her. The guy in the corner bicycle shop actually dropping his wrench to gawk, for instance.

Before reaching the lounge they came upon a small movie theater. An obviously pornographic film was advertised. The posters were crude. Morton became concerned for Annise's modesty, and playing the gentleman he moved to block her sight. She glanced around him at the lewd marquee.

"Wow! *Four Wicked Witches*. Is this the film we're seeing later?" she said eyeing the posters.

"Well, uh, if you want we can," stammered Morton. "I didn't know you'd be interested in, well—"

~~~

At The Shamrock Annise left immediately for the ladies' room. She was gone a long time, but when she returned she was blisteringly lovely in the bright red lipstick and fanned out hair. Nighttime makeup, the counselor reminded himself, was supposed to be more dramatic.

To Morton's delight she'd changed earrings to the purple, swan-shaped ones made of glass he'd found in one of the Simi Valley souvenir shops.

Annise pulled up her stool. "Just think, Morton, we'll have hundreds of places like this to explore. Even better than this."

"Yes. Yes, we will, Annise."

She tossed back her head. "What a wonderful challenge. I mean, what could possibly be more delightful than talking and drinking and having such a wonderful time together?"

Morton thought about it. Yes, there was one other thing. If he was going to be straightforward he ought to come out with it. It had to do with their... well, intimacies.

He took a moment to examine her. Doleful, profound eye carriage like the saints must have had. Cigarette burning seductively at her earlobe. The small glass of tequila turning round and round between her long red fingernails. Add the rawhide lace holding her blouse together, the humps majestically bared to the maroon bar light— No, not yet, he decided. This wasn't the time for a tiff. After all, hadn't she said in the Recreation Room they could have as much they wanted? On the other hand, so far they hadn't had *any*. Still, the future was all before them. There'd be time for these things.

Annise enjoyed her cocktails, that was clear. She hardly flinched as she snapped back a series of shots, chewing the lemon with relish after each one. Morton checked his watch. It was getting late for the movies.

"Maybe we ought to turn in early," he suggested casually. "We'd be fresher if we wanted to do something tomorrow."

"But I thought you were taking me down to *Four Wicked Witches*!" she objected. She sipped her tequila. "I mean, it *did* look like an art film, didn't it?"

Annise wasn't your pushy sort. She finished her drink, blinked her eyes a couple of times, and handed him the keys.

* * *

Chapter 13

The entrance to Annise's apartment was on the second floor. At the base of the metal stairs Morton slipped his arms around her small, tight waist. He could hear her little brown beagle barking in short nervous bursts.

"Don't mind Sassafras. She gets upset with all my men," soothed Annise.

"All your men?"

Her hair was windblown from the ride, loose and tousled. She went one step up and turned to face him. The extra height gained by her hot red pumps leveled her sea-green eyes with Morton's. A ghost-like thrill of conquest passed through the counselor, for she reminded him of those sexy spike-heeled bombshells you sometimes saw strutting their stuff down Hollywood Boulevard, irresistible as Cool Whip topping.

"I've been very uptight today. I guess you could tell," muttered Annise.

"No, I couldn't tell," said Morton.

She stroked his head affectionately.

"Your hair is so soft. Look." She held out a lock. "It's almost as light as mine. And it's getting so long."

A moment passed.

"Listen, there's something I feel you should know about me. But only if you promise not to laugh," said Annise.

"I won't laugh."

"Follow me," she said.

She led him up the stairs, through the front door and into her bedroom.

A copper plaque of praying hands, like the kind kids made at Vacation Bible School, was on the south wall. Beside it hung a group photo of twenty or so of her friends drinking beer at Filthy McNasty's down on the Strip. On the night table was a small plaster statue of Mother Mary cradling infant Jesus. Against the far wall was one of those New Age vanities, the ovaled, copolymer kind where the plastic gleamed like a jewel. Red and white bulbs ringed the mirror and designer makeup vials lined the edges. Above this monster hung a giant calendar. In the squares were many handwritten notations, apparently tracking her social life.

"That's one hell of an agenda," observed Morton.

"Not really. I have lots of friends is all."

"Friends? Are you sure those initials aren't for all your guys?" He smiled.

Annise lit a cigarette. "So what if they are? Most of my friends happen to be guys," she answered.

"Like Joseph Schopen?" he said too quickly.

"Loving your neighbor, Morton, is what life is all about. Not fear of macho men, like Joseph. Jesus himself said that."

"He did?" said Morton surprised.

"Uh huh."

Annise pulled out the chair to her vanity and eased open the wide bottom drawer.

"Promise you won't think I'm bad?"

Morton sat cross-legged on the bed as she brought out a large metal box fitted with a stout brass padlock. He watched as she fetched the key from a hidden compartment in her purse, and inch by inch the metal case creaked open.

First came the magazines. Sideways across the front was the title, *Swedish Sins!* She handed him one.

"Whew!" said Morton thumbing through.

Next were the metal ball bearings tied together with fishing line. Hmmm, what could *they* be for?

She rummaged past the tubular plastic items, the long-life batteries and whatnot, until she came to a tiny black square of silk. Daintily she unfolded it, and with the tips of her fingers contoured the fabric to her torso. It was a negligee. Morton could see where the three holes had been strategically snipped out for erotic purposes. Annise lifted the garment and pressed it delicately to her cheek.

"I'll be back in a minute. Then we can have our talk," she announced. She left for the bathroom.

When she was gone Morton slid the box over. Stubs of old lottery tickets were confettied over the various paraphernalia. Those Catholics, gamblers in spite of themselves, smiled Morton. He nudged aside the carved horse's head with the whip-like strands of black leather at the end. There was a stack of green papers with a rubber band around them. Stock certificates, it looked like. Then, under the chrome plated handcuffs, he found the strangest thing of all. A pistol. A small pearl-handled derringer, western style, and apparently the real thing. He broke open the barrel. Yes, it was authentic all right, and fully loaded with two nasty looking .38 caliber slugs, hollow-points, which he knew inflicted greater damage. A small cardboard box with 'Winchester' printed on it held a handful of spare rounds.

Annise returned and stood in the doorway. She'd squeezed into the negligee. Morton was duly impressed in the upright way she held herself as she modeled.

"Well, do you like it?" she asked in a cooing, baby doll voice.

There was an instant of stunned observation as the counselor struggled to take in the critical details.

"Good God in heaven, yes!" he exclaimed.

Annise saw the pistol. Slowly she raised her hands.

"Go ahead and shoot. I've been naughty, Morton. I'm a She-Devil," she said playfully, her voice satiny and hot. "I deserve a bullet to the belly."

But Morton was worried on a different front. A firearm was nothing to toy with. And this one was loaded. What if he hadn't noticed and went ahead and cocked the thing? Risky business, any way you looked at it.

"What's this for, Annise?" he asked breaking the rhythm.

Her eyes cleared. "Oh, nothing," she said sitting beside him on the bed. "I know I'll never have to use it. It's only— Well, if you have to know, it's in case I ever get raped."

"Raped? But how will it help you here in the box? I mean, wouldn't it have to be in your purse to do any good?"

She shook her head. "I could never shoot another person. The Bible tells you to turn the other cheek. But what if I did get raped? Say I got pregnant. What would I do then?"

"Well, uh—"

"I'd have to get an abortion, wouldn't I?"

"You could have the baby," suggested the counselor.

"No way. That's a mortal sin, Morty. It's not a mortal sin if you're married, of course. But if the Courthouse doesn't have a record of it, shit, you're off to hell in a hand basket. I mean, what if a big black—" She took a deep breath. "Abortion," she snorted. "I'd rather die first. I really would."

"But how will a gun help?" he said again.

She stared seriously at him. Suddenly he realized what she meant.

"Are you saying—" he stammered. "Do you mean you'd use this thing on yourself?"

"Of course not. Suicide is a mortal sin too. It's murder, only on your own body. No, I'd have to pay somebody to shoot me. St. Peter stands at the Pearly Gates. He's a tough dude too. He'd know if I hadn't played by the rules."

"But if you pay somebody to kill you you're as dead as if you did it by your own hand," observed the counselor.

"Maybe. But *I* wouldn't have done it. You can't be held accountable for evil in other sources, like a hit man. That wouldn't be my problem at all."

Morton returned the gun to the box. Annise's eyes dampened. He'd touched a nerve. He pulled her close and for the longest time hugged her there on the edge of the bed.

Annise said, "I'm sorry, Morton. I guess all this must seem strange to you."

"A little," he admitted.

"I just want you to know how serious a Catholic I am," she said drawing back.

"How serious a Catholic are you?"

"Well, I'm not saying we can't have sex. We can. Gobs and gobs if we want. Only it's very important you respect how I feel about these things."

Annise stubbed out her cigarette. She went to the vanity, found her leather cigarette case and lit another one.

"You may not be aware of this, but I have a very deep feeling for someone. He's the only person in this entire world I have to be faithful to," she said over her shoulder.

Morton had a sudden irrational fear. He glanced at the inked over calendar. He knew how Catholics could be with authority figures.

"Joseph?" he said weakly.

"Of course not, silly."

"Who then?"

"The Pope," she said, blowing a plume of smoke high into the air. She ran a hand through her hair, twisting the left side into a wild, unkempt look.

"The Pope?"

Morton sagged. He leaned far back on the bed. He was feeling quite tired. When she didn't continue, he said, "But is it OK with the Pope if we have all the sex we want? I thought the Pope was against that kind of thing."

"Oh, hell no. The Pope doesn't give one flying shit about that," she assured him.

"He doesn't?"

"Why should he? The Pope doesn't even have sex."

"I didn't think so," said the counselor.

"Sex is one thing. Like all this we're planning to do. It's really not so evil."

"Oh, no," agreed Morton. "It's not evil at all."

"Intercourse, on the other hand, is strictly forbidden," she added.

"God, don't say that, Annise."

"But it is, Morton. It's been decreed and Holy Water went on it and everything. The Pope says protected intercourse isn't at all fair to the unconceived child."

"But Annise, if the child hasn't been conceived yet—" Morton began, then he halted and squeezed shut his eyes.

She smoked thoughtfully. "On the other hand, there is one little loophole. I won't say I haven't considered it."

"What loophole?" asked Morton.

"Well, it used to be the Pope was infallible, you know. You didn't? Well, he was. But I guess he got tired of being infallible, because in 1956, or '66, sometime around then, he changed his mind and said, 'From now on I'm speaking fallibly unless I say up front it's infallible.' That's exactly what he said, Morton. And one way or another everything he says comes straight from God, so when he declares he's fallible and likely to make a bunch of goofy mistakes, you know it has to be true."

Annise looked around the room. "By the way, did you bring those wine goblets we bought in from the car?"

"Yeah. I put them on the sofa so Sassafras could play with them."

"Anyway," she continued, "the Pope told us we couldn't use birth control. Only there's a big loophole there, because he didn't say it when he was infallible. Do you see what I'm getting at?"

"Kind of."

"This means it's probably OK to use... Well, you know—"

"What?" he asked low.

She leaned toward him. "Rubbers," she whispered.

"Rubbers!"

"But to be honest, Morton, they wouldn't do me any good either. I guess you know why, don't you?" Her eyes searched him.

"Is it because we're not all the way in love yet?" wondered the counselor.

"Love!" she cried. "Love has nothing to do with it. My God, Morton, it's amazing how out of touch with Catholicism you are."

"I'm afraid that's true," he admitted.

"It's because we're not *married*, for Christsake. In the eyes of the Pope we'd be mortal sinners no matter how deeply in love we were. I know it can be mysterious, but all your God stuff has been mysterious from the very start. That's why if you're Catholic you have to have so much more faith than if you're in those other stupid religions."

However, as she'd said, they were free to do this with the toys. The negligee. The vibrator. The leather horse's head whip. All of which the Pope didn't give the first flying shit about.

Annise sat very erectly on the side of the bed, exaggerating the alluring cut of the negligee. More parts were bursting out toward the counselor than he remembered a woman having.

"I'm afraid I'll lose myself if I get too involved," said Annise looking over.

"You're supposed to lose yourself. That's what it's all about," countered Morton.

"But if I go over the edge I know I'll forget myself and do the whole damn thing."

"That's what you're meant to do after foreplay, isn't it?"

"Not us Catholics."

She uttered this with such naïveté Morton found himself genuinely moved. A lot of times you found contradictions in people. You couldn't be an egotist and take offense every time you hit a pothole in the highway.

"So much can be beautiful between two people," she added offering a nimble twist of her torso. "Wouldn't you like to investigate some of *that* with me?"

Morton took a moment to re-assess the three revealing openings in the negligee. "Of course I'd like to investigate some of that with you, Annise. Of course I would."

~~~

And so went the night. First infatuation and the midnight molding of one's dampened Play-Doh made for an intense early period. Soon, however, an edginess began to build between the sheets. It might have been solved with release, if release would have come, but in the end the Pope had his way with them.

Morton groaned and rolled to the side of her queen-sized bed. In their initial haste, the paper Taiwanese lantern had been left on. It cast a muted, Halloween green across the walls. Annise wrinkled her nose, then reached to click it off. For many seconds it jiggled hyperactively above them.

"Does that thing ever get on your nerves?" he asked.

Through the darkness the counselor could make out the whites of her eyes. He was referring to Joseph's comment in the Recreation Room. He felt she wouldn't answer, that she'd been offended. And then, when she didn't answer, he was sure she'd been offended. He was exhausted, yet he had a hard time falling asleep.

~~~

In the wee hours he found himself awakening. Annise was hovering over him.

"I was thinking," she said in a raspy voice. "We could get the gun out. I could point it at myself maybe. That would be interesting, wouldn't it? It might help." She shook her head. "Oh, hell, I don't even know if I'd like that. They tell you to never point a gun at anybody unless you mean to use it." Quietly, she said, "Would you want to point it at me?"

"I don't know," said Morton. He had a sudden thought. "Did Joseph say he wanted to point it at you? Did Joseph try to make you point it at yourself? There's a power in that, you know." He met her eyes, but they were zombie eyes. "Did it excite you, Annise?"

Morton kept waiting, but she never did answer. The next day he thought it must have been a dream, and didn't mention it again.

* * *

Chapter 14

When the counselor awakened Annise was nowhere to be found. The coffee had been brewed, and there was a note on the countertop in the kitchen. She'd gone to Sunday mass.

Sassafras was moping around.

"You haven't been fed yet, have you, girl?" said Morton stroking the little beagle's head.

He put the half pound of hamburger he'd brought over the day before into the dog dish, added a can of Annise's specialty eggdrop soup as an appetizer and went back to bed.

He drifted off to the sounds of Sassafras thanking him with her happy chomping and slurping.

~~~

A couple of hours later he heard the front door open. Annise fiddled around in the kitchen for a few minutes. Then she came into the bedroom and turned on the bright horseshoe of lights at the vanity.

"Pull my zipper, will you, Morton?" she asked picking up her brush.

He went to her and unzipped the dress.

"Boy oh boy, do I feel free," she bubbled stretching her arms. "And so *cleansed*."

"More than usual?" he wondered.

"Yep. I think it might be due to our new Assistant Priest."

Morton helped her step clear of the dress. Annise took a seat at the vanity, flipped a switch and the ring of bulbs magically receded to a soft, pastel red.

Morton began to affectionately stroke her back, by degrees moving lower, to her hips. Finally he reached the sensual little lump at the crease of the buttocks. Quite comely! Her hair was in a long French braid. She undid it and began to brush out the kinks.

"And he's so cute, Morton," she said to his reflection in the mirror. "You ought to see him. The Assistant Priest, I mean. He's the one who gave me Confession today."

"Confession? How do you know it was him? I didn't think you could see each other through the box," said Morton.

"Well, you can't. But a bunch of us had doughnuts and coffee after the service and I recognized his voice. I'm pretty sure he recognized mine. And I knew right when he recognized it too, because his eyes got real big and he turned bright pink."

She brushed and brushed. A million notions ran through the counselor's head.

"You didn't tell him about, uh—" He glanced tensely to the metal toy box left out from the night before. "What exactly *did* you tell him, Annise?"

"I'm sorry, Morton, but I really can't divulge church secrets."

"But I'm the one you did it all with, for Christsake. I'm sure that joker has the lowdown on me by now."

"He is *not* a joker. He's a fine, upstanding man," said Annise. "Just because he's young and good looking doesn't take anything away from a guy being stuck celibate. And on top of it all having to hear some anonymous blonde's nasty little—"

"Oh my God!" gasped Morton slapping his forehead.

"Don't curse, Morty, please. It's Sunday."

The counselor's eyes drifted painfully upward. There was the calendar looming ominously over the vanity, notations scrawled all across the month. He noticed what looked like the printed letters J.S. in certain of the squares. Damned if there weren't a bunch of them marked in on the days he'd been away camping. The counselor felt uneasy inside, similar to the time Perry Barwick told him the dirty sex lie about Stacy Lung, which he later discovered wasn't a lie at all.

A nervous twitch caught in Morton's eyelid. He said, "By the way, did you confess Joseph patting your behind in the Recreation Room?"

"Oh, no," she answered quickly. "Roman Catholics don't have to confess things somebody else does to them."

"I thought so! He did grab your butt, didn't he?"

Silence. Annise said, "Look, did you confess to anybody kidnapping Muriel to the mountains and diddling her in your apartment?"

Morton puffed his cheeks. "Of course not. You know I never—"

"I didn't think so," she interrupted. "I'm saying if you didn't do it, I didn't do it either. We're even. Let's leave it right there, shall we?"

~~~

Annise had a lot to do that Sunday. Among other things she'd scheduled "an evening engagement," as she called it. "Just with a friend though, Morton. Please don't be jealous."

"I'm not jealous. Why should I be jealous?"

In addition, she had an Irish heritage, which she was quite proud of, and she was set on watching the Notre Dame basketball game at 3:00 p.m. Morton made peanut butter sandwiches, and after lunch they entered the living room.

Annise switched on the TV. She lined various lacquers and enamels on the coffee table to re-coat her nails.

"Scoot, Sassafras," she said sweeping the dog off the sofa.

Morton prepared to leave. "Doing it up for evening mass?" he asked as he slipped on his jacket.

"No. Gary said— I mean, the Assistant Priest said he didn't think many would show tonight. You know, with Notre Dame being in the playoffs and all. I guess most of the congregation has money on it."

"I thought gambling—I mean, I didn't realize the church supported—"

But Morton thought better of his comment. He went over to her. "Well, behave yourself, that's all I ask," he said.

He gave her a kiss goodbye. Although she remained sitting Annise responded with a vitality that wasn't merely glowing embers. A great deal of her, he'd learned, was pure beach bunny

'L.A. 2000:' Sex Asylum

flame, a five-foot-four vixen silhouette which men, her Assistant Priest included, by God, saw as the freshest, most untainted soul in all of L.A. Was there competition for a woman like this? Or was she such an anomaly of lust and weirdo virtue her lover might find himself enshadowed by the very lights of her vanity?

Morton got his keys off the kitchen counter. Annise didn't walk him to the door. She seemed terrifically engrossed in the game.

"Who's winning?" he called.

"Those damn Pennsylvania heathens. It looks like I'm going to lose twenty to Wanda after all," she returned over her shoulder.

That Annise Chastain. She was like the snap at the end of a whip where all the sound and fury cracked free. One thing for certain, she was a hard one to ignore.

* * *

Chapter 15

Over the next couple of weeks Joseph and Harvey engaged in loud, marathon disagreements over the running of the Fraction House in Harvey's office, leaving Morton to himself in the sparse room at the far end of the hall. At last he was beginning to feel a little emancipated from the stresses of the place. He even softened toward Joseph when he overheard him pestering Harvey to get additional pain medication.

"I don't want you hurting," insisted the Gestapo. "We're going to spring for better pain pills. Really killer pain pills so we can protect you against yourself. That's the final word."

Joseph the caring nurse? Hmmm.

At mid-week came the delivery from Carney Apothecary of numerous corrugated boxes tightly packed with prescription meds. These deliveries had always been shrouded in mystery. The courier was known to be one of Joseph's drinking buddies, and sometimes he'd bring the shipments in the saddlebags of his Harley. Under the table kickbacks, wondered the counselor? Well, such was the way of the world, wasn't it? Go looking for evil and it would find you. Best leave well enough alone, particularly if you didn't have any proof.

Morton's finances had never been very healthy. He did have a small savings account in the Dar/Neese Credit Union, and what with Harvey's offer of the increased salary he was able to have his electricity and telephone service turned back on.

As for Muriel, she wasn't much improved. But if you had to be there *for* her, never *with* her... Well, in terms of therapy he'd been given his limitations, and each day they were feeling more uncomfortable.

Something wasn't right in his heart, a flutter of insincerity perhaps? And if so, for whom? At home he sat in his green recliner, trying to call it rest, but it felt more like worry. Pain. It was always caused by unfulfilled desire. Where'd he heard that?

'L.A. 2000:' Sex Asylum

Let's see— Yes, it was from Muriel. He was thinking of when he'd taken her and Gordon on a Normalization Field Trip to the Taiwanese restaurant. Morton had been seeing a lot of Stacy Lung at the time, and was disconcerted about their relationship not progressing to the abiding love stage. The clients, with their super sensory perceptions regarding the emotions, were somehow wise to his dilemma.

"There's really no such thing as pain," Muriel informed him in her childlike way. "If you're hurt you're only feeling that a desire you had isn't full. As soon as you quit wanting it doesn't hurt anymore."

Muriel was doing better in those days. People became much smarter when they did better.

~~~

Annise had completed her orientation period. One of the hardest parts of the counselor's new life was adjusting to each Tuesday, when she would pack her bag, as Morton himself used to do, and disappear for another three day, round-the-clock stint at the Fraction House. Even more troubling was the Gestapo's between-the-lines mandate insisting Morton keep his distance from Annise and Muriel.

He'd kiss the blonde goodbye, but within the hour it seemed, that strange L.A. breed of loneliness would set in. A cold, big city loneliness sprawling all around like a smog laden desert, and making a person feel afraid inside. It was an oppression which sought heart warming romance in a very bad way, which sought the safety and protection of another's arms.

As things were turning out, he hadn't been able to see Annise as much as he'd hoped. They'd been meeting for "dates," as she termed their encounters, though from Morton's perspective the time seemed fraught with a lot of coffee drinking and waiting around. When she did at last appear—*materialize* was more the word for it—boundaries and dimensions plain misted away. Her fine *I. Magnus* scent, that atmosphere she carried of the archetypal woman he knew he'd have to hit the lottery to afford—

Yet here she was, leaning provocatively on his shoulder in her favorite Mediterranean style bar, and in a cat-purr voice saying how in her heart the thing she most wanted was a child, an infant in swaddling clothes to nurse in the way a woman was meant to. "A baby, Morton. Like you were as a boy," she cooed. "Exactly like you were. I really mean this."

It was strong stuff.

~~~

That evening Morton worked till five, then dropped by Annise's place. It was a Tuesday. Both were subdued as she packed for the Fraction House.

Subdued? Icy might have described it better. They'd had a few separations of opinion lately. For Morton, apologies and hugs bridged the vexation. Annise though had a wider system of checks and balances. She endured countless emotional black eyes, it seemed, and couldn't get cleansed without a greenish shadow of shame continuing to snap at her heels.

Today they'd had another minor difference. It was over with quickly, but Annise continued to hold the sour, lemony edge.

"Why can't you forget this crap and get on with things?" asked Morton.

She shook her head very far from side to side.

"These aren't the old days," she said by way of explanation. "Because in the old days you could pay your way out of guilt with indulgences. You know what indulgences were, don't you?"

Morton scratched his temple.

"That's when God used to let you do stuff wrong as long as you gave cold cash to the orphans in town," she said.

"God used to let people do stuff wrong?"

"Well, he had to, didn't he? I mean, he knows time both ways. He knows what's going to happen and what's already

'L.A. 2000:' Sex Asylum

happened. So he had to know I'd be paying my evil deeds off somehow."

"Disagreements aren't evil deeds, Annise."

"In a girl's head there's good and evil, Morton. And they *always* disagree."

"How sad," he muttered.

"Anyway, they quit taking money for guilt way back when. It's a pity, really, because my dad's loaded like nobody's business. Nowadays they make you give of yourself."

"Like how?"

"Wanda said if we went to Venice and handed leaflets out with the Harmonic Convergence guy it'd be enough. You know the one. He's got a long beard. Orange on one side and blonde on the other. We could rollerblade and wear our bikinis. A lot of people seem to listen to you if you're on rollerblades."

Her eyes were wide and searching. She ran her fingers up her neck and shook out her great blonde mane. Morton watched the multiple changes in her features as she attempted to balance the Devil's half eaten apple inside her with the Angel's fluttering, gossamer wings. At last she delivered to him yet another of her patented arsenal of looks, but try as he might there was no interpreting it. A few minutes later she drove off for the Fraction House.

~~~

The counselor was left alone in her apartment, a rare occurrence. He and Sassafras wandered into the bedroom and began a dumb stare at her calendar, his nemesis.

Friends? Humph. Friends, friends everywhere, and not a Morton marked down. Yet so many initials! J.S.'s were rampant. L.S.'s were on every other square. What did it all mean? A couple of days ago Morton had confronted her with his suspicions.

Annise replied, "J.S.? God you've got an active imagination. That's Joel Sincowitz. He coached the girl's softball team when I was a teenager. We've been friends forever, Morton. In fact, he's a hot shot Disc Jockey now. And quite a celebrity, I might add. If you'd like, I'd be happy to take you down to the station for an intro."

"Uhhh, well, I would, only the wrist, I mean, the cast... It's difficult to shake hands, Annise, that's all."

~~~

Morton went on home. Throughout the night he tossed and turned. In the morning he had the strangest sensation. He thought of it as aching all over, though nothing in particular hurt. Wasn't this the way Muriel felt when she had bad days? "It's the body that makes the mind sore," she'd said. No, that wasn't it, recalled the counselor. "It's the *mind* makes the *body* hurt." Yes, that's what she'd said. The *mind*.

He telephoned Joseph to say he couldn't make it in.

"Don't sweat it, Allison. Harvey won't know anyway. He's out sick himself," replied the supervisor.

"Harvey's sick? What's the matter with him?" asked Morton concerned.

"He's obese. He's been having heart problems for years, everybody knows it. Plus, he's an old fart," said Joseph.

"Old? He's only fifty-three."

"I'm thirty-six. As far as I'm concerned, he's ancient," replied the Gestapo.

"What's he on? I know he takes Lasix to keep the fluid off. And potassium too, doesn't he?"

Part of Joseph's job description was to inventory each week's delivery from Carney Apothecary, the wholesale pharmacy. Keeping the medications straight for forty-five clients was a mind bending operation, but Joseph was expert at it. Harvey himself took a number of expensive cardiac drugs, and he could get substantial discounts by ordering through Dar/Neese. For legal reasons Joseph had Trina Lopez, the RN, dole out the pills, including Harvey's, but only after the supervisor had checked and double checked the allotments. A mix up in drug combinations, or error in who took what, could at the least put Trina's job on the line, or the Gestapo's, and at the worst prove fatal to the person who got the wrong dose. These high powered medications were nothing to toy with.

"He takes nitroglycerin too, I think," continued Morton over the lines. "Make sure he gets his nitro, Joseph. That's what'll keep him alive in a pinch."

"Thanks for the advice, doc," snorted the Gestapo. "So you're sick, eh? What do I put it down as?"

"I've been feeling a little under the weather. You know, mentally," said the counselor. "I could use a breather."

"A mental health day, you mean?"

"Yeah, that's it, a mental health day." Morton thought a moment. "I just feel like everybody's soul is in a big tomb, Joseph, and no matter what I do this gigantic rock keeps rolling shut across the doorway." He paused. "It's like we're all penned up in there together! It's really frightening."

"You're talking about life in L.A.," said the Gestapo.

"Or maybe the Fraction House," said Morton.

He could hear Joseph blowing out a lung full of cigarette smoke on the other end of the line. Morton ground his fists against the throbbing in his forehead.

"Well, any advice?" asked the counselor, his voice low and directionless.

"Why don't you get drunk and eat a big fried chicken meal? That's what me and Harvey do when we get upset."

Morton almost said, 'Harvey and *I*, you dumb—' But he held his tongue. He was doing better at navigating these delicate political waterways.

Alcohol therapy? With a juicy cholesterol side order? This didn't sound right for a three hundred pound Freudian with heart problems, did it?

"Hmmm, maybe I'll give it a try," said Morton finally.

Joseph said, "By the way, Allison, you missed one back there. It's supposed to be Harvey and *I*, you stupid son of a—"

Joseph went on, of course. But at the sound of that last Morton hung up.

* * *

Chapter 16

Later that day, after a nap, Morton found himself steering his pickup down the long east to west thoroughfare of Hollywood Boulevard, known as the Strip. He needed time to himself, he felt. Interior privacy, call it, as opposed to the exterior life he'd been leading in the Fraction House Administrative Offices, and with Annise too, for that matter.

Every now and then, from one of the side streets, a limousine with some hot shot movie star in the back swung out, cutting off the working men trying to get home. Between the stoplights and fast-food chains Morton got a glimpse east to the faraway peaks of the San Gabriel mountains. There was a freedom up there. A good rain in those mountains could wash the sticky glitter dust of the city right off a person. He'd been trying to bolt this place for years.

Los Angeles, the City of Angels, it meant in Spanish. Well, maybe, but of whores too. And of all the mid-level lunatics in between who made for the phoniness and the criminal sizzle vibrating in your ears like burning cellophane. The populace was a lot like nature herself around here. Raging wildfires. Mudslides that took the houses of fat cats right off the hills. Earthquakes!

The mountains? Colorado was pretty, he'd heard. The Rockies. But no, they banned campfires there a couple of years ago. Oregon maybe? There had to be someplace left, some *natural* asylum for the soul.

His truck growled and bounced as he made his way deeper into the city. He came to Filthy McNasty's, the bar Annise and her friends had been photographed in. In fact, this was an area he knew.

In his early days at the Fraction House, before he and Joseph had gotten fully acquainted, the supervisor organized an after-hours outing with Perry and a couple of the other guys. Morton tagged along. They'd gone to Joseph's favorite titty bar, The

Green Room, it was called. The Gestapo was obviously tight with the barmaids, and before they knew it all of them were half looped on Snakebites, which was a shot of whiskey with a layer of peppermint schnapps floated over the top.

"This stuff's electric, Allison," Joseph said, smacking his lips. His eyes bulged. The veins at his temples throbbed. "Reminds me of when I used to toot the white stuff."

"The white stuff? What white stuff?"

The Gestapo didn't answer. Instead he waved for another round, lit one of his long black cigarettes, then began his odd habit of stripping matches off a cardboard match pack and crumpling them onto the bar top.

What a night! Until Joseph buddied up with one of the hot-to-trot tattooed barmaids, or boob dancers, or whatever they were called. Morton and Perry and the rest were forced to scramble for a way home. Well, sometimes it was good to leave the old days way back there in the past where they belonged.

Morton waited for the light to change. As he might have expected there on the Strip the ladies of the evening were already strolling the sidewalks. Very beautiful ones too, he observed, and each trying to catch his eye as he slowly accelerated. Bad to the bone weren't they, hair all teased up and wearing those high stiletto heels? This wasn't a shallow studio version of whitewashed blondes and scrubbed down streets. No, this was the *real* L.A. tour.

Farther along... Wow, if it wasn't The Green Room over there on the right! Morton slowed. The door was propped open with one of those dingy vinyl bar stools. There wouldn't be any dancing this early in the evening, only a few locals taking a quiet moment for themselves. He parked.

Morton wasn't the most seasoned of drinking men, but recently Annise had been showing him the ropes. She'd been helpful in pointing out ways to relieve oneself of idle time while simultaneously gaining an aura of strength and psychological productivity in the lounges. An inner smile for Annise Chastain washed through him. Their relationship? Perhaps he'd leaned a

'L.A. 2000:' Sex Asylum

bit to the cool side. One of them had, for sure. He needed to remember how when two chemicals met there was bound to follow a by-product radically different from what either of you were individually. Yes, he'd go in and have himself a beer, do a bit of thinking.

~~~

Morton had been inside thirty minutes or so when the shift changed and the evening barmaid came in. She was a woman about forty-five or so, he decided, though her hair was still bright blonde. He watched as she mixed herself something in a small paper cup. Really, she was a marvel. Voluptuous breasts. Beautiful oval hips. He kept imagining Annise Chastain reaching that age and wearing those same tight fitting jeans and plunging leotard top. It made him feel proud.

She stepped over to him. "Another beer?" she asked.

"Yes, if you don't mind."

The floors weren't varnished. Dust hovered in the strips of light filtering in through the open doors. She returned with the beer.

"Pardon me for saying this. I want to tell you what an attractive woman I think you are," volunteered Morton.

She fluttered her eyelids. He'd embarrassed her.

"I'm sorry. I didn't mean that," he said.

"It's all right," she answered with the slightest parting of her lips.

Morton noticed a peculiar flaw in her smile, odd for such a beauty. Several small teeth protruded from her upper gums, sprouting out over the incisors in a way he'd seen only once or twice before. Well, so what? She was still lovely. He certainly wasn't going to take back his compliment.

The Green Room was all green inside. Behind the long semicircle of the bar hung a gigantic mirror and mock-up vanity, which acted as props for the exotic dancers. Gallon-size jugs of pretend makeup ringed the wooden stage. Along the side walls of the place were grainy photos of famous old-time movie stars. Outside of a few particulars the decor was startlingly like Annise's bedroom, reflected Morton, except for the missing Taiwanese lantern.

After a few minutes the barmaid came down to his end and started washing glasses.

"I really didn't mean to be so forward before," apologized the counselor. "It's just you remind me of someone."

"Oh?" she said looking up.

Morton explained about Annise. How attractive she was in the physical sense. "And yet she's so genuine and upbeat with everyone she meets, or so it seems anyway," he said.

"How old's this girl?" asked the barmaid lighting a cigarette.

"Twenty-three," he said.

She took his glass and slowly drew him another beer. "This one's on the house, friend," she said.

She stepped aside, and from a special bottle under the counter mixed her own in a paper cup.

"Twenty-three?" she echoed.

Morton nodded. The woman pulled up a stool on her side of the bar. The soft afternoon sunlight was drifting lazily through the open doors. They sipped placidly at their drinks and by degrees began a conversation. She was really a specimen, and the more they talked the friendlier they became. They were changing, opening their minds with the tranquil, alcohol closing of the day.

Morton finally relaxed. An authentic rapport began to develop between them. Her leotard top was accentuated by bright yellow tiger stripes slanted diagonally across her chest. He couldn't restrain himself from admiring her figure. And on a woman that age!

"I used to be a showgirl before I bought this bar. You know, Vegas style dancing. Not super big time or anything. I actually knew a few of these guys," she said waving around at the pictures. "Not any more. But I used to. I met Bogart though. I met Clark Gable once."

'L.A. 2000:' Sex Asylum

As they talked the barmaid became more and more animated.

"You seem so real. You're not like the twisted crap slopping around out there," said Morton. He thumbed over his shoulder toward Hollywood Boulevard, the infamous Strip.

"Why do you say that?" she asked taking a drink.

"I can just tell. Aren't there things in life you can know without exactly knowing them?"

She smoked and the smoke came up into her eyes. Without answering, she turned back to her work.

As the time passed Morton couldn't keep from sneaking glances, though he knew she saw him. A fresh notion popped into his head. Before the Fraction House he'd come close to becoming an accountant. You could make potent money in that field, he thought. You could afford the things you needed to survive with any kind of style in L.A.—a sleek sports car, a hot blonde.

Drifting back to his first night at The Green Room he realized how off balance he'd been in those early days at Dar/Neese. How he'd brought a truck full of raggedy mental baggage to the job without the slightest inkling of how heavy the load was. The place was a bona fide asylum, and at first he didn't think he'd last a month among the nuts and the whacked out fetishes of the staff members.

Morton always had trouble starting things. But he had even more trouble quitting things. At night he couldn't stop the day and sleep, so he had insomnia. After getting to sleep he couldn't seem to quit sleeping in the morning and start the day. Psychologically, the counselor suspected this meant something. Harvey said it was a binge personality, but Morton decided that was because Harvey went on so many binges.

Many times though the bad turned out good, for Morton found he achieved more balance, in a personal sense, from being spun in many diverse mental orbits. Maybe he wasn't a hundred percent sound upstairs—who was?—but he'd discovered a smidgen or two of equilibrium. For much of this, he thought pursing his lips over the beer foam, there was Muriel to thank. Sweet little Muriel Gonska, the schizophrenic. In a way she was the only real friend he'd made in L.A. No, he mulled, she didn't pilot a sleek sports car. In fact, she didn't even drive.

Morton continued to steal looks at the barmaid. This went on. Morton looking, then looking away. Then she'd look and he'd look away. It became rather nerve racking.

Finally she came and stood across from him for the longest time. Leaning there, about to say something, but not speaking. There was one other customer a few stools down. He pushed away from the bar.

"See ya t'morrow, Roxanne," he slurred.

They watched as the fellow, thin and unsteady on his feet, swayed out into the day's aging Chablis sunlight. Morton laid a twenty down. "Can I buy you one?" he asked the barmaid when they were alone.

"No," she said offering a smile. Then her face changed. She was frowning. There was a psychological term for this abrupt shift in affect, but at the moment Morton couldn't recall it.

"You know what? You remind me of someone too," said the woman. Her eyes opened wider. "How could I forget it? You were in here once with Mad Dog Joseph. That's what his dealer calls him. And us girls too once we got to know him. He's one of our, uh, gold-plated customers, I guess you'd call it."

Morton pressed his lower teeth thoughtfully onto his upper lip.

"Remember? You were very gallant. Joseph was all over me and you did everything you could to stop the crime."

"I did?" said Morton.

"You sure did. You stepped right up and volunteered to cold cock the guy."

Morton struggled to piece together the events of that foggy, Snakebitten evening.

"He probably deserved it," suggested the counselor.

"He probably did," she agreed. "But he's such a good looking S.O.B. There wasn't a dancer here didn't want to shake the sheets with Mad Dog Joseph. As a matter of fact, there's hardly one in here hasn't."

Morton grimaced at the picture.

"You were so sweet," she went on. "You said, 'Honey, you're not like that shit out there. You don't have to be with that paw happy womanizer if you don't want.'"

Morton wagged his head at his own audacity. Regret? Well, not so far.

"Thing is, I did want," she went on. "I didn't need rescuing. Us ladies in The Green Room are pretty tough cookies."

She picked up her cigarette. She smoked. She drank more. Morton noticed how intent she was on keeping her lips together so as not to expose the wayward upper teeth. She stared into the distance, and he could sense a shadow crossing her, a sweep of melancholy much like he'd found with Annise's flash alterations in mood.

"Joseph." She shook her head. "I guess I should have listened to you that night. He left me in a bad way."

"What do you mean? Did he rape you? I get the feeling he's capable of that."

"Rape's a hard word. A man can rape even when the woman agrees," she said.

Morton's mind fled to Muriel, to the way she looked the night he returned from the mountains, all curled up on his rug, her face so battered and puffy. The hospital found sperm in her. That was a fact. Voluntary sex? Like a prostitute with a sleazy john? Morton's heart gave a sudden flutter. Knocked around by Wojeck, her father, then raped? It had happened in the past, no question. But Morton knew Wojeck. He was a bad man once, yes, but he'd been full of remorse every time they'd met. Was he reformed? Had she even gone there? The scary thing was her being in jeopardy of losing her sanity to these new traumas. She seemed bent on wreaking havoc against herself, and then keeping the lunatic's eerie silence. Why?

Goddamn if she wasn't a goopy web of stickum all her own, that Muriel, only with a helical whirlwind of love-me/love-menots lassoing the poor groaning bee as he was about to shove off to another flower. A paradox, she was. A sage insanity walking around in a pubescent body, a body perfectly obedient to what the mind had been telling it for the last twenty-five years. Which was refuse to mature. Girl or woman, this was the great question. And moreover, if she found the answer what would she do with it?

"Yeah, the Mad Dog does pretty much what he wants," offered Roxanne. "It wasn't just me. A few of the other girls got hurt too. Now he finds pigeons someplace else and brings them in here. A few weeks ago he had one on each arm. A bombshell blonde and a foxy little redhead. All drugged up, looked to me like. Who knows what the three of them were up to? It's not my business though. I know enough to steer clear."

"You're smart," said Morton.

The barmaid met his eyes. "What you said before has been bothering me. You said I'm real. You said I'm not like that crap out there." She nodded toward the Strip.

"Yes. It's something I can feel about you," returned Morton.

She leaned very close to him. He could smell the perfume and the tobacco about her.

"I want you to do something." Her eyes scanned the place. Empty.

She reached out and touched at the hand in the cast. She stroked his other hand, slowly took hold and started moving it toward her. Morton could see what was about to happen. He considered trying to stop it. Her eyes though had gone sweet and lonesome. Well, it *was* a boob bar, he reflected. Probably she was salty enough not to be embarrassed by this sort of thing. What would it hurt, he wondered, as she very deliberately lifted his good hand and placed it inside her leotard top?

"It's OK. Feel," she said soothingly as she guided his fingers under the flesh of her breast.

She was older, yes, and there were those teeth. Nevertheless an inadvertent arousal washed over the counselor. The barmaid's hand covered his. It was warm. She moved his fingers all around. After a moment he began to notice a line of tiny knots beneath the skin.

"Those are from the stitches," she said looking Morton in the eyes.

She made him grasp the entire thing. It wasn't merely firm, it was outright hard. Not like a breast at all. Her top was stretched far down. Across her cleavage were small red and blue tattoos, faded over time.

"They put silicone in a plastic bag. They cut me open and stuffed it in here," she said.

He was so close the gray roots at her hairline appeared as if in magnification.

"See how smooth my face is?" she went on. She eased Morton's hand out of her shirt. She pulled back hard on her hair. Along the temples were tiny suture holes.

"Touch here. I really want you to," she urged.

Morton ran his fingers along her forehead and cheekbones. "I had my face lifted. Those are the scars it left. This one over the eye, by the way, is different. It came courtesy of the Mad Dog." She stepped aside and reached for her cigarette.

"Do you still think I'm real?" she asked taking a drag.

Morton was quiet.

"I'm sorry, I didn't mean to—" he began. He was feeling uncomfortable and headachy. He slipped off the stool.

"You think I'm a shell, don't you?" she said.

Morton hadn't previously considered such a notion, but it occurred to him now that maybe, just maybe she thought this about herself. He didn't respond.

A shell? He wondered for an instant if Annise, like the barmaid, would remain a teenager in her head till age forty-seven—or was it fifty-seven?—still wearing skin tight jeans and carrying the flashy cigarette. We all had our faults, he reckoned, our guilts, little or big. Somehow they had to be neutralized, didn't they?

He'd become aware of Annise's Saturday night custom of sitting anxiously at her vanity and drafting a quickie diary of the week on her slim-line Imagineer 3000 notebook computer. He tried to peek over her shoulder as she typed. "Oh, no you don't!" she objected, blocking his view.

Sunday morning her printer hummed out the pages, which she quickly stuffed in her purse before heading off to church. Preparation for the Confession Box, he wondered?

"You said you liked me before. Do you still like me?" pressed the barmaid as he stepped back.

Morton put a ten dollar bill on the bar top. A moment of indecision split them, a free instant when neither knew what to do. Spontaneously he leaned and kissed her on the cheek, but at once regretted it.

"Of course I still like you," he said. "And I still think you're better than that miserable bullshit outside."

Like before he thumbed over his shoulder, but his gut wrenched. Did he really mean it?

"I like you too," said the barmaid very low. "But remember, if that twenty-three year old is anything like me, she's phony too." The woman did not smile.

"What?" said Morton. "What do you mean by that?"

* * *

Chapter 17

It was dark in the streets now, except for the violent jumping swords of halogen lancing across the flooring from the passing headlights. The room felt dreamy, kind of mystical in a cold, hellish way.

A group of females appeared at the door. Blondes. From the roots out anyway. They were dressed for work, it appeared, in their skimpy tiger-striped miniskirts and low-cut Lycra tops. One kicked the stool with the side of her high heel and the door swung shut.

The barmaid rounded the counter and hugged Morton warmly around the neck. It was not a phony hug, he could tell. Yet it frightened him, for while he could feel her underlying angelic soul cooling his fevered brow with her cheek, from below the belt rose a subtle base force, the cloven footed beast secretly mingling in the marrow of a hot female heart— And the counselor the reluctant recipient!

"If you ever get a chance, maybe you might stop in again. The Mad Dog could use a good whipping, if you've got a mind," she whispered.

"He could?"

"He's in here most every night doing his nasty thing. Remember us the next time you're feeling gallant."

Morton was rattled. All this was more than he'd bargained for. He wheeled to leave. In his haste, however, he bumped smack dab into one of the approaching dancers.

"Oh my, you're wounded!" cried the busty young woman, spotting his cast. Coyly she wrapped her arms around the counselor's hips, pretending to help him keep his footing. She was very aggressive with her hands, only in a practiced way which warded off the sense of insult.

"What have you done to this man, Roxy?" she said.

The girl wobbled, and with a sudden flash of intuition Morton met her eyes. Yes, his hunch was right. The pupils were threaded down to mere needle points. Probably she'd popped Ecstasy, or one of the other designer downs. He hadn't been doing much homework on recreational drugs. The last he'd heard crack had been all the rage.

Morton felt shaky and claustrophobic. He pulled away and made for the door. Outside, the blast of crisp ebony air caused him to pause momentarily on the sidewalk. From behind he heard one of the girls say, "Where you been hiding *that* hunk, Roxanne?"

The strobe-like whites and inkwell blacks of the L.A. night shivered around him. He found his keys and moved off down the sidewalk. Rape, he kept thinking as he walked. Even Annise admitted it was a small death for a person. A kind of perpetual movie reel of pornography, only living and breathing in the shape of a human monster you could never elude inside your mind no matter how long or well you lived, or how hard you tried to forget it. No, it wasn't simply on the glossy magazine page of *Swedish Sins!*, or the flickering video screen. It was a recollection of the flesh, a memory you would always be prey to. Because it was etched on your *self*, on your *soul*, for those who had one.

Morton scratched his chin, and all at once he realized how lonely he was. Despite what Stacy Lung had been to him in the old days, even despite Annise Chastain and all her feminine wiles, he was lonely inside. He considered Muriel for a moment. Wasn't this her problem as well—loneliness? Maybe, pondered the counselor, all insanity amounted to in the long run was a core sense of isolation, of fearing no one would ever understand why you were such a nut. Least of all yourself!

* * *

Chapter 18

Morton started back toward his apartment, but when he came to the intersections that would lead him there he couldn't bring himself to make the turns. Like the single man he was he went ahead and stopped here and there around town. In The Amazon he ordered one in honor of Annise, as she'd recommended. The night though was already old.

Finally he put down his glass and drove to Vera's Russian Diner. As was his custom he paused to get a copy of the *L.A. Times* from the vending machine out front.

Vera was there as usual serving late night eggs and bacon to the people straggling home from the multitude of L.A. clubs and lounges. Morton was lucky to get a corner booth near the window where he could be by himself. He ordered a hot dog and a cup of coffee. Isolating, he wondered?

A good bit of time must have gone by, because when he at last glanced up from the newspaper he saw the crowd had thinned out.

Vera came over. She said, "You know I close 1:00 a.m."

"I know," said Morton.

"You don't look so good tonight. You look, I think, funny," said Vera.

"Funny?"

"You been maybe too long with those kooks up the street. They even eat crazy. They bring them down here. I see what they do."

She turned Morton's good wrist and tapped at his watch crystal. "Five minutes, you go. OK?"

Vera was short, stout and silver headed. She was nice, too. Morton smiled.

"OK," he said folding his newspaper.

"Nyet," she said changing her mind. "I want you stay. I lock the door in a minute. You stay though. We talk."

"Thanks, but I've got to get on home," he said.

Morton met Vera at the cash register. "You ever hear of a person having a bad soul? That's what I think I have today, Vera, a bad soul."

Vera nodded. "You need work with shoulders. With back. You need man's job. Long as I been alive soul never lifted nothing."

"Maybe not. But it can spin a mighty thick web. It feels like I'm about to fall in and get eaten alive. You ever feel that way, Vera? Like you're about to get eaten alive?" asked the counselor.

Vera glared around as the final patrons, half in the bag it seemed, trudged out into the wee a.m.

"Every single day, my friend," she said handing him his change. "Every single day."

~~~

Back at his apartment Morton found a note thumb-tacked to the door. He stood in the moonlight and read it.

TO A FRIEND

I ask this, Morton. What should a lonely woman do to get tenderness and love? And not the most beautiful woman either I know. Have sex with someone? At first I sometimes think so. Later I think this is wrong because I never get tenderness in such a way. But how, Morton? Since I haven't got any friends, any real friends I mean, I sometimes get sad and feel tears starting. I do not even have a good smile anymore. So a girl looks at the bed and thinks maybe that's the way.

Do you think a woman who does it with other men is a bad woman? No, Morton. She is a female woman. She is afraid if she cannot have you she will not stop making believe she can have you.

Why not let me feel you? This is all I ask. The hard days are over for us, I promise. I don't ask for love

'L.A. 2000:' Sex Asylum

exactly. But will you please hold me? You are a good man, Morton, and you and me both know not everyone in the world knows this about you. People say you aren't good because they are bad fools and don't know you like I do.

I am not trying to fake you either with this letter. You know I don't write letters so you know I am not trying to fake you. I only say will you please squeeze me like you've done so many good times when I was lonely?

Doesn't it make sense for two people to do a nice thing like this when they do not have a friend?—

There was no signature. The language was halting, yes, and the penmanship was off. Well, maybe that was the way it went when your troubled blondes got around to making amends.

Morton folded the note and put it in his shirt pocket.

He heard a horn beep. Down the block a yellow cab was parked by the curb. He could see the silhouette of a woman in the back seat through the purple slant of the streetlight. Her long hair was down over her shoulders, rather than in the ponytail Annise had taken to wearing lately. Ah, things were looking up. She'd seen fit to sneak away from the Fraction House for a little late night delight. But what was this cab business when she owned that cool little Mazda? That Annise Chastain was clever. It'd be just like her to leave the car at work as a decoy for some sexy truancy.

She emerged, and they moved toward the dark place between the streetlights where the lawn had been worn down. The moonlight was a pale icing on the bushes. So still. So deathly quiet there in the courtyard, yet even from that distance she seemed open and accessible.

The dust was moist with dew, kicking up the smell of a bygone era, of nature and old-timey farm life, not of glitzy L.A. at all. It was a gentle, romantic smell. And for once none of her high priced *Heroin* perfume splitting the air. Quite refreshing.

Buck Buchanan

They drew nearer in the darkness. The counselor put his arms out.

"Hello, Morton," said Muriel. She remained a few feet away.

"Muriel!"

She wore an over-wide grin. A full minute of silence elapsed as the two sized each other up. Which was quite like Muriel, really. Wait till the thing that must be said formed instinctively on your lips, otherwise offer only those blue volcanic eyes for communication.

Paranoid of rapists, the neighbors, policemen, Priscilla Daddio, the Fraction House—paranoid of L.A. itself—Morton snatched her wrist and led her swiftly into his apartment. He went to flip on the light.

"It'd be safer with candles," she suggested serenely.

He lit a candle.

"You're tired, Morton. I want you to sit in your chair and rest."

"But Muriel, you can't be here. You're going to get in such trouble. At this rate you'll never make it into the apartment."

She went downcast, kind of weepy-eyed and self-indulgent, a sharp contrast to the huge smile she'd greeted him with. "You worry too much. Try to take it easy for a few minutes. Here, I'll take your shoes off for you," she said.

She made herself into a small coil on the floor, nuzzling her chin against his leg as she patiently set about untying his shoe laces.

"Did you read my letter?" she asked.

A second passed.

"I pinned it on the door."

"*Your* letter? You mean—" Morton looked at her in astonishment. Muriel gazed back Bambi-eyed. There came a crude banging at the front door. Fearing the worst, Morton shot to his feet.

"The lady didn't pay yet," said a man through the screen. The yellow cab was idling at the end of the sidewalk.

"Oh. Well, no problem. How much is it?" Morton reached for his wallet.

The driver had a tally sheet in his hand. "I'm giving her a break. But it still comes to a hundred and eighty dollars," he said.

"A hundred and eighty dollars!" cried Morton. He turned to Muriel. "Where in the hell did you go?"

Muriel shrugged. "Just from the Fraction House," she said meekly.

The driver said, "We've been sitting out there four hours, buddy. The meter runs whether we're moving or not."

That Muriel. No, she wouldn't have been aware of meter rates or cash flow problems. She'd be learning it soon with her independence, but up till now her counselors had seen to the day to day details.

Morton went to the closet and pulled down the alligator-skin briefcase which contained his elaborate document collection. He rummaged through until he found an old Fraction House 'Travel Voucher.' This was a common form used by hospital Emergency Rooms, Nursing Homes, etc. allowing taxis to pick up the slack when their vans weren't accessible. Cabbies were well acquainted the procedure. Morton filled in the blanks and signed it.

"Dar/Neese?" observed the driver.

"Right."

"The supervisor over there authorizing this?"

"He'll clear it as soon as I call him. When you get there ask for Trina Lopez. She's the acting Night Sup."

~~~

When the cab driver was gone Morton said, "This running away you keep doing really worries me, Muriel. I have to notify Joseph. You understand, don't you?"

"He's the one told me to come visit," she returned.

"He what? To come here?"

"Sit down, Morton. I'll rub your feet."

"But you escaped again. You don't seem to grasp the weight of all this."

"I didn't escape. Joseph went over to Harvey's house and had him sign me off from being grounded. Harvey's very sick, you know."

"I know. But you being here is what I'm getting at," said Morton.

"I can be here. I can be anywhere with you."

The counselor swallowed hard. "That's a sweet thing to say, Muriel, only—"

"Don't you remember?" she interrupted. "They gave you Temporary Custody of me when you got hired back. I even didn't know until Joseph told me."

Morton recalled his office visit with the supervisor. Yes, he'd been given Temporary Custody, which he was invoked never to use. It was 'a formality, rather than a reality,' as Joseph explained it.

"I've got to call Trina, at least," said Morton. "I'm feeling squirrelly undercurrents going around these days. It's as if everything adds up right, only none of it seems all the way true."

He eyed her. The dark mascara she'd put on her eyelashes cast a tiny comb-like shadow onto her cheeks. Muriel with mascara? Hmmm.

Morton dialed the number of the Staff Lounge at the Fraction House.

"Dar/Neese," answered a female voice. It had a comforting familiarity.

Morton discretely cupped the receiver. "Annise, it's me. I was hoping you'd answer," he whispered enthusiastically.

"It's about time I heard from you. After our last deal I thought you'd hop right on the phone," she said.

"I probably should have."

"At least you're repentant, that's something."

"Yes, Annise. Yes, I am."

"So how have you been, Rodney?" she asked.

'L.A. 2000:' Sex Asylum

Silence.

"Uh, this is Morton, Annise."

"Morton? Oh! Hah!" she laughed. "Just playing around. You know how I am."

"I'm learning, Annise."

"Look, I'm glad you called. Before you start I need to tell you about Muriel. Something's happened."

There followed a commotion on the other end of the line.

"Allison? Is that you?" It was the Gestapo.

"Joseph? Christ, it's two in the morning. What are you doing at work?"

"Busting my ass as usual," he replied. "Haven't you heard? Harvey signed me over a Power of Attorney while he convalesces. He'll get it back of course, but as of 6:00 a.m. today I become Director-in-Chief of all Dar/Neese affairs. Ain't that a kicker!"

Morton's lower jaw jutted forward. "What's up with Muriel, Joseph? She says you told her to come over here," stated the counselor getting down to business.

"You've had Temporary Custody from the beginning, Allison. We're relaxing the formality part where I said you couldn't hang out with her."

"You mean I can hang out with her now?"

"It's been brought to my attention by one our of rising star staff members that letting her free before she's free would be good for the normalization process."

Morton perceived an instant of discontinuity in the lines as he envisioned bosomy blonde and bulked up Gestapo smiling grotesquely at one another.

"So she didn't run away?"

"No. I told you, she's free as a bird. Why don't you go ahead and keep her overnight. You've got Guardianship right now. In terms of the paperwork it'd be more kosher if she turned up under the wing of her Legal Guardian rather than moping around Dar/Neese all the time."

"Keep her overnight? Is that what you're saying? You must have gone crazy, Joseph."

"You're sounding so much healthier than when we talked before," soothed the supervisor. "Why don't you take the next couple of days off too. I've finally realized you're going to need time to work on Muriel. I mean, you know, work with her. She's had a few, er, difficulties this last week. We'll go over it all on Monday."

"Well, OK, I guess," said Morton.

"Me and Annise really missed you today," added Joseph warmly.

Morton considered replying, 'You really ought to do something about your grammar, Schopen.' But why be harsh? Thinking better of it he said, "You missed me?"

"Quite a lot. Didn't we, Annise?"

In the background Morton heard Annise pipe up, "We sure did, Morty. We missed you something terrible."

Morton put his flutters aside. He had to trust somebody sometime, didn't he? Well, why not Joseph? And Annise too, for that matter. His bad soul began to ease. Perhaps he'd been mistaken after all about the supervisor's ill will. The guy could be very charming when he wanted to.

"Give me credit, won't you Allison? Your Temporary Custody was designed for something like this. The kid shows up on your doorstep a second time without it and we all go to the dogs. Well, for you I suppose it'd be jail for twenty years, but of course none of us want that."

"No, we don't want that," agreed Morton weakly.

The counselor was exhausted. This day felt like a hundred days, and all in the desert without a scrap of shade to douse the flaming blood in a man's brain. As if there had never been any other days, only this one, bleached out and transparent, a web the size of Hollywood itself with its knee-deep layer of flypaper enveloping you. The grimy rumble of the autos, the smoke and the tattoos, the clinging satin shirts of the club goers. Christ, it was too much.

"You're beat," noticed Joseph through the lines. "Have a couple of Snakebites and turn in. We'll straighten this out after the weekend."

"Thanks, Joseph. That's very thoughtful. Sometimes I think I've misestimated you."

"I forgive you," said Joseph. "This time."

Morton hung up. Muriel was in his recliner. She was sporting her super wide grin once again, and wearing—could it be?—a sheer orange chiffon nightgown which reached barely to mid-thigh. Where did she come up with that? Her right heel bobbed rhythmically against the footrest. He noticed her small overnight bag on the coffee table. Had she been carrying it before?

The counselor knuckled at the sleep in his eyes. Muriel stood, diaphanous and surreal. A stray gust of moon wind skittered through the screen door. The candle flame cast a quivering, twig-like pattern across the walls.

"It's late, Morton. Come, I'll tuck you into bed," she whispered.

Slowly she extended her arms. Morton let himself be helped to the bedroom. It had been a long hard day. But all things came to an end. This craziness too would pass, he told himself. Vaguely remembering the Custody details, he muttered groggily as they walked, "And no legal hassles either, babe."

"No," agreed Muriel softly. "No hassles at all, babe."

* * *

Chapter 19

Morton sat on the edge of his bed. Muriel left and returned with the candle. The room was black except for where the light flickered.
"Aren't you going to undress?" she asked. She sat down beside him.
"Wait now. This isn't right, Muriel. I'm going to go out and sleep in the recliner. You take the bed."
Muriel lounged back on the pillows. "OK. But relax a minute with me first. I'm afraid to be alone right now," she said.
The counselor yawned. He eased down as far as an elbow. They didn't speak. For some reason there seemed nothing to say.
Muriel lay flat on her back. Snow-colored moonlight fell through the window onto the fully visible arcs of her body. Her arms were tucked along her sides like an Egyptian mummy. She wasn't fossilized though by a long shot, but communicating a super-alive vibrancy through the transparent nightie. She was a finely formed specimen of womanhood, no question.
Morton lowered his head drowsily to the pillow in contemplation. He really ought to have felt complimented. She could have run to— Well, where? Her letter mentioned "other men." It said she looked at beds and thought maybe lust was the way. This seemed so unlike the Muriel he knew. And whose bed was she looking at anyway? Gordon Theodoricus? Well, Gordon was a nice guy maybe, but he only had the standard Fraction House cot...

~~~

When Morton next opened his eyes daylight was pouring through the window. He was still on his bed, only under the covers now. Quickly he glanced over. Muriel was there beside him. She too was beneath the covers. He felt a chill below the waist. Gingerly, so as not to disturb his guest, he lifted the blankets.

Jesus God in heaven, he was naked! He looked over. Muriel was wide awake, her eyes trained on his.

The counselor sucked his breath and jerked the sheet over his chest like he'd seen actresses in soap operas do. Muriel began to titter at his modesty. By degrees Morton too opened up with a soft morning smile. It was nice to at last see her cheerful. Maybe those bad days of breakdowns and heavy-hearted tears were over for them after all, as she'd suggested in her note.

Muriel tossed the bedclothes aside and went to the window.

From outside came the racket of the Thursday morning garbage pickup. The blinds were open from the night before. If the garbage men looked the correct way they'd have been rewarded with a real working man's feast. For yes, sweet little Muriel Gonska was naked as a jaybird.

Morton was feeling much clearer today. He thought back over the past evening. He hadn't been drunk, just tired. And no, nothing immoral had happened, thank God.

The counselor shook his head at Muriel's impetuousness. The mentally disturbed, he understood, tended to be oblivious of their body language. Still, he was rendered dumbfounded when she planted her elbows and leaned far out the screenless window, affording him an extraordinary view of her aft physique. Well, you had to excuse your nut cases their naïve curiosities, didn't you? It wasn't really lewdness or exhibitionism. More like random acts of disquietude, he decided.

Morton sat up against the headboard and put a thoughtful hand to his face. Inside him, a spring was uncoiling. For the first time in months he felt simple in his heart. Quite a relief. After a minute, though, he realized he was fingering his eye, his nose, and his mouth all at the same time. And amazingly, his ear too. Damned if this wasn't Muriel's own blocking of the senses mechanism! Blocking? Hmmm. It seemed natural enough. Plus you could still look over to the window if you felt the urge.

Muriel lowered the blind. The sunlight, refracted through the sharp white slats, painted a body glove tattoo over her high breasts and her smooth flat stomach. Now, as before, she showed no shyness about being naked. Perhaps she'd always been this open, it was hard to know. No longer was she curled up in a pool of blood and vomit on his rug, zebra-striped with cold moonlight, like a weary convict. She was in her prime. She'd go far. He knew she would.

Morton had mixed emotions, but at last he said, "Muriel, you really ought to put something on. I'm not sure this is what they mean when they talk about normalization."

She was smiling gently. She seemed not to hear him. "I wish I could always feel this way," she said walking toward the bed.

"What way is that?" asked Morton.

She found her gown and slipped it on. "Like I'm not going to fall apart in the next instant," she said.

"Me too, Muriel," replied the counselor genuinely. "Me too."

~~~

Morton dressed and went to the kitchen to start breakfast. Muriel trailed behind.

"You need to bathe," he reminded her.

"They always put me in the tub at the Fraction House. But you only have a shower," she replied.

"You're not at the Fraction House. Tub or shower, this is something you have to do every day."

"All right. In fact, I love to take showers!" exclaimed Muriel throwing up her arms exuberantly.

Morton put the sausage on. He opened the back door to check on his tomato and pepper plants, which were in boxes along the side of the building. They were young still, beginning to sprout their small green leaves. The telephone rang. Joseph

'L.A. 2000:' Sex Asylum

changing his mind about Muriel's Custody situation, wondered the counselor?

"Hello," he said.

"It's Annise, Morton."

"Annise! What a pleasant surprise."

"Listen, the weirdest thing happened. Wanda Novice and Stacy Lung took sick together. They stopped in yesterday to pick up their paychecks, and they were perfectly healthy. In fact, they were all decked out to go clubbing. Now they're sick as dogs over at Wanda's. See what I'm saying?"

"You mean they have bad hangovers?" wondered Morton.

"Christ you're naïve. Stacy hasn't had a date in a year. She's got to be *more* than ready, if you catch my drift."

"Wanda and *Stacy*? Christ, are you saying you think they might be—"

"That's exactly what I'm saying. You know what Wanda's got on the menu as well as I do, Morton."

Well, yes, he did. He knew Stacy's menu too, and had found it short on seasoning. Hell, these days it was flat out impossible to experience someone in their personal recesses, in those tiny nooks and crannies of the soul where they sought asylum. And once he thought of it, Stacy *had* opted for that quirky avant-garde haircut.

"Incredible, isn't it?" said Annise. "And they're the two strongest workers on the upcoming shift."

Morton chinned the phone and flipped the sausage patties.

"Anyway," she went on, "Joseph wants me to pull another three days in back of the three I'm finishing to fill in for those hussies."

"Do you need the money?" he asked.

"Not really. But I'll feel guilty if I don't do it. I mean, after Joseph already asked me and all."

"OK. But don't forget what you promised last time," he reminded her.

"What'd I promise?"

Morton cupped the receiver. "You know, about the diaphragm."

"Oh," she said weakly. Suddenly the voice sounded hundreds of miles away. "Well, I called and called, but I couldn't get an appointment. They said they're backed up three weeks."

"Three weeks!"

"That's what they said."

Morton was quiet.

"Oh, and one more thing. Joseph told me to let you know about Muriel's Termination Meeting. Harvey had to postpone it till week after next. He thinks he'll be better then."

"Why are they postponing?"

"How do I know? Maybe it's a big setup to fire you and make me Muriel's number one counselor."

Morton was quiet.

"For Christsake, I'm joking. Lighten up, will you."

"Harvey doesn't have to be there, Annise. Trina has the RN credentials. And Joseph's a psychologist. A Ph.D., I mean. Or at least he says he is. That's all the Arbitrators require," said the counselor.

"Look, Morton, something very serious has happened with Muriel. I can't say much right now," she whispered. "It's all highly confidential. Plus, I'm in the Staff Lounge and everybody's watching me."

"I'm her Legal Guardian, Annise. I need to know these things."

"God, you're hyper. Have you ever considered tranquilizers, Morton? Joseph was mentioning this the other day. How you're so high strung. He handles all the medication orders, you know. You wouldn't have to do anything. Joseph could get Harvey to prescribe if you wanted." She took a breath. "I don't know how you feel about it, but I think it'd be a fabulous idea."

"Tranquilizers?"

"Sure. My mother's been on them for the last fifteen years. They do wonders for her. Promise me you'll think about it."

"We were talking about Muriel, weren't we? You said something serious happened."

He could hear her rummaging for her cigarettes.

"I guess you haven't heard yet. You know how good I am though at getting the gossip on places."

Morton clicked the stove off. "Yes, I know," he said.

"Sit down," sighed Annise. "It really hurts to have to drop this on you, Morton. I mean, the way you and Muriel have been so close. Are you sitting yet?"

"Tell me, Annise."

"She went manic, Morton. It came on full force a week ago."

"Manic?"

"You're aware of what Manic-Depression is, aren't you?"

"I think so," he returned. "Happy, then all of a sudden sad and upset. The way you get Sunday mornings right before Confession."

"She's changed, Morton. She really has. Everybody's seen it. You've been up in Administration shuffling those screwy documents all this time. I know it's hard work, but you've got to admit it isolates you from the clients."

"She seems fine to me. Well, not fine exactly..." He trailed off.

Now that Annise had pointed it out Morton became alert to how much reckless giggling and splashing was coming from the bathroom. The euphoric side of manic, he wondered?

"It's like she's been saving up to go off the deep end," continued Annise. "And this last week she went ahead and jumped. She spends most of her time crying in her room. When I start talking to her, or Joseph either for that matter, she bursts out laughing. It's an angry laughter, Morton. You'd really be shocked to hear it."

"I am shocked."

"It's full-blown manic-depression according to Joseph. And that's something he's known an awful lot about ever since his last breakdown."

"I can hardly believe all this, Annise."

There came an awkward silence through the lines. "Are you calling me a liar?" she asked tightly. "People have done that before, and it really gets to me, Morton."

"Of course not. All I'm saying is she doesn't seem very disturbed when she's around me. In fact, she acts almost sane."

"Which is exactly why she's at your place. So you can whip her into shape for this meeting. Why do you think you got Custody? Why do you think Joseph sent her over there? Listen, I'm not supposed to tell you any of this. Joseph's going to lay it all on you Monday. Please don't let on who told you, OK? He'd have my ass for sure."

"I won't say anything, Annise. I promise."

"See you in a few days then," she said cheerfully.

"Uh, Annise, about the diaphragm—" tried Morton.

But it was too late. She'd hung up.

* * *

Chapter 20

A few minutes later, the door to the other room opened. Sunlight hung in the lingering sausage smoke. The rush of air swept eerily across Muriel as she flowed into the kitchen. She was dressed in a brown tweed skirt and a white button down blouse. He'd never seen her so straight laced. What a turnaround from her standard Grateful Dead T-shirt.

"Wow! What a dish! Where are you going?" he said looking her over.

"Wherever you take me," she returned. She removed the spatula from the fingers of his cast hand.

"Ours is a professional relationship, Muriel. Not a date. You've got to get this through your head."

"By the way, I left the water, Morton," she told him undaunted. "Remember how you said you wanted to get in my water? Well, I left it for you this time."

The water was Joseph's thing, not Morton's. Something suspicious here? Or was he just hyper, like they all said? And anyway, how much water could there be in the bottom of a shower? He was about to answer, when Muriel said, "Who was on the phone?" She put the sausage patties on their plates, neglecting, he noticed, to blot the excess grease. "I thought it might be the Fraction House. Maybe Annise checking up on you. I mean, checking up on me." She frowned and whipped her head side to side at her misstatement.

"What's all this about you swinging manic, Muriel? You're not that far gone, are you?" blurted the counselor.

She hung her head. The corners of her small, oval shaped mouth slumped slowly downward. Morton could see she intended to stonewall.

"No psycho-babble now. Are you manic or not? I want to know," he pressed.

"Joseph says I am," she muttered low. "But Harvey says he's not really sure yet. On the other hand, Harvey can be a very wishy washy dude sometimes."

"Dude? You don't say that kind of stuff, Muriel. When did you get so racy with your vocabulary?"

The counselor put milk and cereal on the table. They sat down to breakfast.

"I think they're pinning manic on me. That's how come they stuck me with the dizzy blonde."

"Dizzy blonde? Stacy, you mean?"

"Not Stacy, Morton. I'm talking about the one with the sports car and the big tits."

"Annise?" he realized.

"Uh huh. Because if I went manic with somebody strong like you the blame would go smack dab to the Fraction House. On Joseph, I mean. Especially with all the publicity about me being raped."

"Raped! What publicity, Muriel?"

Her neck reddened.

"Not raped. I didn't say raped, did I? I mean about going into this apartment. Publicity about that."

An awkward moment passed.

"I'm not making this up, Morton. Sam Lorenzo told me he saw a memo about it on Wanda's desk. And Gordon said Harvey let something slip during their Therapy Session."

"Let what slip?"

"I'm not sure. But he was very huffy with Gordon, and that's not like Harvey at all."

Morton scratched his chin in thought. "So they're making Annise look responsible for you going crazy? Is this what you're saying?"

"Uh huh. Why else would they hire a dopey counselor for me? And it's true, I am doing a lot worse," she said.

Morton shook his head in dismay. "Secrets. Dirty secrets everywhere," he grumbled.

"They have to fire somebody over it," she went on. "Otherwise Joseph wouldn't be able to get me alone all the time. I mean, therapy-wise." Muriel's cadence took on a stammering quality. "That's why he was going to fire you— Before your wrist got broke— They had Annise all picked out— Joseph knew he could make her look bad real easy—"

"Joseph was going to fire me? What for, for Christsake?"

"I was getting too healthy. He had to fire you, Morton. He knew that was the only way they could screw up my head and keep me from leaving the Fraction House."

"But I thought he wanted you to leave. You're their prime time pupil, Muriel."

"Maybe I'm Harvey's prime time. But Joseph isn't going to let me go anywhere. He wants my funding. He wants my father's blood money so he can do his coke and dine and wine his dancer friends."

"Joseph really does coke? How do you know? I realize he pops those Dexies, and comes down with Snakebites."

Muriel shrugged. "He wants me to stay at the Fraction House forever. He's got his video camera— He keeps me in the tub all the time—" She gave a shiver.

"So it's a prison for you over there? And with that lecher breathing down your neck!"

"Yeah," said Muriel sadly. "My only other way out is Roselawn. If Priscilla wins with the Arbitrators I'll probably end up there."

"You're sure a lot smarter than you let on," observed the counselor. "Are all you nuts like that?"

She looked him in the eyes. "Yes," she said.

"So Joseph was going to fire me, huh?"

She nodded. "He couldn't though. You were hot stuff with me and Gordon. And it all got recorded in the Progress Reports. That must be why he pushed you down the steps."

Dead silence. Muriel seemed flabbergasted at what she'd said. Her face hung strangely slack. It was as if someone else had spoken through her, a devilish medium maybe, rather than those last being her own words.

"Joseph pushed me!" cried Morton.

"I didn't mean that, it just came out."

"But you said it."

"I couldn't have meant it though. Everybody says you slipped."

"I did, I guess. Only something clipped my leg, I've maintained that all along. I thought you stumbled and knocked my leg out."

"I didn't stumble. I was behind Joseph, remember? When you fell, Joseph screamed, 'You tripped him, Muriel, you stupid bitch!' So I thought I must have done it."

"But you couldn't have done it," said Morton staring at her. "Not if you were behind him. You couldn't have kicked me if you'd wanted to."

Muriel shrugged dispassionately. For people troubled psychologically one event tended to equal another in their heads, despite the second one being violent, or even deadly. Their response was invariably a sort of amused, leg bobbing neutrality.

Morton recalled Joseph's special mix of wax and silicone which he used to buff the upstairs floors. He remembered how the supervisor had switched from his leather-soled jodhpurs to high-top neoprene sneakers. At the time Morton attributed the change to the Gestapo's Obsessive/Compulsive Disorder, the old OCD. But he was beginning to wonder if this wasn't a premeditated move to insure his footing, and to insure someone else's bad footing, Morton's for instance, should an altercation arise at the top of the steps.

"I might have been killed, Muriel. That plate glass window doesn't even have a two-by-four across it. One slip and I'm a pile of blood and guts in the middle of the Organic Therapy Garden!" he exclaimed.

"I jumped in front of Joseph to catch you, Morton. That's why it looked like I made you fall. He grabbed me around the neck, or else I might have saved you." Muriel's eyes went sad. "And everybody said I did it. Pushed you, I mean."

Morton saw tears welling in Muriel's trembly, sky blue eyes. Neither had touched their food. She began to silently weep.

The counselor pushed off his chair and knelt beside his friend, comforting her with a hug. Joseph a murderer, he pondered? Was Muriel truly a victim of rape, after all? Or had it been one of those "hard questions" as Roxanne, the tattooed barmaid in The Green Room, had called it? A borderline attack, so to speak, where the violence was present, but not positively diabolic? Who was zooming who here?

Over the years Morton had learned what skilled conjurers active schizophrenics could be. True in the heat of a transition, they became false if fixed in a mental time and place, like reality, for instance, which was what institutions like Roselawn insisted upon. Most remained rigid, insane that was, yet living out their days in a curiously vital, though illusory way. Those who improved managed to somehow join lunacy with the glitzy, bombed-out craziness of L.A. and changed. In your better nuts it was similar to a chemical conversion, where two of the hardest elements like steel and bone slammed together and became the high-tensile modeling clay of a real human being. And what greater transition was there than from prison to freedom? From the Fraction House to the acid twisted neon of the city? Or, now that he thought of it, from a bland puberty encased kid to a full-fledged woman lusting after life?

By degrees Muriel's weeping subsided. "Thank you, Morton. Thank you for holding me," she said.

The counselor's face remained smothered in the fragrant dampness of her newly washed hair.

"You're welcome, Muriel," he replied.

She pulled back. She smiled. Meeting his eyes with the genuine, unmanipulating gaze she'd always possessed with him, she leaned and kissed him flush on the lips. For the longest of seconds she did not break away.

* * *

Chapter 21

After breakfast Muriel put Morton's rubber apron on and began to do the dishes. She was rumored to be crying and wallowing in self-pity, but the way she scrubbed so vigorously at the plates Morton didn't see it. Scrubbing, yes, only without the soap. Well, she hadn't been trained in housekeeping yet. He handed her the bottle of Joy.

"Try this, Muriel. It'll go faster," he said.

He headed to the bathroom to clean up. Sure enough, in the bottom of the stall lay a good three inches of Muriel's foamy shower water. Morton smiled and unplugged the drain.

As he bathed he experienced a warmth more intense than simply the running water. He felt flattered. It was obvious Muriel liked him for real, not in a purely nut's way. Whatever she wanted, she was remaining kind about it. None of us could be blamed for having normal human urges, could we?

The counselor noticed a small plastic container, shaped like a clam shell, wedged in the side of his shower caddy. Muriel must have left it. He shut off the water and carefully pried it open. Morton's mouth dropped in disbelief as he saw the prescription taped on the inside lid, written by none other than Dr. Harvey Mueller, the Freudian.

'Koroflex Press 70cm,' it said. 'Use as directed for birth control.'

Timidly Morton poked at the delicate bracelet sized device. Little Muriel Gonska using a diaphragm! It hardly seemed possible.

A tremor of jealousy shot through him. What had she been doing riding around in a cab all night anyway? And what about cutthroat Joseph Schopen? Jealousy? Hmmm, what an odd sensation.

If the Gestapo had thrown him down those steps there was serious evening up to do. And what about Annise Chastain, the hot California blonde who in actuality was cucumber cool, yet constantly shining it on with a French vanilla icing which melted on the spoon before you could sink your teeth into it? Anger began to boil in the counselor. It was time to take these issues to the source, he decided. Get the low down out of these people once and for all.

Morton wrapped a towel around his waist and stormed into the kitchen. No Muriel. He turned and entered the bedroom, but she wasn't there either. On the bureau he found a note.

> *I had a wonderful night. Joseph is coming now to get me for appointments. I have to be back at the Fraction House after lunch. Thank you for letting me stay, Morton. I love you.*
>
> *Muriel*

Appointments? What did this mean? Morton put the note and the diaphragm into his top junk drawer.

~~~

He dressed and strode out the sidewalk toward his truck. He had a second thought, returned and pulled down his alligator-skin briefcase.

Over the years the counselor had collected scores of blank and partially completed documents. It had been a kind of hobby for him. One never knew when one might need an impressive looking affidavit for something or other.

He sifted carefully through the mass of papers. Incident Report forms from the Fraction House, Proof of Loss forms from Insurance Companies, Meeting Minutes forms left in the Therapy Room. Here was a half filled in Marriage Certificate. Where'd *that* come from? He paused. He had plenty of WhiteOut should alterations be necessary, but no, nothing seemed suitable for his current purposes.

Morton drove to the Fraction House. He considered taking Harvey's private elevator to the third floor as a show of independence, but when a couple of the newer staff members rounded the corner he decided against it, and instead marched up the stairs.

Joseph wasn't in his office. He'd still be out with Muriel following up their 'appointments.' Trina Lopez, the active Sup when Joseph was away, was behind his desk. She gave Morton a warm smile. God, but it was hard to remain on the attack when you couldn't locate the enemy.

"Come in," said Trina, rising. "I am so glad you are here, Morton. I was afraid I would not get to say adios to my amigo."

"Adios? I'm not going anywhere, Trina."

"Not you, Morton. I have not had a chance to tell you, but Joseph is letting me go."

"Letting you go? He can't do that. Harvey's the bigwig around this place."

"Not right now. Joseph has a temporary Director-in-Chief position. He can do anything he wants."

"He's firing you?" said Morton.

"He is tired of me looking over his shoulder. I have known this all along."

Morton nodded.

"He is a medical buff, you know. He thinks he can prescribe uppers and downers and evener-outers to anybody."

Trina's eyes began to dampen. Morton rounded the desk and hugged her. He felt her double starched dress crumple between them. "I'll miss you," he said. "You're the sharpest nurse I've ever met, Trina. You'll get a job a lot better than this one, I'm sure."

Trina reached under her coke bottle glasses to clear her eyes. "I am thinking of going with a laboratory in Glendale. Shearer-Kaplan. Not so many problems. I mean, you know, hassles with the staff. I will study new medicines. I will be a chemist, kind of."

"Wonderful! Quality assurance. That's what you've always wanted, Trina." He reached out and straightened her nurse's cap. "Everybody knows Joseph never treated you fairly."

"Do not trust him, Morton. I am not so sure about the new blonde counselor who hangs out with him either. I cannot keep good account of the drugs with Joseph always meddling in. Also he is letting go our two secretaries. He let Henderson, the accountant, go too. He says to keep costs down, but I think it is so he will have no one oversighting him. I mean, watching what he does with the money."

"He's screwed with Muriel's prescriptions from the very beginning," agreed Morton. The counselor turned suspicious. "Maybe he's got something on Harvey, the way he makes him write scripts for whatever he wants. That ever occur to you?"

Trina said, "I do not repeat gossip. But I am afraid something bad may be happening. Muriel is too good a person—" She hesitated.

"Yes?" said Morton.

She took a deep breath. "I cannot tell you how I found this out. But I heard Joseph had an affair with one of our patients a few years back. He never got brought up on charges, but—well, it is only gossip. I checked the files. They were all swept clean. You would expect as much from Joseph."

"An affair? Who with?"

Trina went to the door and looked nervously up and down the hall.

"This was before you came," she said. "I do not know if you are aware, but Sally Featherman was not always echolalic."

"Sally!" cried Morton.

"Shhh," waved Trina. She whispered, "A few years ago Sally was a lot like Muriel. She was doing very well. Joseph was her psychotherapist, like he is Muriel's therapist now. They were talking about her going to live on her own. Then something terrible happened. Some horrible trauma. Nobody knows for sure what it was, but over a few weeks' time Sally broke down. One day she started repeating what people said. You know, the echolalia. She makes sexual innuendo out of everything, Morton. There has got to be a reason."

"She sings sometimes," he pointed out.

"Yes, but she never makes a statement of her own. That is typical of echolalia. She is frozen in someone's world which is not her own."

"How do you know all this?" wondered Morton.

Trina shook her head. "I cannot say. But if you are wondering why Harvey puts up with so much bullying—"

"Harvey knew about it?"

"Harvey is a kind man, Morton. He has always wanted the best for Dar/Neese. If something like this got out the Fraction House would lose its accreditation in a blink. The Arbitrators could even pull Harvey's medical license."

"So he covered it up," sighed Morton.

Trina said, "I do not know. It is possible Muriel could be in jeopardy."

"And Harvey's hands are tied," realized the counselor. "Joseph could spill the beans about Sally at any moment. Sure, it'd ruin him, but it would also bring the L.A. psychiatric world down around Dar/Neese's ears. This place is Harvey's whole life, Trina."

"Yes, Harvey may be stuck—how do you say?—between a rock and a hard spot? Do watch yourself. And for Jesus' sake watch out for Muriel."

"Don't worry, Trina. I've never trusted that scoundrel. He's after Harvey's job, isn't he?"

"The good people are thinning out around here. This much I know," she said.

Morton lifted a sheaf of papers from the desk. "Look at this study Harvey did. He wrote it up for one of the medical journals. Joseph stamps it with the Fraction House seal and adds his own signature. Christ, the Gestapo's looking like a bona fide doctor. See here, he's signing it 'Dr. J.S. Schopen.' He's no M.D."

"He says he is a Ph.D.," said Trina.

Morton pointed to Joseph's fancy framed diploma on the wall. "You can get those certificates out of the back of *True*

Detective for $19.95 a copy. To be honest, Trina, I don't think he's a doctor of anything."

The RN shook her head. "I am afraid I have already said too much. Hug me one more time, Morton. We may not see each other anymore."

They embraced. This time it was the counselor's eye going damp.

* * *

Chapter 22

Morton trotted briskly down to the first floor, glanced behind, then took the laundry room exit into the Organic Therapy Garden, one of Joseph's pet projects.

Ahead he saw Perry Barwick, the Speech Pathologist, and Sally Featherman. They were both wearing their khaki gardening shorts. According to Dr. Schopen millions of negative ions were released when you dug up so many pounds of dirt. Or was it positive ions? And when you planted bushes and flowers and whatnot other particles were also scientifically released. Taken altogether they cast a tremendous calm over unsound minds, particularly if the digging was done after lunch when the clients were full and a little sleepy. Joseph had it all documented.

Morton nodded to Perry, who didn't talk much.

"Working hard, Sally?" asked the counselor as he passed by.

"Working hard, Sally?" echoed Sally Featherman as she copied Morton's mannerism by nodding echopraxically to Perry.

Morton re-entered the main building through the side door of C-Wing. Sam Lorenzo, the Inertial Catatonic, was standing rigidly outside the bathroom door. This meant he'd held it precisely nine and a half days and was timing his entrance to meet the critical moment. He was beginning to do his slow motion dance, which always prefaced a sudden bolt to the toilet. Morton waved, and Sam began a painstakingly robotic wave in return.

The counselor continued down the corridor. Ahead he heard Annise's voice coming from the cafeteria, along with the drone and clatter of the others in there. He paused. She was explaining to Odette Gunner, the 'Neurotic Self-Scratcher,' why she shouldn't tear such bloody holes into her forearms every time she got scolded.

"That's a phobia, Odette. A simple little Self-Rejection Phobia. You're really not trying to *reject* yourself, are you?" said Annise.

"That's not a phobia," returned a voice Morton immediately recognized as Gordon Theodoricus, the Synthetic Paranoid. "I'm the one has phobias. That is a goddamn Bipolar Barrier Fetish."

"Please, Gordon. I'd rather you didn't curse," said Annise.

A few moments later Gordon came hurrying down the hallway. When he rounded the bend, Morton snatched him by the shirtsleeve.

"Gordon, I have to talk to you right away! In private," whispered the counselor.

Gordon's eyes bugged open. Instinctively the paranoid looked over his shoulder to see if he was being followed. No, no one there.

"Certainly. Come this way," he whispered back.

They entered Gordon's room and took seats on the edge of his cot, their heads tilted close, as was the old therapeutic style between these two friends. In the background a tape was playing Chinese restaurant songs, which Gordon listened to round the clock since it was the music he most disliked.

Morton said quietly, "Tell me about Muriel. And don't worry Gordon, this is all strictly confidential, so it's quite all right to talk about it."

Gordon shifted uncomfortably on the cot. His eyes began to wander with the beginnings of Paranoid Strabismus, an indication something was troubling him.

"What is it?" asked the counselor, his voice taking on an added peacefulness.

"Oh, nothing. That blonde keeps hiding my bed hardener. She's beginning to get under my skin." The bed hardener was the stiff plastic board Gordon used to resist the softness of his mattress. He rubbed at the back of his neck.

"About Muriel," Morton reminded him. "I have to know how she's been doing lately. You're the only person I can trust around this place, Gordon. I really need to get your opinion."

"Well, she's not like she used to be when you were working with her, that's for sure." Gordon leaned closer. "This time it's bad, Morton. We've all been very worried about her."

"I understand Harvey let something slip in your Therapy Session," said Morton.

Gordon glared over as if the counselor had a strange clairvoyant grip on this. Then he relaxed, clairvoyance it seemed, being natural enough as far as paranoids went.

"You know how Harvey shows us the coloring book," said the paranoid after a moment.

Morton nodded.

"I was in the therapy tub last week. There was a picture of men in white suits putting a girl in a cage. Usually I know who I'm supposed to put an X over. But Harvey must have snuck in this new picture and I didn't know what to do."

"Yes?"

"I had to X somebody out. So I X'd out the men in white suits. Only I did it too hard and the page ripped. Harvey got real upset, Morton. He said those white suits meant doctors." Gordon glanced behind him. "And he's a doctor too, you know," he whispered.

"I know," agreed Morton.

"Then he said I was sneaky."

"Sneaky?"

Gordon wrinkled his forehead. "Yep. He said I X'd out the doctors because Joseph and him won't let Muriel leave the Fraction House." Several seconds passed. "I don't mind Harvey so much," he said. "At least he's flabby. I can respect flabbiness in a person."

"What do you think they're going to do to Muriel in the long run?" asked Morton cautiously.

Gordon's eyes darted around the room. "Murder her. They're going to murder her, Morton, I'm certain of it. And murder you too," he said shakily.

"Thanks, Gordon. You've been a great help."

Morton shook his friend's hand, then stood to go.

"By the way, why don't you put a few pictures on the wall? Maybe get a rug or something. It'd make it a lot nicer in here," suggested the counselor.

Gordon crossed his hands in his lap. "That has occurred to me," he said, his eyes wandering the ceiling.

~~~

Morton checked his watch. Five after one. Muriel's note said she'd be back at the Fraction House after lunch.

He decided to go down to E-Wing, the women's dormitory. At the double doors he spotted Stacy Lung leading a group of female clients to their second shift luncheon. This time there was no avoiding contact. Morton offered a shy smile. Stacy jerked her head in a way which flipped forward her newly bobbed hairdo.

"I guess you're here to see Muriel," said Stacy curtly.

"Yes," said Morton.

"Better watch out. Rumors are flying about you two."

"Rumors? What rumors?"

"You and Muriel spending nights together. You and Muriel out at bars on Hollywood Boulevard. Everybody's aware of it, Morton."

"Hollywood Boulevard? That stuff's not true, Stacy."

"You're not allowed in here today," she informed him.

"Sure I am. You know Joseph's Dictum. All staff are allowed everywhere except for the Administrative Offices and the Therapy Room."

Stacy said, "I'm talking about Joseph's Dictum that no staff is allowed at the Fraction House on their day off. You're sick today, Morton. It's marked right on the schedule. You better beat the feet out of here before somebody tells on you." Stacy turned to leave.

Morton felt a flash of irritation. "By the way, you're not supposed to be here either. You and Wanda took sick together, is what I heard. Everybody's been talking about it you know."

The group moved off. Stacy wheeled around. She was about to shoot him one of her old venomous glares, but he tugged closed the double doors before it reached him.

Morton proceeded to E-7, Muriel's room. She kept it locked, as was her Fraction House privilege, but he had the key she'd long ago insisted he keep.

Inside, he saw Little Morton, the teddy bear, propped on her pillow. The room was small, and one of the only ones with a window, but done up pretty well, he reflected, on account of all the shopping instruction Annise had been giving her at the mall.

He lay back on Muriel's bed, with Little Morton resting on his chest. Later he heard the supervisor's gravely voice in the hallway.

"And don't forget, you're scheduled for the tub at three this afternoon."

"But Joseph—"

"No buts, Muriel. I'll send someone for you at a quarter till."

The Gestapo's leather soled shoes squeaked into the distance. Muriel entered. Immediately her face lit up.

"Oh Morton, thank God you're here!" She ran over and threw her arms around him. She seemed so happy, but when she drew back he noticed chalky salt streaks on her cheeks from recent tears. He took her by the shoulders.

"Sit down, Muriel. I want you to level with me. Things aren't just evil around here anymore, I'm afraid they're turning dangerous."

Muriel sat gingerly on the edge of the bed. "What do you want to know?" she asked.

"Your letter last night. It was one of the most beautiful things I've ever seen."

"It was?"

"Yes, it was. Beautiful and sweet and everything you are as a person was in there. I have a question about it though. You mentioned—I want to be delicate. You mentioned something about having sex with men. This is what I have to ask you about."

"OK."

"You said you looked at the bed and thought maybe sex was the way. Be straight with me now. I'm your Legal Guardian. Meaning I have to protect you. Now, tell me, have you been screwing arou— I mean, having sex with people?"

Muriel lowered her head. At last she said low, "I heard that blonde gets a thousand dollars a month from her father. And stocks and bonds too." She crossed her arms.

"A thousand a month? Really?" Morton was amazed.

Muriel slapped her forehead. "Uh, oh. Now I've done it. I've made her twice as sexy because she doesn't have to earn her way. Is that what you think being feminine is? Somebody who draws her face on with pounds of makeup and lays around in the tub all day?"

"She lays around in the tub all day?"

Muriel dropped her arms. "I've got a question, Morton. Am I a feminine enough girl? Or am I just another one of those plain jane nut cases?"

"You're a very strong woman, Muriel. One of these days you're going to realize how femininity and being strong go together."

"Strong? What are you trying to say?"

"I'm saying strong. You know what strong means." Morton waved absently.

"Yes, I know what it means. It means you're saying I have like a little bit of Harvey's Freudian penis envy, aren't you? It means you're saying I'm a little bit manly because I'm a natural schizophrenic who doesn't have a red sports car."

Morton still had hold of the teddy bear. He set it aside. Her auburn hair seemed damp and about to kink up, apparently from a new dressing she'd used. In the swirl of morning emotion he must have overlooked it. He moved the locks gently back from her cheeks.

"I'm not so abnormal, Morton," she continued softly. "I want the penis as much as any other woman. Only I want it on a good man where it can be used right."

Morton wiped at his brow. Audacious little thing, wasn't she? On the other hand, this kind of lingo might be expected if she was swinging toward the high side of manic-depression. Strong? Yes, she was definitely that. But there were the bows and ribbons too. And the hurt of course. Always the confusion and the foolish hurt sneaking in, which was the very thing he worked so diligently to prevent.

Morton said, "I found your diaphragm in the shower. I saw the prescription date Harvey wrote on it, so I know this is a new thing for you." He reached into his pocket to give it to her, then realized he'd left it in his bureau drawer. "Anyway, ummm, I mean—" Suddenly he blurted, "Have you used it yet?"

"Only for training. Because I'll be out on my own soon. But I'm sure I won't be needing it. You can keep it if you want."

"Who's training you? Joseph?"

"Stacy."

"Stacy! What the hell does she know about— I mean, have you figured out what to do with it?"

"Not really."

"Did you use it when you ran away?"

"No."

"Then you could be pregnant."

"I'm not though."

"How do you know?"

"Joseph took me down to Cedars for a pregnancy test this morning. I'm negative."

"Pregnancy? *That* was your appointment?"

"Uh huh."

A sudden look of bewilderment came over her.

"Wait a minute. I don't want the penis on *him*, Morton. I promise I don't. He's a bad man, everybody knows that."

"What are you saying, Muriel? Are you telling me Joseph Schopen raped you?" pressed the counselor.

"I get mad sometimes. Sometimes I think bad men should have it cut off. Mount it in the Smithsonian and let those dancers in his boob bars envy it. Not me. I don't want that thing in any way whatsoever."

There came a knock. Before Muriel could answer it the door swung open. It was Annise Chastain. Her hair seemed damp, as if she'd treated it with a high powered chemical. The ends coiled silkily down her back. Impressive!

"Morton! Fancy catching you here," exclaimed Annise.

Morton started toward her, but she pushed out her palms. "No romancing on the job now," she said with a smile.

There was a small love seat beside the closet. Some of Muriel's clothes had been tossed onto it. Annise went over and began to straighten up.

"So how'd last night go?" asked Annise glancing between Morton and Muriel. She opened the closet. "You're quite a lucky girl, hanging out with the most happening cat around."

"Me, you mean?" said Morton.

"Wow, your hair, Muriel!" noticed Annise. "You used my mousse after all, didn't you? It's just so adorable."

She went to Muriel and bounced the ringlets therapeutically. "You're *such* a cute girl."

"Thanks," said Muriel shyly.

"By the way," continued Annise changing to her professional tone. "Joseph sent me down to get you, Muriel. He had to change your therapy time. He needs you upstairs right away."

"He wants me upstairs?"

Morton and Muriel exchanged a frightened look.

"You can take Harvey's elevator. Joseph said it would be all right."

No one moved.

"Go ahead now," prodded Annise. "I need to talk to Morton in private. And don't forget the new terry cloth robe we got for you. Let me see." She went to the closet, pulled it off a hangar and handed it to Muriel.

The three of them entered the hallway. Muriel started to mope away.

"Tootaloo," said Annise guiding Morton the opposite way down the corridor.

Over his shoulder the counselor offered a hurried goodbye wave to Muriel as Annise tugged him quickly out the side door.

* * *

Chapter 23

Annise led them across the enclosed courtyard to the sand paths winding into the jungle-like Organic Therapy Garden. Every fifty feet or so they came to a concrete bench. Here and there small dirt trails led into the more secluded areas where Gordon obsessively planted his prized ferns and Sally Featherman compulsively dug them up.

At the final bench Annise paused, then stepped into the high foliage bordering the back fence.

"Come this way," she beckoned, dipping beneath one of the bushy palmettos. Fraction House antics—they weren't merely for the patients!

Morton followed her to an unlikely opening, a tiny glade with sharp California sunlight striking through the overhead trees from the west. So much like a kitten with a ball of twine, that Annise Chastain, he thought as she scooted onto a small wooden bench.

"Isn't this a splendid hideout? Come, Morton. Sit with me. I want to tell you things," she exulted, her golden hair shimmering in the brilliant bars of light.

The counselor joined her on the bench. It was cool there. Free feeling, yet secret in a devious, childlike way. This was how it always began with Annise. Was today to be another bright Sunday morning turned dim and snowy when the godforsaken Notre Dame game came on? He had to remember his mission. He forced himself to recollect his brewing resentments at the way her torch flared fast and furious, but invariably twisted away chill and cold, smoldering with the last fading heat from his fingertips. This would not go unaddressed forever. No, not by a long shot it wouldn't.

"I've got something important to say to you, Annise," began the counselor.

"Excellent," she replied. "Because I've got something big to lay you too. First though, I forgot to mention that tomorrow's my brother's birthday. I've told you about David. He's on a golfing scholarship at Pasadena Tech. I didn't? Well, anyway, I'm going to have to run out to my parents' place. They're on Linda-Vista Drive. That's a big deal road these days in Pasadena. I'm sure I mentioned it. I didn't?"

"I thought you have to work for Stacy and Wanda the next three days," said Morton.

"I do. Only I told Joseph about David and he agreed to let me have tomorrow off as long I pull two days after that. Christ, and I'm so exhausted already."

"I could rejuvenate you," suggested Morton leaning toward her.

"You can come out to the house if you want. Dad's been dying to meet you. And my little sister, Aphie, will be there. She's flying in from San Francisco. She probably won't like you though. She never likes any of my boyfriends."

Dad? Aphie? David? The counselor's mind drifted away for a moment. He imagined himself in their fancy suburban backyard, relaxing in one of those fan-backed rattan chairs. Giant statue of the Pieta to the left. Stained glass windows of the main house looming high on the right. His pickup truck parked hastily out front, the faded green paint flaking off the fenders. A glass of Sopov in one hand, Annise offering her fine white breast like in a misty Hieronymus Bosch picture to the other. And all the while the gardeners clipping calmly around them...

"Uh, thanks Annise, but I think I'd better pass on the birthday party."

"I thought you might say that. But I do have something big to lay on you, Morton. It really can't wait."

"It can't?"

"Absolutely not." Annise's thigh brushed against his. She had a sleeveless sundress on, and like a child grown hot and sultry in her teens, she hooked her fingers under the hem and unconsciously hiked it up as she continued to speak.

"I was thinking we might be able to squeeze in a couple of hours tomorrow evening," she went on. "I've got to be back at the nuthouse by midnight though. There's this really hip place over on Colorado Boulevard. It's an Irish bar called Samson's Sweat Shop."

She rocked fore and aft on the bench. Her skimpy dress rose by imperceptible degrees to the white gauze covering home plate. Morton saw it in her eyes—yes, she knew what she was doing.

"Meet me in the parking lot at 7:30. I promise it'll be hot," she added.

"Done," said the counselor.

Annise glanced around. "I've got to get back to work. But Morton, I want you to know I'm going to have something incredibly special for you tomorrow."

"Something special? You mean like a gift?"

"Yes, it's a gift all right. I'm going to powder it and wrap it and all," she said.

Morton spontaneously conceived an offering of his own. Damned if it wasn't what they'd both been in such dire need of since the beginning.

"What a coincidence, Annise," he said. "Because I've got something special for you too. I can't wait to see your face when you open the box."

"Great! We'll exchange. It'll be like an early Christmas!" she cried.

A transitional second passed. Annise casually lifted her hand, and in your lusty L.A. fashion fanned back her three feet of hair and let those weirdly dampened ringlets rain forward over her breasts. Before Morton was quite aware of it they were engaging in a long, sensual kiss. For the first time an unaffected passion put sparking coals under their flesh. The Catholic cherub was turning sweet devilish succubus right there in the Organic Therapy Garden.

The counselor's eyes lifted in bliss as he at last began to grasp the fruit of his labor. The overhead petals of the eucalyptus tree drifted apart in the slight breeze, revealing the distant glare of the three windows leading up the back stairwell of the Fraction House.

Firm as it was, the blonde's sumptuous mounds of body melted like heated caramel into Morton's. The kiss was profound. Like thirty kisses stacked together. He felt such a fool for questioning her emotion, when his eyes drifted to the next stage upward between the limbs, and he saw, materializing through the crystal vista of the only non-Plexiglas window in the building— Yes, it was the mug of Joseph Schopen behind a pair of high powered field glasses, steadying down on them from his perch at the base of the third floor stairs.

Morton brought Annise to her feet. Once more she moved flush into the embrace. The counselor's hands moved to her hips. In protection, he rotated her, using his back as a shield against the Gestapo's eavesdropping. It might have been best to stop, but by instinct for that cleft in the center of the heart his palms drew lower. He squeezed shut his eyes, happy at last in the arms of his starlet.

Nothing however was secure at a place like the Fraction House. And this little glen happened to abut E-Wing. He hadn't noticed before, but through the leaves he now saw at eye level the steel-barred hallway window of the women's dormitory. A bit too close for comfort, he felt, gradually releasing the hem of Annise's dress.

He had a sudden hyperventilation, a sort of half-breath phobia. He broke the kiss, and pressing Annise's head to his shoulder angled for a glimpse through the dorm window. His heart sunk like a bundle of decaying ions, for peering anxiously at him, less than ten feet away through the barrier of leaves, iron bars, and Plexiglas, were the blue volcanic eyes, only now turned to brittle, aqua-marine glaciers, of Muriel Gonska, the sweet Incested Schizophrenic.

* * *

Chapter 24

According to their agreement, Morton drove out to Samson's Sweat Shop the following evening. He was to meet Annise at 7:30. At 8:30 he was still in the parking lot, waiting. He felt his jacket pocket. Yes, the special gift was still there. At last he went on inside and ordered.

Samson's Sweat Shop was supposed to be an Irish place, but it seemed mostly Cubans were in there, or perhaps they were Mexicans. He'd never been good at distinguishing one ethnic group from another, which might have accounted for his instinctive lack of prejudice.

At 9:00, when Annise arrived, she paused extra long in the doorway, employing that cat-like habit of hers, as if deciding at the last minute which way she'd go. Morton might have been a hair irked by then, but when he laid eyes on her satiny lavender pantsuit, the gleaming red high heels, part of her hair up, part down around her rouged cheeks in fuzzy little curlets, her beauty as full-blown and enticing as the California skyline— Well, suffice to say his irritation waned somewhat.

"Ah, there you are!" she called.

The line of heads at the bar turned to watch her high-heeling toward him. She placed a tiny kiss in the air beside his ear. "Just give me two seconds," she whispered, and she left for the rest room.

Morton wasn't privy to the ins and outs of your ladies' room transformations, but when Annise returned some later she exuded the spirit of several centuries at once. She seemed more than a female, as if three or four females had gotten into her and were vying for top dog status. Vibes of serendipity surrounded her as she offered her famous Don't-Worry-Be-Happy smile. A person couldn't help but feel comforted.

Morton had already ordered Annise's usual Bloody Mary. They chatted a bit. It was good to warm up after not connecting for a real date in so long.

"How did your brother's party go?" asked the counselor.

"Poor David," sighed Annise heavily. "He's been terribly upset this last week. He was in this big golf tournament, and they say he moved his ball or something. Which isn't exactly kosher, I guess. It's some little bullshit thing, I'm sure. The problem is, they were talking about expelling him. Can you believe that?"

"How far did he move the ball?" wondered Morton.

Annise frumped her lips. Turning serious, she said, "Do you think because a person cheated as a kid they'll cheat as an adult?"

"He cheated as a kid?"

"Well, not any more than the rest of us," she replied.

Annise took a long drink of her Bloody Mary.

"I think he's out of the woods though, thank the Lord," she continued. "The college built the golf course, and Desert Realty—that's Dad's firm you know. You didn't? Well, I'm sure I told you. Anyway, Desert Realty holds the lien on the back nine."

"What a lucky coincidence," said Morton.

"Lucky? Meant to be is what it was. Dad simply phoned up Dean Myers. They met in the clubhouse for martinis a few hours ago," said Annise.

"Wow, fast work," marveled the counselor.

"So you see, as it turns out David didn't move his ball after all. And this way he comes in third!"

She raised her Bloody Mary and clicked it against Morton's glass of beer. Through the lavender pants suit her thigh moved delicately against his.

Their coziness felt somehow inauthentic, intoxicating, yet distracting in a strangely ultra-focused way. Deep inside he felt himself quivering. Tremors of the heart? He didn't know. In Annise's presence he often found himself thinking of Muriel Gonska, as he was now. That would be natural enough, wouldn't it? Annise being Muriel's counselor and whatnot?

The blonde placed her hand on Morton's forearm. Perhaps she'd picked up on his sense of insecurity.

"I wanted to tell you how settled Muriel was after you left yesterday," volunteered Annise. "I know she was shaky when we were in her room, but after supper she turned into a different person."

"That's the way schizophrenics are," returned Morton.

"But she was *totally* different. We actually started hitting it off, can you imagine? We played dress up with her new clothes. We were giggly and girlie all night long. It was *so* dynamic."

"Muriel giggly? The same Muriel I know?" said the counselor.

"Yep. She started following me around like an awe-struck little sister. It was a real trip."

Morton's forehead creased involuntarily.

"Gordon was a dream too," she went on. "He told me you stopped by and had a talk with him. Honestly, Morty, you've been bestowed a powerful gift for dealing with these crazies. It's as if you've got the deepest secret of insanity locked up way down inside yourself. And somehow you know to only let it out exactly when it's needed."

Annise smiled over at him, then leaned back and lit a cigarette. The counselor looked closely at her. Golden. Angelic. Shrouded in warm planes of smoke. A magnificent thing.

"I'm beginning to worry about you. You don't seem quite yourself, Morton. I've been thinking about this. Have you noticed how you're always around women these days? That's a proved way people go bonkers, you know."

Morton's jaw jutted forward.

"Don't you have any men friends? Someone you can sit down and talk things over with?" she asked.

"Gordon."

"But he's a nut."

"He's honest."

"He's crazy."

"He's fair."

They looked away from each other.

"I used to have a best friend," said Morton.

"Yeah?"

"He was killed a few years back."

"In the war?"

"In a way it was a war. It was in the old days. The police shot him for trying to buy pills. You know, like the kind Joseph gives Sally and Gordon and a bunch of those guys on C-Wing."

"How sad. But hard drugs can change the way God made you, Morton. Believe me, you don't want anything screwing around with your absolute self. Unless a doctor prescribes it for you of course."

"So you think it's OK for a doctor to screw around with your absolute self?"

"Oh, that reminds me," said Annise breaking the flow. "I brought something from the Fraction House for you." She reached into her purse.

"The gift? Is it time for our exchange?"

"Not yet. This is something different."

She placed a large prescription vial before him. Morton glanced around the bar, then nervously slid it behind his beer glass.

Annise said, "Remember when we talked about how hyper you've been? Well, a great thing happened. I was able to get a script for Librium. Don't look so alarmed. It's only a mild tranquilizer."

"Librium?"

"Sure. It's short for equilibrium. Which means it restores balance, Morton. God, everybody needs balance. Especially you males."

"You've got a point there. Only I'm not sure I want my absolute self screwed around with," said the counselor hesitantly.

He examined the vial. The label was pre-printed in the usual Dar/Neese manner. Under the heading 'Patient,' Morton's name was penned in. Harvey was listed as the prescribing physician.

"Wait a minute, Annise. Something isn't right here. This is Harvey's name all right, only it's Joseph's handwriting. See?"

Morton showed it to her.

"What difference does it make?" she asked. "Joseph has the Fraction House Power of Attorney. He signs for everything, doesn't he?"

"He's not a doctor," said Morton.

"He's a Ph.D.," countered Annise.

"Maybe, maybe not. Either way it's against the law for him to sign prescriptions. By forging Harvey's signature he's impersonating an M.D. That's big time illegal."

Annise slapped both hands down on the bar. "Morton, you're proving my very point. Can't you see how wired you're getting? I weasel Joseph into doing you this huge favor, and you want to throw him in the clinker for it."

"You weaseled Joseph? I thought the tranquilizers were his idea."

Annise shrugged.

"He's stealing Harvey's scholarly papers too," Morton went on. "I know for a fact he's been signing as 'Dr. J. Schopen' on Harvey's articles to the medical journals. Joseph pumps iron and hangs out at titty bars, Annise. Believe me, he does not write scholarly papers."

By degrees Annise went downcast. When it came to the Gestapo Morton realized he could sound a bit harsh. Maybe he really was a paranoid type, like they said. It wasn't impossible, was it, that Joseph had Morton's best interests at heart? Certainly Annise did, he couldn't question that. She was so giving, and he so overbearing.

The counselor felt bad. He waved for the bartender and bought them another round. Annise eased into a smile. The man bringing out his wallet and paying for things—he'd learned how far this act of social deference could go toward stabilizing her emotional equipoise. Beneath the bar Morton tenderly stroked her knee.

"Do you really think people have absolute selves, Annise? I mean, do you have an absolute self?" he asked thoughtfully.

Annise smoked her cigarette. "I might. If I do though it's certainly not in this wretched body."

"It's not in that wretched body?"

"Of course not. It's in the *soul*, Morton. This worthless piece of flesh is only a measly vehicle."

She rotated on the stool and opened her arms. Together they observed the silken jump suit as it revealed those abstract parts beneath gelling vividly into soft, esoteric angles. As far as sensuality went, let the record show that she came with a body about to burst the return address on her envelope.

"To be up front, Morton, none of this is worth analyzing. It's like David's ball, it's all in the hands of fate."

"Fate?"

"Sure. Isn't it obvious? In the long run you either will or won't take your medication." She snatched the vial and shook it for emphasis. "I can pray for you. Christ, I *do* pray for you. But I'm not the Pope, Morton. I don't have the kind of pull even those dopey nuns get."

Morton said, "I don't understand. I mean, if it's all in the hands of fate what good would it do to pray about it?"

"I'm glad you asked that. Because what God does, you see, is he *arranges* fate."

Annise licked her lips, then polished off the rest of her Bloody Mary.

"He does?"

"Uh huh. And prayer, Morton, is what helps him arrange it."

"How often does he arrange it?" wondered the counselor.

She thought it over. "Every two or three days," she said leaning back.

They were quiet for a minute. Annise tapped the ash off her cigarette.

"Look, how do you think all these people change the future?" she asked him. "Like saving each other from cancer say? And heart disease and VD and all? Particularly if they smoke and drink and screw around and do all the things that cause those things?"

"How?"

"Prayer, for Godsake. Otherwise the whole thing would be a terrible crock!" she cried holding out her hands.

Somehow conversations with Annise seemed to gradually rise in volume. Others were always overhearing. It made Morton feel sheepish, and he resolved to keep quieter in the future. Nevertheless, here she was finally meeting his eyes with that telegraphic way she had of not actually meeting them.

Under the bar her hand found his. At last, it seemed, the relationship was blossoming. His heart calmed. But no, she was slipping something into his palm. It was one of the light green Librium capsules. She gave him a small but firm nod. Hmmm. Internal medicine. Was this really called for in his case? Well, maybe he was hyper, after all. What would it hurt, really, to take a prescribed medication, especially if your absolute self was in need of a change? He placed the pill in his mouth.

"By the way, Joseph's got a new Dictum. We all have to pee in a cup for him."

"A drug screen?" asked Morton.

"Yeah. You'll have to do it too. But don't worry, the Librium's prescribed. As long as no illicit drugs turn up you're OK."

"Why are you staring at me, Annise? I'm not into illicit drugs. For that matter, I'm not much into prescribed drugs either." He sipped his beer.

~~~

"Morton, it's getting late. I was wondering if I could go ahead and give you my gift now?"

"I'd like to give you mine too. Only—" He drew his legs back. "Annise, before we exchange, there's something I feel I have to know. It's extremely difficult to ask this, but I really must have an answer."

"Yes?" she said.

"It's about fidelity. You do believe in it, don't you? In fidelity, I mean? Because sometimes people can get different moralities in life and you can't always tell which kind they've got."

Annise crossed her arms. A silent moment went by. She squinted over at him.

"Well?" he asked peering cautiously at her.

"I absolutely do, Morton. Absolutely, yes I do believe in fidelity. And in all the important shit that goes along with it," declared Annise. She thumped the bar for emphasis.

"What important shit?"

"Oh, marriage, christenings. Those nifty long-term 401K plans."

Morton swallowed. "Well, good. Because you can't always tell about somebody by looking. Say for instance if a person has a lot of men's initials all over their calendar and they're not the same initials her boyfriend has. It can get a guy to wondering is all."

"Sometimes, Morton, I get the feeling you think I might be a little bit of a snake." She pursed her lips.

"Look, Annise, I'd be a fool not to realize men are dying to get their hands on a sexy piece of blonde— Oh, I'm sorry, baby, I—"

She smiled. "It's OK. I think I know what you mean. You're complimenting me, aren't you?"

Quickly Morton nodded.

Annise said, "As a matter of fact, this brings us right up to my gift. Spiritually, it's amazing! This is exactly the topic I was hoping for. It's what this entire night has been about."

Morton scratched his temple as she slipped her hand into her purse and lifted out a small box with a red bow on the top.

The counselor started to remove the silver wrapping paper. Then he paused, reached into his jacket and handed her the palm-sized velour pouch which contained her present. Ahhh, it was going so smoothly.

Annise uncinched the leatherette drawstring. "What a cool little sack!" she said excitedly.

Morton balled his wrapping paper and set it aside. Savoring the moment, he slowly opened the box. Inside he found a thin plastic container. Beige-colored, and rounded at the edges. *'Freefold All-Flex,'* read the outer label.

Annise freed her gift from the white tissue paper. She held it between her fingers, the long red nails adding to the sexy thrill of the moment.

Morton smiled over at her. Carefully, he unsnapped the plastic container. An odor of baby powder and antiseptic filled the air. The counselor's eyes doubled in size. He clapped shut the lid.

"Jesus Christ, Annise!" he whispered shooting frightened looks around the bar. "This is a fucking diaphragm!"

Annise was slipping free the stainless steel clasp on the white plastic case Morton had given her. Timidly she extracted the yellowish, bracelet-sized device. In a flash her cheeks brightened from pinkish Sunday sun to burning Saturday night crimson.

"My God, Morton," she gasped staring up at him. "This is a... a goddamn diaphragm?" Her voice had lifted to a soprano pitch.

Yes, it was a diaphragm. Muriel Gonska's diaphragm to be exact. He realized how discolored it was compared to the newer one. Tested a few times, perhaps, powdery and slightly shopworn perhaps, but not really damaged.

A dead silence fell across Samson's Sweat Shop. No one at the bar, least of all the two of them, seemed able to comprehend it. Annise scooped away the two items. They both drank deeply. This had gone *beyond* good fortune.

They remained quiet, a new quality in their relationship. Gradually the noise level came back up.

Annise took the counselor by the hands. She'd exchanged her little-girl look for one of genteel determination. "Morton, do you realize what's happened tonight?"

He shook his head.

"Here we have two people who hardly know each other turning up in this little Irish bar—"

"Cuban, Annise. It's a Cuban bar."

"Turning up in this little *Irish* bar with any of a thousand gifts. Yet they bring exactly the same thing. Think of the odds. Do you see what I'm getting at? I mean, they bring *exactly* the same gift?"

"Yes?" said Morton.

"It just seems hard to fathom. I mean, if you think of it in terms of..." She trailed off.

Annise lit a new cigarette and took many puffs. She got a small mirror from her purse and embarked upon a fretful adjustment of her makeup.

Morton returned, "Are you trying to say this might be— I mean, it might in some way be—" He hesitated. He could hardly bring himself to utter it. "Fated?" he said.

Annise's mood started to crumble. She began to gather up her things. Morton went to touch her, but she jerked away. Black clouds were forming. A squally cold front appeared. She checked her watch.

"I've got to go," she declared clamoring to her feet.

She did not move away however, but stood there for the longest time, facing him. Morton's soul—what was this, he was now thinking in souls?—trembled with fascination.

As swiftly as the barometer had dropped, the winds subsided. The currents of indecision detailing the fine texture of her face bled away like drying rain, and a new day opened up. No longer was the time 10:00 p.m. Friday night, or the place some smoky Pasadena lounge. The moment had crystallized, and as occasionally occurred at the Fraction House a bizarre history of insanity could shimmer up into the future like Christmas at a department store, bright lights and money everywhere, the promise of health and new desires springing from the heart like so many thrilling pony rides for a ten year old.

Morton felt oddly tranquil. He sensed he had gained, well, yes, a share of equilibrium. Unlike he would normally do, he peacefully, sleepily almost, awaited her next move. It was a slipping away of aggression. Hmmm. He kind of liked the feeling. It was similar to the soporific drugs of the sixties.

Annise's eyes were lowered. Very softly she said, "We've still got a little time left, Morton. I don't have to be back at Dar/Neese till midnight. Would you be interested in— I mean, would you maybe want to come by my place for a little while?"

* * *

Chapter 25

In the parking lot Annise said, "Follow me. I know a quickie short cut."

"Are you OK to drive? I know you've had a long day," said Morton softly.

"Of course I'm OK. You know how careful I am not to weave when I've been drinking."

Morton got into his pickup and followed her along the smoggy freeway skyline. Over the heavily populated basin a spooky maroon cloud hung like a great bloodshot eye in the illuminated ozone. Up ahead he could see her hair whipping like cream out the window into the hot L.A. winds. Off to the left twinkled the purple lights of the skyscrapers and the towering banks he felt certain Annise expected to be drawing from one day, the future glowing all around, from the suburbs to the seashore, in garish streaks of halogen and neon. Expensive! He had a few bucks in the Fraction House Credit Union. Perhaps he ought to get up his gumption, go down to UCLA and finish his accounting degree. Or maybe fate alone would have him drawing from those banks one day. At the current rate it would require serious fiscal intervention, because ambition certainly wasn't getting it. A fear shot through him.

Canada, he wondered momentarily? No, the malls up there likely wouldn't stock those sequined dresses Annise needed for her busy weekends. Each morning as he passed the boutique down the block from his apartment he considered buying her one of those cool Grateful Dead T-shirts with the funky Casey Jones Choo-Choo train puffing into the distance. But that was Muriel, wasn't it? Maybe it was Morton too, a little bit. Certainly it wasn't Annise.

Come to think of it, he couldn't go to Canada. The Muriel mess was in full swing. No, he wasn't going anywhere. Not yet, he wasn't.

'L.A. 2000:' Sex Asylum

Annise was a Type-A driver. Morton's pickup couldn't keep the pace.

By the time he arrived at her apartment she was already in the process of opening the notorious locking box. She set out the miniature riding crop with the horse's head handle. A couple of the magazines. The pistol was there—that nasty little derringer with the ominous words *Smith & Wesson* engraved on the barrel. As she rummaged Morton noticed a crisp new packet of bonds. He sat on the edge of the bed.

"It looks like Santa came early," he said nodding toward the thick, rubber-banded notes.

"Yes. He gave me the greatest gift of all," she said warmly.

"Love?" wondered the counselor.

"Money," said Annise.

Morton frowned.

She gathered a few things and headed for the bathroom. At the doorway she turned and said, "Make yourself comfortable. We want to be as unencumbered as possible for this. Don't you agree?"

Unencumbered? Hmmm. Yes. Yes, we do, decided the counselor. He leaned down and untied his shoes. Absolutely yes we do!

He undressed and stretched out on the mattress. But wait, he thought. Best to show modesty at times like this. Avoid all possible stresses. When in doubt, conceal thyself, that was the religious way to do these things. He rolled the covers down and climbed under.

He heard the water running in the bathroom. Lying around in the tub? he wondered momentarily. She returned in her black negligee with the holes cut out. The diaphragm was in her hand.

Shakily she said, "I couldn't get it to work, Morton. I've never done this before and it won't fit and I don't want to use it anyway. I wanted you to help. I was sitting in there all crooked and I kept hoping and hoping you'd come in. But you didn't. And now I'm ashamed and embarrassed and I don't even want to *see* this damn thing."

She flung it on the floor. It bounced twice like a stick ball pinkie and came to rest in the corner beside the vanity.

"Didn't the doctor show you how?" asked Morton.

Annise batted her eyes. "I told him I already knew," she said weakly.

Her head dipped. She became grave, kind of nun-like. That Annise Chastain—any admixture of ice or heat was liable to steam out of her at the next moment. All the counselor could do was cross his fingers and prepare to shadow box the upcoming apocalypse.

She sat on the edge of the bed. She showed him the tube of contraceptive, which read 'Ortho-Gynol.'

"This jelly stuff, Morton— It kills the little babies, doesn't it?"

"Well, it, uh—"

"It does. I know it does," said Annise.

She tossed her hair far back, then let it roll forward again.

"Can't you understand this, Morton? Murdering all those millions of happy little babies hurts me inside. In *here*."

She put her hands to her mid-section and went to the vanity.

Morton sat up in the bed. He felt the covers drop very low over his hips. Annise didn't seem to mind.

"Maybe I could use a— Well, you know—" he stammered.

"A condom?" she asked delicately.

He nodded shyly.

"Oh, I don't know. I've heard guys don't really like it. Rod always said he never liked it."

"How come Rod used a condom?" he asked.

"What do you mean how come?" she flared. "Wait, now. Are you implying I was unfaithful to Rod? You are, aren't you? You're saying Rod used rubbers because he was afraid I might be screwing around and give him something. That's what all your infidelity stuff in Samson's was about, wasn't it?"

"This is a new Century, Annise. I mean, a new Millennium, or something like that. Neither of us should die of any diseases Rod might have had. Or anybody else for that matter."

"Anybody else!" she exclaimed. "Who are you talking about? Lance?"

"Who's Lance?"

"I told you about Lance. I didn't? Well, Lance is Rod's brother. And don't look at me so weird. Anyway, what happened is—"

Annise went on to elaborate how serious her commitment to Rod had been. When she saw it fading, though, common sense led her to prepare for, as she put it, "a new serious commitment."

"Were you in love?" wondered Morton.

"Oh, yes. Rod and I didn't have very much in the way of sex, but we were definitely in love."

"I see."

"It was his brother who was the sex fanatic."

"Lance, you mean?"

"Uh huh. He's older. And he's extremely, I mean *extremely* motivated." She shivered at the recollection. "I gave myself completely to Lance. All I've ever wanted, Morton, is someone to give myself to completely."

"Whatever happened with Lance?"

Annise waved nonchalantly. "We broke up. We're still friends though."

"Friends?" Morton eyed the calendar looking for L.S.'s. And they were there. Friends? Humph!

"I'm healthy as a cow. I've even got tests to prove it." She snatched a paper from her locking box and tossed it on the bed. "HIV negative, if that's what you have to see."

The counselor checked over the form.

"The problem here, Morton, is a condom only catches those millions of babies. They all get murdered the moment it comes off."

Morton thought hard. "But *you* don't murder them," he returned. "I think I see a loophole in this. Because if you don't kill them it couldn't be considered a mortal sin, could it? I suppose... I suppose it might be considered one of those venial sins. But like you always say, venial and mortal are entirely different matters."

By way of the mirror Annise met Morton's eyes. Her face went open and free as she gradually took in the concept. She stepped over to the bed, and with the negligee working its peekaboo wiles rolled his head lovingly across her torso.

"Do you realize how happy you've made me, Morton?" she said. "God, I'm so grateful you're finally getting it."

"Getting what?" asked the counselor, his voice muffled.

"Catholiscm, for Godsake! Everything about it has to be thought through with a fine tooth comb if you're going to have any fun in this life. It's a very complex doctrine. I'm glad you're with me in the planning."

"I'm with you, Annise."

"Only one thing, the Pope doesn't much go for rubbers," she added. "Unless they're just for disease, of course. But we probably don't have a problem there, since you were with Stacy for so long. As a Roman Catholic, Morton, the Pontiff's women are obligated to use the rhythm method."

"Rhythm? That's pure Russian Roulette," replied the counselor looking up.

"The Pope doesn't play Russian Roulette, I'll have you know," said Annise. "And besides, if you're good at it the one loaded bullet never comes up. Don't you see? We're free. Hot, horny and free!" she cried.

Like the open wings of an angel in the classiest of porn movies Annise descended into the covers. The overhead lantern went off leaving only the torrid red glow from the vanity. Once, Sassafras scratched at the door.

"Bad dog!" called Annise glancing up for an instant. They heard Sassafras pad back into the kitchen by her bowl.

* * *

Chapter 26

At last they'd begun. Their touches on the journey toward union moist and electric, yes, yet in a mysterious way cool and unconfined, an open vista of dreams and hopes finally coming true. The fierce lust the counselor had expected drifted instead toward a narcotic wealth of emotion, the invisible angles leaning one into another like lyrics into the music of a love song. Capturing them. Releasing them. Then, like liquid in the jaws of a vise, tightening again and making its universal statement. The ocean of woman washing timelessly over the city's bold arc of fireworks.

Hands seeming to slide everywhere, easily reaching their destinations. He pressed to synchronize their stride. It was so good. So solid and real.

Until... Well, until in his roamings he felt something at the base of her spine. More there than buttock, it seemed. It wasn't bone, he could tell, but something different. He touched again, cautiously along her backbone toward the fatty little coccyx.

Yes, he was right. A mass apparently. Not so small either, he realized, but close to egg, or maybe golf ball size. It was actually buried there. A tumor imbedded somehow at such a strange spot.

Annise kept the rhythm slow. She really was your psychological type of blonde. Through the dim red light she gazed at him with the sensually sleepy though obviously wide awake look she was so expert at. Morton gazed back with the same narcoleptic eyes.

Annise whispered, "People can be so strange sometimes. But deep inside I'm the happiest person in the world you feel the way you do. Especially after all this."

"Feel the way I do about what?"

"About fidelity. And about all the important shit that goes along with it. You'd be shocked at the thoughts going through my head. I'm paranoid of losing you and I don't even have you."

They resumed the languid pace. The future itself a great lioness beneath him. As happened sometimes when he exerted himself, a tickle formed in the back of the counselor's throat.

He opened his eyes. The vanity appeared, the bulbs muted and shadowy. He placed a light kiss on Annise's forehead, then rolled slowly to the side.

Perhaps he'd been overly serene. Or perhaps, after feeling the tumor, a fear for her well-being had engulfed him. Whatever the cause, he was suddenly impotent.

"Sorry," he said.

~~~

Afterwards Morton was nervous. Annise set her cutting edge Imagineer 3000 laptop on the vanity. Next came an attack on the keyboard, a virtual reality scream of guilt it was. A torrent of tapping only half silent like sin, yet louder in its meaning than a Jew's screech at the Wailing Wall. Well, we all employed our personal methods of therapy when things out of the ordinary happened.

The counselor struggled with his emotions. How did you say this to someone? he kept thinking. That by chance in your passion you happened to cross over a place— Not trying to. Not trying to at all. It simply occurred. And so much worse, really, what with the relationship just starting up... Of course, you didn't want to frighten anyone, but what I think I found... What I think I accidentally found is—

Annise abruptly halted her typing. She gazed into the air, carried the ash tray to the bed, crossed her legs yoga style and lit a cigarette.

"It doesn't always work right at the start, does it?" she said.

"No, not always."

"I liked it though. I guess you could tell."

"Things get in a person's mind. Sometimes it seems like a lot of energy gets used up for nothing." Morton shook his head.

"Like needless energy. Don't you ever feel things should be more—I don't know, fair? Or important maybe?"

"What's important to you another person might not even care about. Even horrible things are good sometimes. Christ, when you think of it, everything has importance," said Annise touching his thigh.

"Like what?"

"Oh, I don't know. Say politics for instance. Otherwise you wouldn't have any government the way it gets mixed in with business and taxes and corruption and all. And the Catholic Church, naturally. Think what would happen without the church, Morton. All that gold! Imagine those huge paintings they keep in vaults just being lost on the multitudes. Honestly, there's a million important things out there. Hardly anything *isn't* important," she said.

"How about cancer? There doesn't seem a damn thing good about that," Morton said.

Annise thought for a moment. "There must be though. Otherwise God wouldn't have made it. So in a way I guess you could say it's as important as anything else. As long as you never get it yourself, of course," she added smiling.

Morton stood and took her hand. It hadn't gone right. What did? Nevertheless, he led her into the bathroom where the light was better and made her feel it. At first she took it as a curiosity. Eyes moving all around as she examined herself. By degrees an intensity gathered.

Twenty minutes later they emerged to a different world. The day had been summer-like. She'd run the air conditioner and now there was a sharp chill in the air. In the bedroom they reached for their clothes at the same time and bumped one another. A hard glare followed. The next instant they remembered they were naked and angled shyly away. The Garden of Eden had gone sour as a cooked grapefruit on an electric eye.

Annise started to dress for the Fraction House, then paused to light yet another cigarette. Morton waved his hands at the smoke. She whipped her head toward him.

"Do you think smoking might have caused it?" she asked quickly.

"I don't know, Annise."

"What about drinking?"

"I doubt it."

"Do you think I'm going to die?" she asked. "That's always possible you know."

"No, of course not. You'll have to have it checked out, that's all. I'm not sure anybody really knows what causes these things. Maybe it's like you said before. Maybe God causes it and it'll all be for the good."

She spun around. "God? Don't be ridiculous. The Devil, Morton, is the one who causes this shit!" She gave him an ominous stare.

"The Devil does?"

"Yes. And God is the one who *heals* it. That much I know."

"Maybe. But you'd better see a doctor anyway."

Silence.

"God and all's fine, Annise. But you've got a lump and it has to be seen to."

"Will you please stop it, Morton? I'm going to be late for work as it is."

She was hurrying on with her clothes. He went to her.

"Annise, please listen to me. You might have a malignancy. You need a surgeon. That tumor, or whatever it is, will have to be taken out and biopsied and—"

She wrenched away.

"Leave me alone. I have to get back to Joseph— I mean, to the Fraction House."

She stubbed out her cigarette. She found her overnight bag, jerked the old clothes out of it and began stuffing new ones in.

She put her hands on her hips. "Look, half an hour ago I didn't even *have* a problem. You're the one who found it. You're the one who *told* me about it. And doesn't it strike you as strange that all this comes on the very first day in a person's life she's decided to go through with—"

Annise shook her head violently. She grabbed her purse. "Oh, to hell with you. You don't even know what the fuck I'm talking about!"

She stomped to the front door. He heard it slam behind her, leaving him alone in her bedroom.

* * *

Chapter 27

That night was tough for Morton to get through. Everything felt so flimsy and off track.

The following afternoon, a Saturday, he was out driving, alone. Soon he was absently turning onto Hollywood Boulevard. The Green Room, he pondered as he took in the garish sights? Roxanne and her flock would be congregating about this time. Like the mentally disturbed drivers he'd seen in cars alongside him, he whipped his head angrily back and forth as he waited at the stoplight. The Green Room, what a joke! The way things were going he'd likely run into the Gestapo there anyway.

Finally he meandered back to his place and sat in his green recliner. Shit, he thought, he knew what the fuck he was talking about.

~~~

On Monday, at work, he remained upstairs in Administration all day, hoping Annise would drop by. She didn't.

There ensued a great deal of hubbub in preparation for Muriel's Termination Meeting. Harvey still wasn't back, and Joseph seemed everywhere at once. Signing this. Setting up that. Disciplining staff. Snapping closed the Therapy Room door as his clients, Muriel included, skulked lackadaisically in. It crossed Morton's mind that Joseph's frenetic energy could be coming from the Dexedrine he regularly popped.

By now the supervisor had flip-flopped so many times on Morton's visiting rights the counselor felt the need to tiptoe down to the women's dorm to see what was up.

He managed to locate Muriel, sometimes escorted by Stacy or Wanda, but couldn't seem to pierce the Fraction House smoke screen of needless overprotection. He'd been hired to help stabilize her, yet they wouldn't let him within a hundred feet of her.

From a distance however, the counselor could see trouble brewing. As in the old days Muriel was ignoring the outside world. She'd begun to sink deeper and deeper into the bizarre isolation of the Fraction House.

Days passed. What was he doing at Dar/Neese anyway? His role had been to orchestrate the complicated paperwork for Muriel's Termination Meeting. After all the red tape delays and big wheels gumming up the gears, her day arrived.

That Monday morning Morton snapped open his alligator-skin briefcase. In the top half were compiled the necessary documents clearing Muriel to enter her small apartment in Culver City. If she could only toe the line a little longer she'd at last be living on her own—not as a nut anymore, but as a normal human being pretending like the rest of the screwed up population to be a sane occupant of the great city of Los Angeles. It was an exciting thought.

Everything ended, Morton knew. Even heavy Freudian rebonding relationships where the counselor was supposed to become the surrogate parent would have to ultimately terminate. Endings. Was it really like Harvey said, finishes made room for new starts? That Harvey, he'd be an optimist till the day he died.

Pensively the counselor closed his briefcase, cramming the overflow of his own rumpled collection of forms in around the edges. No, he was not a neatness freak, like some around the Fraction House.

At work Morton ascended the familiar steps toward the third floor. He came to Joseph's Plexiglas—no, *real* glass peeping Tom window. He paused at the landing and surveyed C-Wing, the courtyard, the tree tops and the exotic flowers of the Organic Therapy Garden. In a funky way the place had charm. So few understood the shadowy, asylum sensibility of those troubled individuals who were forced to pass their nights here. A nostalgia entered him. He'd made friends, a mystical kind of union with those who were suspended halfway between their hearts and their heads and not sure which way to lunge when they needed a handhold. And there were the others, the witless and the semi-addled, the daffy and the clearly harebrained who came to work during the day, called themselves 'in the swing,' then trudged back to their own personalized madhouse at night. These, of course, were the counselors.

Morton squinted into the morning sunlight. Joseph was right, the glass was crystal clear.

He was about to turn away when he observed a movement in the bushes near the far fence. One of your secret rendezvous, it looked like. Hmmm, even the furthest gone could manage to weed out an alcove for their off-brand mating rituals. Some things never changed.

Morton cupped his hands to the glass. He could make out two heads. Above them hovered an unlikely plume of smoke. Sam Lorenzo showing Sally Featherman how to set slow burning fires again?

There was an opening in the tree limbs. Yes, he realized, he was having the same view Joseph did the day Morton caught him eavesdropping with the binoculars. The counselor squinted. By degrees he was able to make out Annise's distinctive blonde tresses. A cuddling scenario? He looked harder. It was eight-thirty in the morning, yet the Gestapo's Hitleresque five-o'clock shadow was identifiable even at that distance. No, it wasn't a fire. They were smoking cigarettes. Morton angled in front of the glass, but try as he might he couldn't verify a dirty deed.

They began to move toward the path. The counselor ascended the final stairs. His wrist had been out of the cast a couple of weeks now, yet at the top landing a déjà vu of pain assaulted him. He paused and grasped his wrist. At the rate of his tumble, he ruminated, he could easily have plunged through the plate glass window, falling another two and a half stories to the concrete below. It wasn't a pretty picture.

The floors, he noticed, weren't slippery anymore. What was it Joseph said, he didn't need them super-lubed with Morton out of his hair? Yet the counselor had been hired back. It was almost as if Dar/Neese was planting a thorn in their own side. It was fishy to the max.

Morton strode down the hallway toward the Conference Room. Joseph's office door was open, as it always was these days. To the counselor's surprise the three large drawers of the Gestapo's metal cabinet were cocked open.

Unlocked files! This was the rarest of occurrences. Documents. They were to the bureaucracy what flour was to roaches, or greenbacks to greedy stock brokers. He pulsed with alertness. Joseph would be arriving any second for the meeting.

Morton rounded the austere desk with the medicine vials arranged in long rows and began to rifle through the forms. Ridiculous, the medications not being locked up. Could it be more than just sloppy organization, what with Trina gone?

He noticed one of Harvey's meds, the hydromorphone, set aside from the others. 'Take one capsule as needed every 4 hours. For severe pain only,' read the label.

The counselor turned back to the file cabinet. He wasn't interested in the confidential 'Histories,' nor the personalized 'Therapy Notes.' No, his need was of forms that *weren't* filled out. It could not be termed stealing if you rounded up affidavits of the public domain before the doctors and lawyers rubber stamped them 'private.' He didn't know what the future might call for, but people sometimes needed bailing out of their predicaments, and a stray page of prevention, he'd discovered, could amount to a briefcase full of cure.

Stealing? Hah! What Dar/Neese and Roselawn had been doing with Muriel, with a person's life blood—*that* was stealing!

He found the forms he wanted, was out of the office and three steps toward the Conference Room when Joseph's voice boomed from behind.

"Allison!"

Morton slowed.

"You're early. Go on in. I'll join you in a minute."

* * *

Chapter 28

The Conference Room had a plush, over-saturated feel to it. Everything in there was of a rich black leather, including the frames for Harvey's colorful paintings of the brain. These, the Freudian insisted, were the finest pieces of L.A.'s New Wave art movement, but to Morton they looked more like sad clown faces with stringy gray matter drooping around the eyes.

The sofas and easy chairs were arranged in a circle for the big meeting. Joseph came in. Morton opened his alligator-skin briefcase and handed the supervisor the thick sheaf of papers he'd been working on for so many weeks.

"Atrocious piece of luggage you got there," said the Gestapo turning up his nose.

With no other comment, Joseph took the mass of papers, walked to the corner of the room, and with a sly smirk dumped the entire bundle, neatly tied manila envelope and all, into the wastebasket.

"What's this, some kind of prank?" started the counselor.

The door adjoining Harvey's office swung open.

"Morton! So good to see you," called the physician hurrying over. He took Morton's hand and pumped it warmly. "My man! Well, we're both back on the job. You as counselor and me resuming as Director. This is great, isn't it?"

Morton patted the Freudian's massive shoulder.

"How are you feeling, Harvey? I've been worried about you. Joseph said we'd bother you if we called."

With an acute motion of his head the Gestapo signaled Harvey to the back of the room. In the interim Morton went to the wastebasket and lifted out Muriel's emancipation papers. Joseph eyed him like a hawk, all the while whispering into Harvey's ear. From the corner of his eye the counselor watched as the Gestapo used his back for a shield and secretly passed something to Harvey.

The usuals began to trickle in. The Social Worker, Wanda Novice. Roselawn's tough Clinical Sup, Priscilla Daddio. The two State Arbitrators, always male and never the same ones it seemed, entered in their starched blue suits. Trina Lopez, the longtime Dar/Neese RN, was noticeably absent. Morton missed her. Joseph said Emily and Wojeck Gonska were supposed to attend, but when the meeting convened they were nowhere to be seen.

"We're ready," announced Harvey.

The Freudian opened the side door leading to his office, waved his pipe, and in marched Muriel Elaine Gonska, the schizophrenic.

Upon her entrance a communal gasp went up, for she was wearing racy high heels and exceedingly short leather culottes. Her top was a black form-fitted leotard, cut daringly low. The look on her face was of fear, but the rest of her jiggled and swayed like old movie reels of Marilyn Monroe. Annise came behind her attired in a striking turquoise jogging suit. Monday wasn't her day to work, but apparently she'd swapped shifts with Stacy or one of the other counselors to make this meeting. This juggling of shifts was a common practice around the Fraction House.

The two ladies waited in the center of the circle for Harvey to bring the place to order.

"You all know Muriel," he said. "And this is Miss Annise Chastain. She's Muriel's prettiest—excuse me—*newest* caseworker."

This was an icebreaking attempt at humor. The group offered timorous grins.

"Join us, ladies. Both of you. Sit anywhere you'd like," said Harvey.

Annise immediately sat beside Morton, leaving an appropriate leg of space between them. She tapped lightly at his thigh.

"I've missed you," she whispered. She offered a secret smile.

"I missed you too," he returned low.

Annise continued looking at him. Her eyes betrayed the lack of grace which had plagued their last date. She altered position on the cushions. Morton winced for her discomfort. She couldn't help herself, and he watched as she reached around and covertly touched her coccyx. Yes, the tumor was still there. Her eyes sunk. Praying for a miracle, he'd noticed, didn't always bring one.

As might have been expected Muriel clammed up. She glared suspiciously around the circle.

"You're the person of the hour," urged Harvey. "Pick a spot you feel safe. This is what we're all about at Dar/Neese, security of the self."

Muriel walked toward Morton and Annise, then suddenly wedged awkwardly into the space between them. Very bold! The counselor gave a tiny shake of his head. Not a good start.

"Let us try to establish a perspective," suggested Harvey setting aside his pipe. "Muriel is a lovely young woman. Her life is all ahead of her. She's progressed so beautifully, and now, as most of us here are aware, she's begun to fall back into her old ways."

He glanced to Muriel, but she lowered her head. Annise gave her a motherly pat on the shoulder.

"We at Dar/Neese do not want to see her back in Roselawn," continued Harvey.

Much nodding, except for Priscilla who frumped her lips.

"The problem is she has such a short time left on her contract at the Fraction House. As you know, Joseph has taken the initiative and rented a tidy little apartment for her in Culver City, not far from here. I think we all hoped Muriel would be fully normalized by now."

More nodding. More frumping. The Arbitrators remained stone faced.

The physician lifted his pipe, struck a match and held it. "The main issue is this, ummm... Well, this recto-sexual thing, as Freud terms it."

Morton shifted uneasily. Something wasn't aboveboard here. In terms of closure with the Fraction House, he couldn't understand this sudden harping on Muriel's painful history. They'd gotten way beyond that dopey recto-sexual bull by now, hadn't they? He kept silent. He possessed her freedom documents. Later he'd be given his turn.

Harvey pressed on with the nasty, underhanded scenes concerning Muriel's father, which took place, it was claimed, when she was around six years old. This was where the Freudian came into his own. He went on for many minutes, ultimately declaring Muriel's mental illness boiled down to one obvious issue: Penis Envy.

"And why does Muriel desire a penis of her own?" said Harvey.

Everyone shrugged their shoulders.

"Forced oral copulation, if you will," he climaxed. "As we've learned, this was perpetrated upon her by the father. In addition to Penis Envy, she developed this, ummm, nasty business of anal retentiveness. In the field, we commonly see these problems surfacing as self-induced constipation, ala Sam Lorenzo. Records show Muriel became quite famous for this at Roselawn."

Priscilla interjected, "Sometimes the reverse occurs, does it not, Dr. Mueller? Joseph's schizophrenics can swing to the *other* side and go loosey-goosey when they get upset, can they not?"

This went on. It was tough going. In fact, it wasn't even fair. Termination Meetings, in Morton's experience anyway, had never called for such elaborate personal muckraking. Psychiatry and overblown credentials began to inflate all around like a Mickey Mouse parade float.

"At this point I'd like to turn things over to Joseph Schopen, Dar/Neese's esteemed Clinical Supervisor," said Harvey.

Joseph stood and adjusted his tie. "I hate to differ with the good Dr. Mueller. However, in her therapist's opinion, Muriel's is a case of forced sodomy by the father. This, over time, lead to what I call *acquiescent* sodomy. One might even go so far as to call it, ummm, agreeable."

Muriel winced. Morton scowled. Annise uncrossed her legs. On the other side of the room Wanda Novice gazed wanly out the window at the passing traffic.

"This was the causal factor in Muriel's periodic loss of bowel control," continued the Gestapo. "I need to qualify what I'm going to say next. Her occasional untoward releasing of her bowels feels to Muriel, in her therapist's opinion, like a sort of, well, simulated orgasm. It all adds up to a bizarre chasing after her painful, though sensuous past. You see, she's been seeking to relive the seediest moments with her father. Through extensive regression in the tub— Or rather, I mean, using the vehicle of Hydro-Therapy and thereby reducing her defense mechanisms, her psychotherapist has been able to verify much of what he already suspected was her slimy past."

Big words and bogus psychology, that was your Joseph Schopen in a suit and tie. Given half a chance he'd turn even whitewashed Disneyland into a picture of filth and naked boob bar decadence.

"Her *sensuous* past? That's ridiculous, Joseph," interrupted the counselor.

Muriel had been pretty stiff. She now hardened to granite.

"May I *please* continue?" chastised Joseph staring Morton down.

The Gestapo went on. "We've used certain of the so called Transference Techniques with Muriel. This is where the therapist takes on the behavior of a client and acts it out in a more reasonable way so the disturbed can see themselves in the light of another person. For instance, appropriate use of the toilet... uh..."

Joseph trailed off. He was in a bit deep here. Psychotherapist. Hah! This was one of those fancy titles refined out to mean anything the mad scientist said it meant.

"Thank you, Dr. Schopen," said Harvey. "Thank you so much."

He motioned for Joseph to sit down, then called on Wanda for her two cents.

The Master of Social Work cleared her throat, and said, "The opinions I've heard are forgetting very crucial factors." Wanda pushed back her cropped brown hair. "I am absolutely certain it had to have been flat out heterosexual intercourse with the old bastard that drove the poor girl batty. What in the world, I ask, could be more damaging to a budding young woman than a brutish male— I mean, you know, the father doing these things?" Wanda wrinkled her nose in revulsion.

The physician didn't look well. He made an effort to cross his legs, but couldn't quite manage it. He was sweating profusely. As Wanda talked on, the Freudian began to slap impatiently at his pockets, likely searching for his medication. Morton watched as Joseph eased over and passed Harvey a small vial. The Lasix? The nitroglycerin maybe? Nitro meant heart pain, didn't it? Whatever it was, the doctor slipped one under his tongue.

"Harvey, are you all right?" said Morton, once again interrupting the meeting.

Joseph fired Annise a special look, and right away she reached around Muriel and shook her palm to shush Morton.

"He's sick. He needs help, Annise," whispered the counselor around Muriel's back.

Harvey was gasping for breath. Morton started to his feet, but the blonde caught his shirtsleeve and tugged him down. Poor Muriel was jostled shoulder to shoulder in the tussle.

When Wanda completed her assessment she smiled over at Muriel as if she'd rescued the girl from some machismo hell. In return, Muriel blinked a couple of times.

Harvey began a violent fit of coughing.

"Joseph, can you take over?" he hacked. "Please forgive me you all. I guess I'm— I guess I'm not well enough to do this yet."

Harvey attempted to push up out of his chair, but couldn't and slumped heavily back.

No one seemed willing to do it, so Morton rose and helped the Freudian into his office.

"Thanks," grunted Harvey settling onto his sofa. "Please though, don't make a big to-do about this, Morton. I'll be OK in a bit."

"But, Harvey—"

"I think this nitro must be getting old. It's not working like it used to," he mumbled. He pointed at his desk. "The ones in the envelope are new. Joseph picked them up this morning."

"Picked them up? Is Joseph driving to the pharmaceutical house now?"

"I don't know, Morton. He might be. He's been in charge of everything."

Joseph trying to swipe Harvey's Directorship? Why? In order to control the incoming drugs from Carney Apothecary? In order to get his hands on Wojeck's annual fifty thousand dollar contribution? Or was it a power trip for sex with hot blonde staff members? Hell, for all Morton knew, the Gestapo could be after sex with the clients. His OCD was bound to drive him into a corner. Find an obsession. Get compulsive about it. Then over-do every aspect and pray like the Devil the sandcastle cemented up solid around you. Which of course it never would. Sooner or later the tide was going to rise.

Morton opened the packet and Harvey slipped one of the new tablets under his tongue. After a minute he began to change color for the worse, a washed gray taking over from the bright red. Morton was concerned. Maybe Harvey was fat, but big people could be so kind. And he was mighty damn handsome with that brown and white mix in his beard. Old? Joseph was always saying so. But Morton only thought of him as good, or generous.

"Won-der-ful," sputtered Harvey. "Now you go back in there, Allison, and take care of our girl."

"All right," said Morton.

"I'm afraid for her. She's such a perfect child. She deserves the best. The very best. I wish I could have done more for her."

"It's not over yet," said Morton. "We'll rescue her. With your love and my counseling I know she'll come around."

"She needs to be out of here. And I mean out of here immediately. If you knew what I do—"

Harvey stopped abruptly.

"What do you mean, know what you do?"

The door opened. It was Joseph.

"You're going to have to sign me back as Director-in-Chief, Harvey, else the Arbitrators won't let us proceed," declared the Gestapo with sudden authority.

Joseph had the forms in his hand, already typed in, it looked like. Was there a typewriter out there in the Conference Room? Harvey seemed exhausted. In a woozy daze, he signed where Joseph indicated.

"Excellent," said the Gestapo.

Joseph pivoted, and with a Third Reich spring in his step returned to the meeting.

* * *

Chapter 29

When Morton re-entered the Conference Room he found Joseph in firm control. He was busy naming each of the twenty-two Program Goals Muriel had achieved at the Fraction House. "Speaking cordially to others during meals," or, "Dressing appropriately without supervision," were questionable successes. He showed graphs and told percentages proving, he claimed, how well normalized she'd become.

"She was almost there," he grieved. "Almost there."

With a strange look in his eye Joseph outlined Muriel's recent changes. "Intense anger. Withdrawal. The extreme mood swings which mark manic-depression. And lately we've even seen evidence of paranoia."

"Paranoia!" cried Morton.

"She's scared to death of me and Annise!" exclaimed Joseph.

"And for the record, of coming back to Roselawn with Priscilla," added Dr. Daddio quickly.

"The patient needs exposure to reality, Priscilla," said Joseph. "The clinical picture here at Dar/Neese is about the beauty of the larger group."

"Roselawn maintains over four hundred and fifty long-term clients, Dr. Schopen. That is an exceedingly large group," said Priscilla.

"I'm talking about the mass of *society*, Dr. Daddio," replied the Gestapo. "About the great diverse culture we all live in every day we're free. And with us Muriel *would* be free. Free to normalize. Free to change. This, really, is what a successful Fraction House setting is all about."

Priscilla puffed her cheeks. Joseph gave a breezy, 'Now we're into the groove, boys,' nod to the Arbitrators.

It was suddenly clear that Joseph was making a pitch to keep Muriel at Dar/Neese. Not to release her, as Morton had been led to believe. Perhaps they meant to extend her contract another couple of years. This was done now and then if extreme circumstances could be substantiated. Very convenient, for they all knew her state funding would jump up triple next year when she turned twenty-six. In the long haul this could amount to hundreds of thousands of dollars.

But the real gold mine for both Roselawn as well as Dar/Neese came from her father. Wojeck had struck it big with his genetics firm in Burbank, Dynasplice, and each July wrote Harvey a personal check for fifty thousand dollars, buying off his sins, according to Muriel. Call it what you would, the cash went straight into a special Fraction House escrow account, accessible only by the Director-in-Chief. Since it was a personal donation not even the Arbitrators could point to where it ought to be used. It was a free wad of cash, so to speak.

It occurred to Morton how many Snakebites the Gestapo could buy for a lady like Roxanne if he could get his hands on that kind of green. And he could, couldn't he, with this new Power of Attorney Harvey had signed over to him?

And what was all this with Muriel's new sexed-up attitude? She'd never been so flamboyant in the past. Yet here she was with her culottes hiked up to the rim of her stockings. Anyone who cared to look could see where the garter fasteners met with the dark ends of her nylons. Clinically, Morton knew that sharp turns of sexuality were typically sparked by lewd pressures from outside the patient's own heart and soul.

The counselor's eyes swept to the Gestapo. Muriel and *Joseph*, he wondered? What was it she'd said that emotional, sunlit morning in Morton's kitchen? Something about the lecher breathing down the back of her neck, video camera purring away in his free hand? Or was this the counselor's fertile imagination turning paranoid for his friend? God, but it was hard to distinguish between the reality you recalled and the one which actually took place out on the street.

He waited patiently. Oddly, neither Joseph nor the Arbitrators asked for his opinion, though he had a glowing report all written up and ready to deliver. The truth of the last two years alone would have liberated her. But no, he was being silenced.

Morton felt his composure bleeding away. He counted slowly to twenty, as Harvey had taught him. He breathed deep. So this was the reason Joseph threw his files in the wastebasket! Now he understood why he hadn't come across the mandatory G-F document in his work preparing Muriel to split. This was the single most coveted form known to the mentally ill. The clients dubbed it the 'Get-Free' paper. Morton had queried Joseph about it, but the Gestapo simply said, "Harvey's handling that," or, "Don't give it a second thought—me and Trina got it under control."

But Harvey was ill. He hadn't been handling anything. Trina never dealt in Administrative affairs. And anyway, she'd been fired. No one, not Dar/Neese, not Roselawn, not even the Arbitrators were about to unshackle the poor girl. It was clear as a bell. The whole thing was a ruse, just like Muriel tried to tell him that morning in his apartment. Christ, it seemed so long ago now.

"One second, Joseph," intervened Morton. "Isn't someone supposed to be writing up the Meeting Minutes? Where's the stenographer? This going into her old ways isn't protocol for a Termination Meeting, you know that. Everyone here knows that, don't they?"

Morton looked around at the group. No answer. Even Wanda Novice, his old friend, wouldn't meet his eyes. Instead she rustled in a small paper bag and distractedly munched a handful of freeze-dried bananas chips.

Morton exclaimed, "What's going on here? This is a goddamn *Retainment* Meeting, isn't it? You're not letting her out on her own. You're all planning to keep her locked up, aren't you?"

Morton glared at Priscilla Daddio. Then he glared at the Gestapo. "Why wasn't I informed of this, Joseph?" he demanded.

"God, you're hyper, Allison," snorted the supervisor. He pointed to the machine on the table beside the Arbitrators, the reels slowly turning. "We're being taped, thank you. It *is* all official. But you're quite right. This is a Retainment Meeting. Someone will get Custody, but believe me, it won't be you. Interfere again, Allison, and I'll have you ejected from this meeting."

Hyper, did he say? Here Muriel's future was being decimated with a bunch of outdated psychological nonsense. Annise and Joseph were playing eyeball footsie across the circular shag carpet. Priscilla and Wanda sitting there like two rock encrusted snowballs, pretending everything was fine and dandy when the ax was obviously poised to fall across Muriel's tender neck. The counselor's heart raced. Hyper? That was an understatement.

He recalled his prescription, legitimate medication for times like this, it was. He quickly swallowed one of the light green Librium capsules.

"Look, Joseph, this isn't right. There's a hundred reasons—"

"Cap it, Allison," snapped the supervisor. "You got no pull here."

"I have as much as the next person. I've been her counselor for two years. I've even been her Legal Guardian, for Godsake."

"Her Guardian? Show me the papers," shot the Gestapo. "I wouldn't let you be Guardian of the roaches around this place." Joseph's lips puckered at his poor choice of phrasing.

Morton opened his briefcase and lifted out the blue Temporary Custody form he'd signed in Joseph's office almost a month ago. He passed it to the Arbitrators. Slowly, they shook their heads.

"That's the blue form," said Joseph. "It's our new Custody Repeal document. You better look close at it, Allison. You signed away all past and future Custody of Muriel. Everybody knows pink means Custody."

"But Joseph, you told me—"

"I don't even know why we're tolerating your presence here. The new Fraction House Dictum states all Dar/Neese employees are required to have at least a college degree. Most of us are Ph.D.s."

Muriel sprung to her feet. "He's practically an accountant!" she burst out. "He would be an accountant too by now, but he came here to save me instead."

This from the patient was far too aggressive. It would surely go against her with the Arbitrators. Morton reached to pull her down. In the process his fingertips inadvertently caught the strap of her leotard top. As she dropped onto the sofa the elastic material stretched southward off her shoulder and unluckily extended beyond the high chuff of her breast. All at once she was topless to the world.

Across the room small bosomed Priscilla Daddio emitted a high pitched gasp of shock. The counselor was himself taken aback. He waited a moment, but Muriel did nothing to conceal herself. She merely sat there, exposed but placid, like some nymphet in one of those ancient paintings, smiling as if nothing but pipe dreams were on the line here.

Morton blushed. He craned his neck toward Annise hoping for assistance. One hand was covering her mouth. Her eyes were wide with a frozen disbelief. As with Harvey earlier, no one seemed to have the courage to help the girl. It was the old hang back and stare routine, like a crowd of jaundiced New Yorkers too paralyzed with their own backdrop of fears and scrambled psychology to stop a rape.

Morton waited another moment, but Muriel was out to lunch. No, she wasn't going to fix this herself.

At last the counselor took the initiative. He reached gently to her shoulder. He could feel her rigidity. He took hold of the silky, leotard fabric and moved it upward over her torso, adjusting here and there like a fussy mother until she was safely covered. As he did this a velvety heat traveled down his spine, so different from the sharp, lustful chills he'd experienced with Annise.

Muriel met his eyes. A kind of ultimate privacy walled them off from the spectators. A euphoric, drug-feeling calmness enveloped him as he tended to her. He found himself smiling. Only a second had passed, hadn't it?

"There, we're all back to normal," he said smoothing the final wrinkles out of the leotard.

Morton didn't give a rosy hoot about the others. He stroked along Muriel's neck in the soothing, paternal way he'd done so many times before.

The room began to hum. The tape recorder spinning? No, it was the lonely chatter of their voices, gossip amongst the masses. Then, so low as to be under the decibel level of identifiable words, Muriel leaned close to him, and whispered, "I love you, Morton. I love you more than anything."

"What?" said Annise. "What's she saying?"

Joseph flapped a handful of papers. The meeting was back in swing. So loose and wavy, the vibes in there. Too many things happening perhaps. Twirlings in the brain. Funky thumps of the heart. The gut and the knees trembling in a nervously dispassionate way that made him know he cared.

* * *

Chapter 30

The meeting moved ahead. Joseph's penetrating line of attack made the Fraction House case look better and better. At least until Priscilla reached into her Armoralled, kid leather briefcase and unrolled a long blue-lined scroll, like a double-wide cash register receipt.

"This is a computerized list of the drugs, controlled substances is what they are—shocking, really—which Muriel was put on and taken off while under the care of Dar/Neese."

Priscilla tapped her glasses lower on her nose and began to read. "Seconal. Nembutal. Mellaril. Thorazine. Tofranil. Navane. Effexor. Wellbutrin. And this is just a start. These are powerful psychotropic drugs, gentlemen."

Priscilla passed the list to the Arbitrators. They examined the document with great care, and in turn handed it around the circle.

When the paper came to the Gestapo he leered up and said, "This is highly confidential information, Priscilla. How'd you get your hands on it?"

Confidently, Priscilla slit her eyes. "Harvey asked for Dr. Daddio's consultation regarding these prescriptions. Dr. Mueller was concerned someone handling the dosages might be jeopardizing the young lady's health."

They all knew she meant Joseph himself. But the Gestapo said, "You mean Trina Lopez, the RN? She signed off first on all the scripts. That's been taken care of. She's no longer with us."

Priscilla stroked her chipmunk cheeks.

"The patient is perfectly fine," continued Joseph. "Anyway, it's her *mental* health we've been focused on."

"And that's all screwed up. Muriel is paranoid, schizophrenic, and manic-depressive, or as we now say, bipolar," countered Priscilla.

The momentum began to swing toward Roselawn. Priscilla smugly tucked her straying fronds of pitch black hair up around her ears. She made no bones about being hot for Harvey's job. With him sick, and already in a kind of pseudo-retirement, she was sniffing hard for a weak link. Joseph however was further along in his machinations for Director-in-Chief status. And so came the infantile snorting and hissing between them.

It occurred to the counselor that only people who thought they were peers felt like fist fighting. Two preachers. Two oldsters stuck in the same cubicle at the Nursing Home. The teen wouldn't swing on the oldster, only on another teenager who'd staked claim to the same urine-sprayed curb. Why? Stupidity! You'd think Priscilla and Joseph would have seen that.

Morton balled his fists. Muriel must have intuited his pressure-cooked agitation. She plied her shoulder soothingly against his.

~~~

There came a period of debate over the patient's social fitness. Joseph addressed Muriel directly.

"I know this is difficult," he sighed. "But we really do need your input, Muriel. We're all deeply concerned with your welfare, missy."

Muriel looked up. "You are?" she peeped.

"Of course we are. Please, tell us where *you* stand. As you know, it's obligatory for the taping."

After a moment Muriel said, "I'm not sure, I think I'm feeling a little... Like a little funny inside."

"Estranged?" asked Priscilla. "Is that maybe what Muriel feels? Like estranged and kind of hateful inside?"

"Uh huh. That's what Muriel feels," said Muriel to Priscilla.

"Estranged from objects? Is that what you're trying to say?" wondered Joseph cautiously.

"Yes, that's what I'm trying to say," agreed Muriel.

"Well, this isn't so terrible," sang Joseph. "Objects aren't in any way alive, you know. It's the *people* we're concerned with. We understand what we're getting at, don't we, Muriel?"

Muriel blinked several times. "Yes, we understand what we're getting at. Except— Well, except I sometimes see people as objects."

Priscilla started writing furiously in her notebooks. There was a round of grumbling.

Morton piped up. "I don't think she's so weird. I feel that way myself a lot of the time. I think most people feel that way."

A lot of shifting in the chairs. Much desultory leg crossing and uncrossing.

"Do you have anything else to add, Miss Gonska?" asked Joseph monotonally.

Muriel shook her head.

"Let the record show the patient defers further comment," said Joseph. "That's a motion, by the way. Will anyone second the motion? If so, this Retainment Meeting can come to an end."

Dr. Daddio lounged back in the plush leather chair. Her chances of snagging Muriel this time around were remote. But Priscilla was your chain-link sort of builder. One day she'd turn up with each of Joseph's incriminating remarks transcribed from the tapes, and like a black widow suck Muriel straight into Roselawn.

"Will someone please second the motion?" pressed Joseph.

"I second the motion," said Annise waving her arm.

Joseph banged the gavel. "This Retainment Meeting is over," he said. "We're awaiting judgment by the Arbitrators. Muriel, we'll forward the verdict to you as soon as possible. Miss Chastain, will you escort the patient back to E-Wing? There's one more item we have to see to. It'd be best if she weren't here for it."

Annise took Muriel's arm. They rose, vibrant blue velour and blood red suede hovering above the counselor in a mist of scent and flutter, like a couple of tropical butterflies.

"Thank you, Morton," said Muriel. She bent and kissed him softly on the cheek. Joseph's sarcastic, "Humph," could be heard all the way across the room.

Surprisingly, Annise too stepped close.

"See you soon?" she whispered. She gave Joseph a nervous glance, then, with a supple arch of her movie star body kissed Morton full on the mouth.

A bit embarrassed, the counselor was nevertheless encouraged by Annise's outward show of affection. Joseph visibly tensed. Wanda frowned. Muriel looked away. The Arbitrators grinned excitedly. With those antique blue suits and stiff upper lips, likely they didn't get much at home. Well, such was your asylum sort of love, thought Morton, as the two ladies with the hourglass figures moved out of the room.

* * *

Chapter 31

When Annise and Muriel were out of earshot, Joseph said, "Despite your outbursts, Allison, I've allowed you to stay in this meeting for one reason. I want Wanda, the Arbitrators, Priscilla— I want everyone present to hear me formally terminate you."

Joseph banged his gavel yet again.

"For the record, let this mark a shift from Muriel Gonska's Retainment Meeting to Dar/Neese's Severance Action against Morton Allison."

Joseph gave Morton a sly smirk across the circle.

"So you see, in a way, it is a Termination Meeting," continued the Gestapo. "It's been apparent for months that you and you alone, Allison, are responsible for Muriel's regression. We've got it well documented how she was driven manic by your sexual advances."

"By my what!"

"On May 23rd of this year, not even three weeks after her rape, Muriel spent the entire night at your apartment. Isn't this true?"

"Well, yeah, only—"

"Where did she sleep?"

Morton's lower jaw jutted forward.

"In your bed?" asked the Gestapo.

Morton didn't answer.

"We know she was in your bed. We know too— Well, let me put it this way, was she clothed?"

"Clothed?"

"Clothed. Dressed. Were her sexual organs covered, is my question? Or was she wearing a certain sheer orange gown much of the time? That chiffon one with the little see-through tassels?"

Damned if that Joseph Schopen wasn't a mighty fashion conscious supervisor. The Arbitrators came quickly to life.

"I want the record to show our information came directly from Muriel, who blabbed about it to Stacy Lung like a manic on the upswing would."

The Arbitrators nodded.

"Stacy confided it to Annise Chastain, Muriel's primary counselor. Annise confirmed the reports with the patient herself, then notified Muriel's therapist, me."

"This is all hearsay!" cried Morton.

"Do you deny it?" asked Joseph.

The Arbitrators wrote and wrote.

"But Joseph, you sent her to me," objected Morton. "And anyway, I had Temporary Custody. I mean, I thought it was Temporary Custody. I got home late. She just turned up. I talked to you about it on the phone that night, remember?"

"It was kidnapping, short and simple," said Joseph. "Don't worry, Allison, we're not looking to prosecute. I've already discussed this with Priscilla and the Arbitrators. We all agree Muriel would be hurt more if we dragged it into court."

Morton stroked his chin. So this was Joseph's scheme. Send Muriel to his place with a phony Temporary Custody so he'd be implicated as the lecher. It fit snugly with the first setup, when she'd been planted in his apartment the night he returned from the mountains. Morton lasered the Gestapo. It was becoming clearer how Muriel had gotten so battered during her absence from the Fraction House.

Another day Morton would have found himself violently angry over such a chain of events. Today, however, he felt a kind of narcotic ease, though the circumstances were no less desperate. The Librium, he wondered momentarily?

Joseph said, "You knew full well you were supposed to be there for her, not *with* her. A stabilizing presence only. Didn't we have this agreement?"

"Sure, but—"

"We rehired Mr. Allison because the patient *appeared* to improve with his presence," said the Gestapo addressing the group. "The fact was he'd been abusing her sexually all along.

A smiling, stable client, as we know, often indicates someone masking a severe trauma."

Joseph rustled his papers. "When she was discovered in his apartment the Cedars-Sinai Emergency Room found semen in her." He held up a photocopy of the lab test.

"She'd been out two weeks for Christsake! I wasn't even in L.A.," objected Morton.

"Do you have proof of your whereabouts?" asked the Gestapo scowling.

"If semen was found why didn't you test me? You knew goddamn well it wasn't me. That's why you wouldn't do the test. For all I know it might be your sperm, Joseph."

The committee shook their heads in disgust, even Wanda. Morton had lost all credibility.

"The police were there," continued the counselor. "Why didn't they go to the hospital with you if you thought I'd done something? Why wasn't I arrested right then?"

"As Dar/Neese's Agent, and Muriel's Legal Guardian, I take full responsibility for what happened at the hospital. I probed her very carefully. I mean, you know, discussed this with her. She refused to admit the rape or to prosecute. I did what I thought best, under the circumstances."

"That's old-time thinking!" cried Morton. "Nowadays justice is what's important. Nowadays women *face* their perpetrators, Joseph, and put the blame where it belongs!" He glared at the Gestapo.

"As I've said, we're not browbeating ourselves with the *material* evidence," persisted Joseph. "Muriel's mental well being is our foremost concern. We *could* prosecute. We have loads of so called circumstantial evidence, Allison. But each of us, including Muriel herself, believes that course would be detrimental to all involved. Which includes Roselawn, by the way, in case they get her back."

Priscilla closed and re-opened her eyes indicating her agreement.

"No, we won't be prosecuting. We can terminate you though. And this is why we've taken such pains to assemble these witnesses and to formally tape record these proceedings. As of now, this the 3rd day of June, you're history, Allison."

"You're firing me? But I didn't do anything, Joseph."

"It is Dar/Neese's position that Muriel needs three months with only healthy Fraction House encounters," continued the supervisor. "She may still be capable of going on her own, but we won't know for certain until we give Annise Chastain and her therapist a crack at her."

Priscilla said, "Dr. Daddio would like it noted that it is precisely these *un*healthy Fraction House encounters which have worsened the patient's condition. Roselawn wants Muriel's funds at Roselawn where the state can keep a tight leash on this kind of volatile sexuality."

The Arbitrators nodded. Bureaucrats. They'd accept any version of the truth as long as it was stated in a sufficiently squirrelly way.

"Severance Action adjourned," announced Joseph. The gavel banged for the last time.

~~~

The group prepared to leave. Morton lingered behind in a stupor. How many hours had gone by? Was it time for another Librium yet?

Slowly the counselor closed his briefcase. He wouldn't be needing it for a while.

Joseph stepped up. "Here's another document for your collection," he sneered. "Your Severance Declaration. All signed and rubber stamped the way you like them."

Morton looked wearily up. Yes, it was official. The imprint of Joseph's Fraction House Power of Attorney was pressed into the paper.

"This one might be hard for you to get over, Allison. I recommend a few Snakebites and another Librium."

Morton looked up. "*Another* Librium? I took one a short while ago."

"It doesn't hurt to double up. Particularly in times of need," recommended the Gestapo.

"Uh, thanks. Maybe I will," said Morton, confused.

"No hard feelings, Allison, but if I never see you again, it'll be too soon. I want you off the premises immediately. And don't try to sneak back either. We've got a legal injunction against you showing up here. Now get the hell out."

The supervisor turned and disappeared through the door to Harvey's office.

* * *

'L.A. 2000:' Sex Asylum

Chapter 32

One by one the participants filed out.

Morton remained on the sofa, his knees close together. This was one of those occasions when he suspected he belonged in a Fraction House. Nobody felt sane all the time, did they? Yet others were always telling him how grounded he was, a real regular joe. He thought about his comment to Annise the time they'd gone to the wine country. "Sometimes I feel out of step at the Fraction House. Like I don't exactly fit in," he'd confided as they sampled one of the burgundies in the Tasting Room.

"You don't fit, Morton. It's not because you're nuts. It's because you're too damn normal," replied Annise. She threw back her hair. "Now me, I blend right in. The more problems a person's got, the more comfortable people with problems are going to feel around them."

The counselor picked up his briefcase and began to shuffle down the hallway. Outside the usual sirens were ringing, mixing with the roar of the incoming jets and the droning cloverleafs of the freeways. So unpredictable, the times when that piercing L.A. loneliness chose to enter a person.

He came to the Therapy Room. The door was ajar. Inside he could see the infamous tub, now drained of water as it was the lunch hour. In the absence of a patient, Joseph's recently installed mood lights had been cranked up from low yellow to beaming white. Morton noticed how well worn the inner doorknob was, evidence of Joseph's OCD hallway checking fetish.

The counselor wandered in and sat in the brass framed chair reserved for the therapist. In his pocket the Librium capsules rattled in their vial. Another one might really turn him inside out. Possibly divert him from what he needed to do. There was always an imperative, wasn't there? Something only you knew was called for, something that needed doing in a purely subjective way.

He felt weak, as if he were Muriel's stuffed Little Morton and Joseph had kicked the insides out with his fancy jodhpur boots.

In the early days, before the Gestapo gained such thorough control of the place, Morton had been the one to escort Muriel up to the Therapy Room. At the time Harvey was her psychotherapist, and he allowed for the first twenty minutes of the Session to be private between the primary counselor and the patient. Muriel had worn a pleasant one piece bathing suit, not stripped naked the way Joseph's new Dictum required. Those had been such fine, candid moments. Muriel had helped him out as much as he'd helped her. He recalled the day he'd been depressed about needing to end it with Stacy.

"I don't have the courage to confront her on this. She'll be devastated. But then again she's been cold as ice for months. I feel paralyzed. I feel like a child, Muriel," he'd said.

"A child?"

"Harvey tells us to listen to the child inside ourselves, doesn't he? Well, my inner child doesn't have the guts to tell her it's over. I think he wants to suck his thumb and have somebody else talk to her about it."

Muriel patted the top of Morton's head. "You're not listening to your inner child," she said. "You're listening to your inner baby. Deep in her heart, Stacy knows the same things you do. You won't be telling her anything new."

"I won't?"

"No. Just take your thumb out of your mouth and lay it on her straight."

This, of course, had been the right advice. Another pill? Or jerk the Librium pacifier out of your inner baby's mouth and take action?

Morton had an idea then. His jaw jutted forward as he opened his briefcase. His head was clearing. If he moved quickly he could get on top of this. Time was of the essence now.

'L.A. 2000:' Sex Asylum

He fanned through his document collection. On top were the G-F forms, along with the triplicate Sanity Verification forms he'd acquired from Joseph's office. They wouldn't do. There were Organ Donor applications. A few Living Will Declarations.

Hmmm, here was one, and it was bright pink to boot, a real find!

Morton examined it closely. It was the Temporary Removal form Gordon Theodoricus had swiped the time he hid in Harvey's office during the annual fumigation. Gordon nearly perished that weekend trying to get pesticides into his blood stream so he would be protected from the cancers pesticides in the blood stream caused.

When he got out of the hospital the paranoid slipped Morton the wordy Temporary Removal form. "Here is a keeper, my friend," he said. "If you ever need something temporarily removed, flash this. It's vague. It's a weird color. It'll work for anything."

Well, the bad really could turn out good sometimes.

Using his briefcase as a tabletop Morton worked meticulously over the form, then placed it in one of his legal-size manila envelopes. He got out his trusty stencil and inked the word PERSONAL across the front. He had another thought, folded his new Severance Declaration at the signature line and slid it into the envelope alongside the Temporary Removal document.

~~~

The counselor went out to his truck and put the briefcase under the seat. He drove around the block, parking along the curb at the backside of the Organic Therapy Garden. He eyed the fence. It was topped with barbed wire, but the place where Odette Gunner, the Self-Scratcher, illicitly came and went in the wee hours was shoved down in a U at the top.

Morton tucked the envelope into the front of his pants, and like a large house cat with worn Nike jogging shoes, struggled over the barrier and into the jungle like de-ionized area. He made his way to the secret alcove where he and Joseph had been with Annise.

The counselor shaded his eyes and panned across the Gestapo's viewing window until the glossy reflection cleared. No, no one there.

He maneuvered through the courtyard and shoved open the door to E-Wing, the women's dormitory. In the foyer was a black plastic bench shaped like a mini sliding board, one of Harvey's New Wave art donations.

Morton took a seat and checked his watch. It was 12:45 p.m. Annise and the others would be returning from lunch any minute now. In the distance he could hear someone singing. It was Sally Featherman, who sometimes recited risqué songs to annoy her counselors.

When Morton was first hired Sally didn't talk *or* sing. He discovered however she would copy him when he hummed. By degrees his humming graduated to singing, which Sally began to imitate. She never did start talking, but eventually she began to sing all on her own. It was a bit of a shock to the counselor as well as to the passengers when she began to wail out those filthy ditties from the back seat of the metro lines. Over time she developed an uncanny knack for getting her opinions across by carefully choosing the songs she sang.

Now she was into the coarser verses of *Down By The River*: "Down by the river where nobody goes/There lay a young blonde without any clothes," she sang.

Annise bumped open the hydraulic doors and entered the E-Wing foyer. Her hands were tight over both ears. Slowly she removed them.

"Sally, please, will you hush!" counseled Annise.

Gordon and Muriel followed. The men, except for staff, were off limits to the women's side. Gordon remained at the door.

"Annise, I've been looking everywhere for you," said Morton rushing up to her.

He drew her aside.

"I've come from the big meeting with Joseph and Priscilla and them. They're deeply concerned about Muriel's condition these last weeks. You know, the manic issue."

"I know, I was there," said Annise.

"Right. Well, anyway, they asked specifically for my help." Morton glanced toward Muriel. He whispered to Annise, "Joseph thinks you and I might really be able to do something for her. He wants to get her away from this place. He doesn't think it's healthy around here."

"Joseph said that?"

"I mean Harvey. Harvey said that when we were in his office."

"I see."

"Look at this. They gave me a Temporary Custody for today. You know, to see how it might work out."

Morton pulled the now crumpled manila envelope from the front of his pants.

"Boy, it says 'PERSONAL' on there. It must be important," observed Annise.

"Oh, it is," agreed Morton.

He withdrew the pink Fumigation form and pointed to the darkly underlined place which read, 'LEAVE SAID FACILITY FOR A PERIOD OF EIGHT (8) HOURS.' He showed her the fine print at the bottom. 'ANY AND ALL RISK, PHYSICAL, MENTAL AND OTHERWISE, WILL BE ABSORBED BY THE SIGNER, NOT BY THE COMPANY.'

"What's this?" asked Annise.

"It's a Temporary Removal form so patients can leave the Fraction House. Legally, I mean. Haven't you come across one yet?"

"Well, no—"

"They're used all the time around here. See? It's pink and all filled out and everything, like it's supposed to be."

"Temporary Removal? I thought it was Temporary Custody they gave," noted Annise studying the document.

"Removal. Custody. It's all the same."

"But here it says risk won't be absorbed by the company. I didn't know this place was considered a company."

"Oh, yes. Has been for years. Ummm, I'd kind of like to get rolling," he said nervously.

"Where's Joseph's signature and his Power of Attorney seal?"

"You're exacting, Annise. I like that in a woman."

Morton reached into the envelope and brought out his folded Severance Declaration. He nodded toward the bottom half, which showed Joseph's fresh signature and Power of Attorney stamp. Annise tightened her lips.

"Yes, that's definitely Joseph's chicken scratch handwriting. I guess it's OK."

Morton quickly slid the papers back into the envelope and bent the brass ears of the clasp to lock it.

"You know how these people are, Annise. They change their minds every ten minutes. Especially Joseph."

"You're certainly right there. One day he takes you by the hand and the next he completely ignores you."

"He takes you by the hand?"

"I mean figuratively, Morton. I'm agreeing with you."

"Be careful of him, Annise. He's got that OCD problem. You don't want to turn into one of his obsessions."

"That's not likely. Frankly, I don't mind his OCD. At least it tells me what to expect out of him."

The counselor checked anxiously over his shoulder. "We've got to get going. I've only been allotted eight hours, like it said on the form."

"Where are you going to take her?" she asked leisurely.

That Annise Chastain, always carrying on at her own supple, unrushed pace, even if the mission was about to burn to the ground.

Muriel had been listening to all this. Morton could see her sneaking looks from under her hair. Sally rocked in place on the art nouveau bench. Gordon hung in the doorway, looking fearfully behind at prescribed intervals.

"I was thinking of heading out toward Venice," said Morton. "Joseph would never suspect— I mean, you know, maybe to one of those sidewalk cafes. Have a cappuccino or something."

"Venice!" cried Annise. "Oh, how I love that place! The beach? Is that where you're thinking of? The boardwalk area with all the vendors and kooky rollerbladers?"

Morton thought a moment. "I have an idea," he said. "Why don't we all ride up there. I've still got the Dar/Neese insurance rider on my pickup, so liability's not a problem. And you're authorized to sign Sally and Gordon out."

Annise looked troubled. Quietly she said, "Don't you think you should ask Muriel? This is supposed to be your special time with her, like Harvey said."

"Yes, yes, of course I should. Wanna go, hon?" he called.

She didn't raise her head, which was one of Muriel's traits, but they all heard the tiny "Uh huh," squeak out.

"Gordon?" asked Morton.

"Sure, I'll go," said his friend the Synthetic Paranoid.

"Fabulous! Then we're all set!" exclaimed Annise.

"You've got to invite Sally too," said Morton low.

"You've got to invite Sally," echoed Sally. She had omitted the "too," noticed the counselor. This was known as 'Selective Echolalia,' which allowed for a certain amount of implied communication. It was one of the first steps toward talking on her own. Morton experienced a chill of excitement.

"There's no point in asking her anything," said Annise. "She always repeats everything anybody says."

"Maybe so. But she deserves to be invited. That's only fair," said the counselor.

"She deserves to be invited," repeated Sally selectively. "That's only fair."

"All right, for Christsake," huffed Annise. "But when she doesn't repeat, Morton, she's mute. You've read the Anecdotals. Joseph's worked so hard with her, and still she hasn't uttered a word of her own in thirty months. It's the kind of thing can really get disgusting."

"It's the kind of thing can really get disgusting," agreed Sally in a sarcastic sounding voice.

Annise put a hand on her hip. "Sally, do you want to go with us up to Venice?" she asked.

A few seconds passed.

"You see," said Annise.

Out of nowhere, Sally Featherman shot to her feet. With her echopraxia she placed a hand on her hip the way Annise had done. "No!" she blurted, plopped back down and resumed her rocking.

Morton ripped his head in disbelief.

"An act of will! I've got to get this documented," cried Annise. "I'm going to fill out an Incident Report and change clothes real quick. I'll sign us out and meet you at the truck."

Annise started running down the hall toward the Staff Lounge.

Gordon and Morton looked over at Sally, shaking their heads in amazement.

Muriel went to the bench. She held Sally's hand and was whispering softly into her ear. Damn, if Sally wasn't on the path to actually talking on her own. What a thrill, felt the counselor, to see such changes unfolding right under your very nose.

Sally calmly raised her eyes to meet Morton's. It struck him how normal her affect was, not so different from his neighbors at the apartment complex. Not so different from many of them at the L.A. malls and football games. A hair cross-eyed perhaps, but not completely incoherent. Yes, she was on her way back.

This was a stressful moment for the echolalic. She was perspiring heavily and shaking at the shoulders. Muriel patted her on the back, and they started off in the direction of Sally's room.

"Morton, call Stacy on the intercom right away. She's up in the Recreation Room. Sally needs someone with her during this," directed Muriel. "And you better get your truck from around back where you hid it. Gordon, you get Annise from the Staff Room. I'll meet you all on the steps out front as soon as Stacy gets here."

That Muriel Gonska. Intuitive counselor to hurt echolalics. Clairvoyant about hidden trucks. And now dynamic supervisor of the upcoming trip to Venice. Morton was moved by her ability to instantly rise to the occasion. He couldn't help himself. He went to her and hugged her tightly.

Sally was close by, and as if divinely timed Muriel and Morton simultaneously opened their arms and enclosed her in the embrace. Gordon came over. He too wrapped his arms around them.

Across the circle Morton could see tears streaking down Sally's face. Gordon reached to wipe them away. Morton looked to Muriel. She also was weeping, the teardrops wiggling down her cheeks in silver threads of joy. With the back of his fingers Morton dabbed at the dampness. Muriel's lips quivered. All at once she laughed. Crying and laughing together. At the same moment, in fact. Funny, it seemed quite reasonable.

Muriel caught her breath. "This is really wild," she said shakily.

Very slowly, the way Sam Lorenzo might do it, their eyes ranged one to the other and they began to minutely nod their heads. Sally too nodded and met the eyes of the others.

"Yes," said Sally all on her own. "This is really wild."

* * *

Chapter 33

Morton, Annise, Muriel and Gordon scrunched into the front seat of Morton's pickup. Annise had changed into a pair of snug fitting maroon shorts. Her blouse was satin with small rubber shamrocks on the shoulders. She smelled like daisies and heather, her cheeks milk and strawberries around the slightly parted carriage of her lips.

Though he'd just been fired, Morton felt remarkably uplifted. Accidentally he squealed wheels as he double clutched onto the freeway loop.

"Whee!" exclaimed Annise, nudging the counselor approvingly with the side of her leg.

Venice was a crowded, hipster-style beach town on the fringes of L.A. There was always a circus-like throb of excitement in the air, particularly along the boardwalk. When they arrived he motored slowly around looking for an unoccupied meter in one of the sardine packed lots.

"Oh, Morton, stop a second will you? I think I see someone I know," said Annise.

Muriel and Gordon stepped out and watched as Annise hurried across the parking lot toward a white sports car with the top down.

"Excuse me a minute," said Gordon. He set out in the direction of a chrome vendor wagon shaded by a Cinzano umbrella.

Muriel climbed back into the truck. "Gordon wants the cotton candy," she said, looking over her shoulder.

Dangerous levels of sugar, artificial coloring, carcinogenic preservatives—ingesting these synthetics by way of cotton candy helped Gordon maintain his high level of poor health and therefore remain strong and resilient to the diseases he was so paranoid of.

Morton found a parking space and pulled in. He killed the engine.

"You're looking good, Muriel. Especially around the eyes," said the counselor. "They made you sound pretty bad in the meeting. But to me you don't seem crazy at all."

"I wish you wouldn't use that word, Morton. And anyway, I'm a certified manic now."

"Are you really?"

She frowned. "My heart feels horrible when I'm at the Fraction House. But sometimes, like now, I feel great. I can get so excited about not being depressed."

"Don't feel too good Muriel. You need moderation. Too good or too bad and you won't be considered normal."

"Normal? Isn't that a word the nutty Fraction House staff made up so they can have each other for company? To be honest, I don't think there's such a thing as normal."

Although they were sitting next to one another Morton twisted the rearview mirror so he could see Muriel through it. This was a trick Harvey had taught him to put space between counselor and client when the going started to get emotionally murky.

Muriel sniffled. "I guess I have been jittery lately. I'm so tired of this. All I want to do is get well. That's all I want out of this rotten world."

"You might get better, Muriel, but you'll never get well. Just look at Joseph."

"Don't you think he's getting better?" she asked.

"How can he get better if he already thinks he's well?" said Morton into the mirror. "All of us need help. We all have parts we want drawn out of ourselves."

"Annise doesn't seem to want drawing out," she returned after a moment.

"Maybe she thinks she's already out," said the counselor.

"Sometimes I feel like certain parts of her might need putting back in," said Muriel. "Maybe Wanda can help. They're tight as bugrugs these days."

"Bugrugs?" said Morton.

Schizophrenics periodically scrambled their metaphors, often turning the meaning more poignant than the clichés they were trying to imitate.

"They spent the weekend together. In Pasadena or someplace where Annise grew up," added Muriel.

"Annise and *Wanda*? I wasn't aware of that."

Hmmm. So this was why she hadn't been coming around.

~~~

Gordon had taken his cotton candy over to the white car where Annise was talking to a young man with one of those new razor haircuts. Morton remembered his cast, what an effective social separator it could be when used properly. He retrieved it from the bed of the pickup and lashed the Velcro in place around his forearm.

Muriel and Morton walked over to the white car.

"This is Rodney Stonesipher," said Annise introducing them. She touched Rodney affectionately on the arm. "I'm sure I've mentioned him to you, Morton. I have? I thought so. Rod and I went through the Jesuit school system together. We were like boyfriend and girlfriend for years. Anyway," she said to Rodney, "that one there is Gordon Theodoricus. That's Muriel Gonska. And this is Morton Allison. Morton has very unique ideas on, ummm—well, psychology I guess you'd call it."

"That's hip," noted the fellow holding his hand upward for the trendy brother shake.

Morton raised his cast. "Sorry," he said.

"Wow, looks bad," noted Rodney.

"One of the nuts I used to work for—I mean, with—busted it for me," said Morton.

"I've heard they can be quite dangerous," said Rodney sneaking a glance at Gordon.

"Not if you don't hit back. If you ever run into a problem remember, don't hit back," said the counselor.

"Really, Morton? I don't think I've heard that," said Annise.

"Sounds East Indian," pondered Rodney. "Sounds somewhat like Yoga. Is that your philosophy? Like Yoga or something?"

"In certain ways it probably is," said Morton.

"Yoga is heavy duty shit," agreed Rodney. "I was up in Frisco a couple of months ago, and I got a hold of this really like hefty book. I mean that sucker was big, man. I was like reading along and out of the blue I came to this page said, 'Meditate on Experience.' That's all it said on the whole page, 'Meditate on Experience.' I closed the book and schoom—that was it."

Annise took the counselor's arm. "Isn't Rod something?" she said smiling.

Muriel stepped up, cradled Morton's cast and leaned her forehead against his shoulder.

So there he was—Annise on his left in her maroon short shorts, hair tossed by the sea breeze over the satiny gel of her copious chest. On his right, Muriel with her low-cut leotard top and suede micro-culottes, all propped up on those sexy Hollywood Boulevard pumps.

"Wow, are you doing good," said Rodney to Morton as he took it all in.

Annise smiled. "Well, Morton and I have been seeing each other," she said blushing.

Rodney leaned against his car. "Do you have a brother by any chance?" he asked Morton.

The counselor shook his head.

"You're lucky. Because hot babes always run off with the brother, you know. It's a curiosity trip. Me and Lance are different as night and day. He's my brother. This is one thing Lance doesn't have," declared Rodney. He made a motion over his car which looked a bit like the Catholic sign of the cross. "He drives a beat up old Chevy. It's full of dents where people keep running into it when he goes drinking."

Annise was listening closely.

"I think women go for opposites, don't you, Morton?" continued Rod. "I'm the upper crusty type, you see. But Lance, he's a live in the basement shave once a week cat. Anyway, we don't talk much these days, ever since he got out of jail for safecracking. Now there's something he's really good at. It's a lot like picking the lock on a hot blonde's chastity belt, wouldn't you say? Get her high, talk to her about God, she'll do anything."

Annise grinned. Rodney gave her a wink. "Come see me sometime," said Rod to Annise. He quickly pushed his palms toward Morton. "Hey, don't get me wrong, I mean as a friend."

A friend, thought the counselor? That word hovered around the blonde like a twisted aura. Morton started to leave. Annise and Rodney embraced, smooching the air beside each other's cheeks.

Muriel guided the counselor across the parking lot.

From behind Rodney called out, "Watch yourself, my friend. This little animal is a fast highway." He squeezed her to him. "And she's smart too. Don't end up road kill on pretty Beaver Boulevard like a lot of us did."

"A lot of us?" replied Morton. He shuddered. Muriel walked quicker.

~~~

Annise's good-byes to Rodney stretched out a little long. Morton and Muriel made their way to the boardwalk.

"I'd never do such a thing," uttered Muriel low.

"Do what thing?"

She looked him in the eyes. "Screw Lance," she said matter of factly.

* * *

Chapter 34

On the boardwalk it wasn't long before Harmonic Convergence approached. He was the guy with the waist long beard dyed half orange and half yellow who passed out freaky New Age religious literature. He offered Morton one of the leaflets.

"No, thanks. I don't quite know what to make of this stuff. There's so many wackos out here," said Morton.

"You're here. What does that say?" noted Harmonic Convergence.

"He's not a wacko," said Muriel. "He's here with me. I'm the wacko."

"Good for you!" exclaimed Harmonic Convergence clapping his hands. "There's a powerful Astrological Pulling Effect occurring right now, my friends. A great Magnetic Confluence of the heavens. I can feel you've both been drawn here for a very important reason, like ball bearings to a magnet."

"I don't feel it," Morton told him.

"It's OK. Not all of us do," said Harmonic Convergence.

Morton said, "I thought that the big Magnetic Confluence already went by. That's what I read in the *Times*."

"Might have. Might not have." He smiled yellow and orange, then reached to shake Morton's hand.

"Sorry," said the counselor flashing his cast.

"Damnit to hell," cursed Harmonic Convergence. "That's a very bad omen, that wrist. I sense stress to your inner magnetism! I feel a blue and purple Chromosomal Osmosis going into effect!"

Harmonic Convergence continued to talk as Morton and Muriel moved off the weathered boards onto the beach sand.

They paused to remove their shoes. The day was radiantly sunny, and the girls so young and sensual, their hair all teased and ribboned up, Day-Glo bikinis strung on like a couple of rubber bands. Morton kept cutting his eyes as he and Muriel threaded the beach blankets. Amazing. For as delectable as they were not a one, he decided, was as fetching in a physical sense as Annise Chastain.

~~~

As they proceeded Morton noticed Muriel trying to synchronize with his steps, an imitative behavior from her insecurities of the early days. But the sand was uneven and they kept bumping hips. He remembered the time he'd taken her hiking in the Santa Monica mountains. They'd been out in the heat, and Morton only had a small pint bottle of water. He offered it to her.

"Have some," he said.

"Not yet, thanks. I only want a certain amount," she returned.

"How much do you mean?"

"I'm not sure. Take yours first, then I'll know."

Sweet kid, that Muriel. She had qualities you didn't often see in Venice. Whether she got them from being locked up in Roselawn or the Fraction House, or from her rare shots at freedom wasn't clear. Nevertheless there glowed a sincerity about her, causing those in her purview, particularly Morton, to abandon desires for the trivial or the double-faced. It had happened earlier with Sally.

"Listen," said Morton stopping and taking her by the elbow. "The meeting this morning was a big ruse. I think it's obvious they meant to keep you at the Fraction House all along. I got the feeling Priscilla was in on it somehow."

"I've known this for a long time," returned Muriel.

"They didn't vote on it today, but the Arbitrators will do what Joseph says. It looks like you'll have to be at the Fraction House a while longer."

Muriel shrugged with resignation. "For the rest of my life probably," she muttered.

"Another thing. And don't get exercised about this. I have to tell you though. Something very ugly happened after you and Annise left the meeting. Remember how we used to talk about detachment? Well, I want you to remain completely detached as I explain this."

Muriel smoothed the sand under her foot. "They fired you, didn't they?" she said.

Morton squinted at her. "Yes. They even got an injunction against me coming to the Fraction House."

"I knew they were going to do it. Joseph gets me all to himself now. Why do you think I've been so scared?"

"Why *have* you been so scared? It was Joseph's semen they found in you, wasn't it?"

Muriel dropped her eyes. The answer was entirely unexpected. "Uh huh," she said.

"Jesus Christ," groaned the counselor. "What does this mean? What exactly did he do to you anyway?"

Morton clenched his fists. Muriel ground her teeth.

"I'm going to see Joseph right now," he said starting back toward the boardwalk.

Muriel grabbed him. "No, Morton! That's what I've been afraid of. He'll kill you, I know he will."

"I'll kill him."

Muriel lunged into his arms. The manila envelope, which Morton was carrying under his shirt, crunched between them.

"What's this?" she asked. Observant to a fault, that girl.

She lifted his shirt and removed the envelope.

"'PERSONAL?'" she read. "What does that mean?"

"It doesn't mean anything. Go ahead, take a look," said Morton.

Edgy and frightened, as Muriel tended to get when faced with important documents, she glanced briefly at the Severance Declaration and returned it to the folder. She then studied the Temporary Removal form. After a moment she gave a giggle.

"This is from when they sprayed the bugs."

"Right," said Morton.

Muriel's eyes darted in thought. "It's pink, like the Custody forms," she noted. He could hear the emotion trembling in her voice. "You— You used this to steal me?"

Morton nodded. "I had to. There's a possibility I might not get to see you again."

"You're wonderful. But don't worry, you'll see me plenty, I'm sure of it," she said.

"I'm making an investigation, Muriel. There are a lot of loose ends we haven't tied up."

Her eyes lit with terror. "But Morton, they've already got a junction against you."

"Injunction," he corrected.

"Injunction against you. This is very bad. You might have to go to jail if they find out you stole me. Annise is going to flip her lid when she realizes you snuck us out of there."

Morton's jaw jutted sternly forward. He examined the twists of Muriel's face. Was she about to cry? No, that wasn't it. She was laughing. Laughing and crying both? Well, such was the modern manic. At least, pondered the counselor optimistically, there were no traces left of the blasted out schizophrenic. That was something.

"Hey, knock it off," he said taking her by the shoulders.

"I'm sorry, Morton. I don't mean to laugh." She looked up teary eyed. "See, I'm crying again."

~~~

Annise and Gordon were coming, dodging the flying Frisbees and the beach bunnies. The four of them regrouped and headed down toward the water.

Annise maneuvered alongside Morton. She was finishing off the Gordon's cotton candy. "Green, my favorite color," she said gleefully waving the cone.

Morton smiled.

"By the way, I was talking to Harmonic Convergence," said Annise. She showed him her handful of pamphlets. "This stuff isn't so quirky after all. It's Wanda's religion you know. You didn't? Plus, Wanda says Harmonic Convergence takes in all religions."

"Even Catholicism?" wondered Morton.

"Especially Catholicism. In fact, Wanda lives up this way. And she's hardly quirky at all. Maybe we could visit her on the way back."

Morton raised his eyebrows.

"What'd you make of Rodney?" continued Annise. "He's a trip, don't you think?"

"I guess so," said Morton.

"My sister Aphie never liked Rod much. We have such different tastes in men."

"Really?" said Morton intrigued, for he hadn't seen much in Rodney either.

They tiptoed into the tide and gazed out over the ocean.

"Isn't it gorgeous?" said Annise working her red toenails into the sand. "Life can be so perfect sometimes."

"No good to swim in though," grumbled Gordon.

"But why not?" objected Annise. "God made it all so wonderful here. The weather. The water. Just *feel* it, Gordon."

Gordon made a face. "I guess you don't know all the toxic waste is down by Huntington and Long Beach. This water here is too clean to be any good."

"You're a bizarre man, Gordon," enjoined Annise adjusting her sunglasses. "Don't you realize things in this world can be changed and made good? Can't you try to see the beauty *in here*," she tapped her forehead, "instead of out there?"

Gordon shook his head.

"All you've got to do is use your mind's eye. That's where you see God and Jesus and St. Vitus and them. That's where truth is. And salvation too," persisted Annise.

"Where?" asked Gordon.

"In here. In the mind's eye," she said.

"You mean there's an eye inside your head?" wondered Gordon frowning. "A *real* eye?"

Buck Buchanan

"There is in my head," said the blonde ambling casually off along the surf.

* * *

'L.A. 2000:' Sex Asylum

Chapter 35

They returned to the boardwalk where they came upon the Lady Astrologer with her turban and her giant charts. They passed the Tarot Card Reader and the rollerblade rental van.

Gordon, Morton could tell, was acting odd. Annise still seemed timid around the clients, and when Gordon slipped on his bicycle glasses with the small mirrors at the temples so he could see behind—one of his bad triggering fetishes—she didn't have the heart to object. Harvey at first sanctioned this practice under the theory that seeing behind him might reduce Gordon's sense of paranoia. One of the difficulties however was sunlight flashing in the tiny mirrors, which caused a strobe-like effect on the retina. This in turn precipitated the weird blinking which tended to induce his so called fits.

The paranoid strutted into the distance. Morton didn't say anything. From now on insanity would have to be someone else's ball game.

Annise's tanned arm pointed ahead to a group of Hare Krishnas. They were being heckled by a rival group with a sign. 'BIBLE BOB'S JESUS FREAKS, TOLEDO, OHIO,' it said. Both factions had their tambourines, their robes, their finger cymbals. Bible Bob's people wore long greasy locks, while the Hare Krishnas were bald except for a thin ponytail coming off the napes of their necks.

As they passed Annise was lured into debate. Morton pulled her along. "But they don't even *know* about the saints, Morton. They need my help."

Finally they came to the counselor's favorite exhibit—the chain-link cubicles where the professional bodybuilders from Gold's Gym performed their weightlifting routines. There was always a crowd of gawkers there. Gordon had wedged in among them, his fingers twined rigidly into the fence. Already he was in the first stages of eye-flitting and those strange mechanical head jerks.

Buck Buchanan

The problem was that he was paranoid of the bodybuilders due to their contamination with good health. Gordon's glasses had come off. The nervous looks over his shoulder were beginning to spin him around as he tried to see who might be sneaking up from behind. It was looking like a full scale attack of Synthetic Paranoia. Morton remembered the time Gordon had explained, "I realize I'm sickly. I'm dying more and more every day I'm alive."

"Who isn't?" returned the counselor.

"The difference is, I'm extremely powerful! Illness gives strength, Morton Allison," insisted Gordon holding up a finger.

Clinically, this was known as a Delusion of Grandeur, where the nut decided he was a big wheel. According to Harvey this malady afflicted about half of all the mentally ill. The other half were battling the dreaded Delusion of Worthlessness, where the nut was too weak to punch out of their own paper bag.

Morton looked over to Muriel—her head down, feet shuffling sadly along, sorrow and helplessness written all over her. A lot of them though, considered the counselor as he paused by the benches, felt worthless and powerful *at the same time*. These were the truly dangerous ones—your Richard Nixons and your Joseph Schopens.

~~~

Annise and Morton took seats on the bench. Muriel came over and sat next to Morton. On the far side of the weight cage a line of foxy young ladies in Lycra shorts and halter-tops were flirting with the weightlifters. California girls they were, extraordinarily striking and voluptuous. The blonde evil-eyed them.

"I don't think I've told you this, Morton," said Annise. "But I haven't worn a bra on days like this since I was thirteen years old."

Morton and Muriel looked over at her. She seemed very serious.

"We had a pool you know," she continued. "You didn't? Well, I'm sure I must have mentioned it. God, the memories I have. Anyway, I started wearing bikinis under my clothes so I could tan on the way home from school. In fact, I've got one on right now."

Muriel and Morton watched, their mouths open in dismay, as Annise began to unbutton the blouse with the shamrocks on it. Leisurely she peeled it back. Beneath was a tiny red bathing suit top studded with sequins.

She leaned close to Morton. "I knew we were going to the beach so I slipped this on underneath. I'm wearing the bottoms too. By the way, it's a T-back." She winked. "You've got to remember, Morton, in California it can get *terribly* hot."

Annise fanned under her arms, folded her shirt and put it in her purse.

Morton noticed how intently Muriel was observing Annise's behavior. The bathing suit top. The sexy flips of her hair. The woman was a tourist attraction of her own, all pink and a thousand yards of lace. She arched around Morton to address Muriel.

"Hmmm, memories. Now there's something you ought to think about young lady," said Annise.

"Young? I'm two years older than you," countered Muriel quickly.

"I wouldn't be bragging about that," suggested the blonde fluffing out her hair. "Memories, Muriel, they're everything in life. You don't have much if you don't have your memories."

"I've blocked all my memories, Annise. They hurt me, so I blocked them."

"You've still got so much though. Take me for instance. Even if I blocked everything I'd still have all the benefits of a really true sense of faith."

Muriel blinked. "Except I don't have any faith," she said.

Annise scratched her hair at the part. "Are you trying to say you don't have any memories *or* faith? Good God, girl, what *do* you have?"

"Friends," said Muriel. "I've got good friends." She pressed against Morton's shoulder.

"But don't you want to stand on your own two feet? Don't you want to be your own woman?" asked Annise.

"Not really. I've always wanted to be somebody else's woman."

"Muriel," said Annise. "Muriel, Muriel, Muriel. You've got to know *yourself*, young lady. That's the first order of business."

"But don't you find yourself through another person? Through, well— Through your lover?" she said low.

~~~

Over by the bodybuilders Gordon was about to lose it. Morton knew the symptoms: Elevated pulse rate. Ocular Strabismus. Dangerously high blood pressure. The synthetic's nervous looks over the shoulder were swiftly evolving into a series of dance-like turnabouts, like a dog lost in the chase for its tail. The danger was of certain neuro-hormones firing all at the same time and causing a seizure similar to the Grand Mal convulsions an epileptic might have.

"Shouldn't you do something?" whispered Muriel to Morton.

But Annise was already on her way. As sometimes occurred with these sorts of public interventions the rubberneckers swarmed in close for the freak show. The last Morton and Muriel could see was Annise attempting to position herself between Gordon and the weight cage so as to block his view of the bodybuilders. Whatever happened next was obscured by the melee.

"I've seen you studying Annise," said Morton nudging Muriel back to reality. "What do you think you'll discover?"

"Knowledge. Women gain knowledge by watching each other."

"Really? What have you learned from Annise?"

Muriel scratched her cheek. She gazed thoughtfully into the sky similar to the way Morton had seen Annise do. "How to undress," she said.

In a kind of torpid slow motion, Muriel lifted her culottes over what Morton recognized as a garter belt. She popped the snaps, hooked her thumbs into the top of her nylons and began to carefully roll them down. There were runs in the heels from the beach walk. "It's hot, Morton. I'm cooling off is all," said Muriel by way of explanation.

A short while later Gordon and Annise came walking up to them. Perspiration was beaded on the paranoid's forehead, but otherwise he appeared to have miraculously recovered. Muriel took Gordon by the arm and walked him down the boardwalk.

"What the hell happened over there?" Morton asked Annise.

"Oh, nothing. We had a little talk, is all," she said.

"A little talk! My God, Gordon's never come out of one of those spells so fast."

"I thought he might be feeling kind of hopeless. I mean, with his synthetic thing and those guys so strong and all. I get that myself sometimes with religion. Like all of a sudden thinking you might be wrong about everything you've ever believed in, and then feeling miserable and paranoid about it."

Morton nodded.

"So I explained it wasn't hopeless at all. Actually, he has everything to look forward to."

"He does?"

"Sure," waved Annise. "I mean, there are going to be a lot more synthetic poisons around in the future, aren't there? More cancers and weirdo diseases and all."

"I suppose so," said Morton.

"And the more synthetics the more we'll all get in us every day, right?"

"Yes, I guess so."

"I told him to be optimistic. Because every day the world gets worse for everyone else it gets better and better for a backwards guy like Gordon." She smiled.

"You told him that?"

"Uh huh. I told him he could feel good about being the way he is."

"But Annise, I'm not certain you should—"

Morton held his tongue though. She was giving it the All-American try, he had to accept that.

"Do you know what he said?" she went on.

"What'd he say?"

"'Thank you,'" returned Annise. "He said, 'Thank you very much, blondey.'"

She put her arm into Morton's. They started to walk. On the exterior she seemed so calm, so confident, yet he could feel her fingers quivering on his biceps as a shaky fear slowly won out over her first burst of gallantry.

* * *

Chapter 36

They caught up with Gordon and Muriel outside a fancyish looking Bavarian style restaurant. Annise cupped her hands to the window.

"Maybe we could get a cocktail," she suggested pointing to the long mahogany bar inside. "The textbooks say it's an OK thing. I mean, the Wulf Wulfensburger book says it's normalizing and mainstreaming and all." She looked at Morton. "Well, it is, isn't it?"

"Wulfensburger?" wondered the counselor.

"Well, maybe it was the B.F. Skinner book. You know the one, *Wet Mind*, I think was the title."

The lounge was called The ManTrap. Gordon and Muriel both tended to be shy of dim, claustrophobic places like this, but by now they seemed anxious to get free of the boardwalk crazies.

"I know how important it is for you to be alone with Muriel. I'll wait a few minutes with Gordon at the bar," whispered Annise. She gave the counselor a quick hug.

Muriel and Morton found a table in the corner. Her eyes were slit from all the smoke in the air. "You always smell like her nowadays. You used to smell like yourself," she said.

Annise had Piña Coladas sent over to them. Morton slid Muriel's away. "I'm sorry, but you're still on drugs. And drugs and alcohol don't mix."

"Oh bullshit," said Muriel reaching for the straw. "Anyway, I quit taking the Tofranil. If it was Tofranil. The way Joseph is, it might have been opium. Besides, Annise is my counselor now. She thinks cocktails are fine."

So, he decided, she hasn't gone entirely around the bend!

The two of them talked quietly. About her future. About her parents. About her fears of returning to Roselawn.

"I'm not sure I can handle any of those places," said Muriel. "The Fraction House is even worse, Morton. I'm so sick of that joint. And this apartment business. I've never lived on my own. Not even once."

"I won't let you get hurt. We haven't come all this way for something ridiculous to happen. I really mean this," replied the counselor.

"There's nothing you can do."

"There's plenty I can do. I've got a briefcase full of answers. I'm still young. I'm strong."

"You're forty-three, aren't you?" said Muriel. "I mean, twenty-three?"

The kid wasn't much for calculations. She scratched her head in confusion.

"You're close. I'm thirty-three."

"But they've got the junction, Morton. And Joseph's got pills and spies and everything. Plus a bunch of my father's money. I guess he makes Harvey take it out of the escrow account and give it to him," said Muriel.

"The fifty thousand?"

"Yeah. It's not illegal either. My father makes a personal check straight to Harvey every year, but Joseph always ends up with it."

"How do you know?"

"From his bankbook."

"His bankbook? When did you see his bankbook?"

"Over at his apart— I mean, I just know this stuff. Like how he drives those Jaguars and buys a million drinks for his titty dancers."

She touched Morton's hand. "I'm so afraid," she said low. "What about you, Morton? Aren't some things just too much for you to take?"

"Well, yes. There was the time Stacy went up to Yellowstone for three weeks and I wasn't getting any— Oh, Muriel, I'm sorry. I didn't mean—" He halted.

"Oh, quit it," she chided. "I'm not a child anymore. I know what these things are about."

"You do?"

"Of course I do. I watched you with Stacy. I see you with that—well, with Annise. Don't you think I realize everybody has to have a mate?"

"Do you really think so?"

"Of course. Otherwise we'd all have two heads. But we don't have two heads, because we use the other person's head when we hug and kiss and, you know, make love together. Somebody needs to watch over your shoulder for you when you're vulnerable."

"I feel like I'm vulnerable all the time these days," mumbled the counselor.

"Maybe you need another head. A head who can see more than two feet in front of her," suggested Muriel.

"Who's your other head? Joseph's?" asked Morton.

Muriel could be enchanting, but she had a stubborn streak as well. He had to remember his purpose.

"So Joseph raped you after all! And he keeps on raping you in the tub, doesn't he?" he blurted.

Muriel was silent. She was capable of clamming up hard and blotting any possible truth out of the picture. Morton knew he couldn't press her any further. His patience was wearing thin. He started tearing his napkin into little bits.

"He tried to kill me. Isn't that what you said? I got pushed. I know I did. You didn't push me. Joseph's black as sin, Muriel. Why is everybody protecting him?"

No answer.

"If only I had evidence that he shoved me, you know, meant malice—"

Morton pushed the pile of paper bits aside. He picked up Muriel's napkin and began ripping it into long strips.

"I know how you could find out," she said. "When you fell Harvey was coming down the hall from his office. He was the first one helping you, remember? He had to have seen the whole thing."

Morton slapped his hands flat on the table. "Harvey!" he cried. "Of course. That's where the answer is."

At the bar Gordon and the man next to him were into a conversation. Amazing. Annise came to the table. "I've ordered hors d'oeuvres. They'll be up in a minute," she said.

"Good. I'm hungry," said Morton.

Annise eyeballed the shredded pile of confetti. "Hungry? Looks to me like you're hyped up again. You're probably due for a pill. Which reminds me, I've got a new script for you."

She handed Morton a fresh vial. It was double the size of the old one. He shook a few of the capsules into his palm.

"They look like the others," he said.

"They're the same. The first ones had a borderline expiration date. Joseph brought it to my attention. These are a lot fresher."

"I'm not sure about this, Annise. I don't have much faith in the Gestapo these days."

"Harvey wrote this one. See, his signature's right on the label."

Morton lifted the old vial to compare it to the new one. Yes, it was Harvey's own handwriting this time. 'One hundred count,' read the inscription.

Annise plucked the original, smaller container from his fingers and rattled it by her ear. "A bunch of the old ones are left in here. I'll get them back to Joseph right away," she said. "Or Harvey, rather. I'll get them back to Harvey."

A dark notion scampered across a corner of Morton's mind. Joseph knew what a suspicious thing he'd done by falsifying Harvey's signature. The counselor's notion was—and he hated to think this way—but maybe, just maybe Annise was assisting the Gestapo in getting back the incriminating evidence.

"Why are you so hesitant? Harvey understands your personality as well as I do, Morton. Trust me, we both know you need a little helper."

Annise passed him his Piña Colada, took one of the capsules from his palm and deftly thumbed it between his lips. "Cheers," she said.

Muriel's eyes grew wide.

~~~

Annise went to the bar for the food trays. Muriel rose to give her a hand.

When they were gone Morton took a moment to survey the place. A curious perfumy odor was floating around, though Muriel and Annise appeared to be the only females present. Hmmm.

Side by side at the bar the ladies awaited the sandwiches. Morton noticed how sleek Muriel's auburn hair had become, really shimmering in the amber light, and down almost to her shoulders. Not hacked off like she used to do, but growing now, finally growing. And right next to her the long golden lanes of Annise's tresses stretching well past her waist.

Morton's eyes wandered across the many feet shuffling under the bar, then back to Annise and the great oval shock of her hips. Such appeal she had with as little as cocking a foot on the railing to get balanced. Those red shorts accentuating her languorous femme fatale sway. Those heart shaped cheeks beckoning like the ladies in The Green Room! They seemed to be speaking to him. It was the old 'hearing voices' routine. "Come here, young man! Come immediately to this woman," they were saying.

Trays aloft, the two turned. Morton looked higher to their faces. A terrible scare raced through him then, for he realized he had made a drastic mistake. He'd been watching... Yes, he had been watching *Muriel's* hips, *her* red shorts, not Annise's after all! It had been Muriel's foot cocked lustily on the railing.

Morton wiped the perspiration from his brow.

* * *

Chapter 37

The three of them munched their food. Gordon remained at the bar with his new friend. Annise observed them over her sandwich.

"Do you think it's all right for Gordon to be talking to that guy so long?" she asked.

Morton shrugged. Annise looked to Muriel.

"Yes, it's all right," said Muriel.

"I don't know," countered Annise. "I've got this funny feeling. Like there might be something fishy in here. You don't think that man could be— Well, gay or something, do you?" Annise pushed her sandwich aside. "I mean, I'm in this bikini bathing suit top and nobody has even glanced at me. It kind of gets you thinking."

Morton looked cautiously around. She was right. It *was* a gay bar. Obvious once you paid attention. Such was your Annise Chastain, always shining through with a glittering piece of perception when you least expected it.

"I've got to think of Gordon. I feel he should know places like this aren't exactly, well—" Annise whispered, "Normalizing."

"I'm not sure that's a good idea," said Muriel softly.

"I'm his counselor. I've got to do something. My God, think what might happen to his mind if the guy tried to give him a— I mean, Christ, it's unthinkable."

"But, Annise," tried Muriel, "Gordon—"

"My Lord, girl, use your head. We're talking about a very unusual thing here. I can't have Gordon thinking all this gay business is OK."

"You can't?" said Muriel.

"Of course not. It would contradict every decent aspect of psychology. Especially the religious aspects."

Muriel bit her sandwich.

"Do you see what I'm saying?" asked Annise.

"I think so," replied Muriel.

"Good. I'll go straighten it out." Annise started to her feet.

"But Annise," said Muriel putting a hand gently on her arm. "Gordon is gay."

Annise froze. Slowly she looked over to Morton. He gave a small nod.

"Ohhh. I seee," she said taking hold of the chair.

~~~

It was almost dark when they left the ManTrap, and though the winds were whipping off the whitecapped water everyone seemed more relaxed. What a day it had been!

Things kept happening, not so much in a flow, but like this or that point coming out of a super clean mirror. At last the counselor felt tranquil. A joy in the moment enveloped him, as if he'd been granted a coveted third wish from the genie—inner quiet, a dreamy peace he seldom experienced. It was nice hanging out with his friends in the sweet California breezes.

But Morton was no fool. He was aware his mood might be attributable to the updated prescription. This medication seemed stronger than the first batch. Not likely though. The pills looked identical.

The establishments along the boardwalk were now aglow in blue and red neon, each a bright, gleaming oasis in the midst of the hot dog vendors and the heavyset sightseers. They came to a gift shop, one of those tastefully laid out tourist traps with an abundance of chrome and leather in the windows.

Annise paused. "Let's run in, Morty. My sister Aphie's coming to visit soon. I need to have something for her. It'll only take a minute," she said, slipping back into her shamrock shirt.

The four of them moved through the aisles, checking out the knickknacks. In the back of the store Morton came across a dusty bottle of Pouilly-Fuisse, a fine French wine. It was marked at $7.99, three times cheaper than usual. It was the only bottle there, apparently a promotion item for the expensive redwood wine rack it was stored in. He'd be alone tonight with his thoughts. Why not a glass of white wine to ease down after a big day?

The counselor checked his wallet. Three dollars left. He'd paid the entire bill at The ManTrap.

He found Annise in the religious icons section. Muriel was nearby. They were scrutinizing a plaster statue of the Buddha.

"Isn't he cute, Morton?" said Annise. "He reminds me of the little Madonna in my bedroom."

The counselor hesitated a moment, then he said, "I was wondering if you could do me a little favor, Annise? I wasn't able to get to the bank today. I'm a bit short on cash. Would you consider loaning me a couple of bucks until tomorrow?"

"What for?" she asked.

He thought of several ways of putting it, but none seemed quite appropriate. He said, "Well, it'd be for a bottle of wine. I found a really great deal in the back there."

"Wine?"

"Yes."

"For us?"

Morton thought it over.

"Uh, well—"

"You're being awfully presumptuous, don't you think?" she said. "First of all, I can't get away tonight. And even if I could, how do you know I'd be willing to visit you?"

Annise wasn't opening her purse. She seemed distracted, and edged backwards as if to put space between them.

"Look, about the wine," she continued. "It's not because I don't want you to have it. I do. But it's not right for the woman to be giving the man money."

"Christ, that's the old days," sighed Morton.

"I'm an old fashioned girl," said Annise.

The gift store turned out to be window-shopping only. None of them made a purchase.

When they reached the parking lot Muriel said, "I'm sorry. I forgot before, but I need to use the restroom. Don't worry, I'll be fast." She started off toward boardwalk.

"It's dark," said Gordon. "I'll walk along with her."

Morton and Annise were left alone in the parking lot.

"We're in private now. Remember what you told me about the bathing suit?" said the counselor.

"What'd I tell you?"

"You said we could take a gander at the bottoms. You know, at the T-back."

Playfully Annise hit out at him. "You're dirty," she said.

Morton flared his eyes. He arched his arms pretending to be a monster and shuffled toward her.

"So let's have a look," he teased. "It's all right. We're at the beach, remember?"

"Hey, you're acting up again. Better take another pill," joked Annise backpedaling.

"Give me T-back," growled Morton hunching over. "I need T-back."

"How about on Thursday? I'll give you T-back then."

"Now!" he said closing in on her.

Without checking behind Annise scrambled away in reverse, one of the problems with your sexy blonde drivers. She bumped into the fender of a nearby Mercedes.

"Ouch!" she squealed.

Her face contorted with pain. The tumor again. Morton took her in his arms.

"Are you OK?" he asked softly.

"I think so. It really hurts though. It might— It might even be killing me, Morton." She bit her lip.

"Have you seen a doctor yet?" he asked.

"No. But I talked to Gary. I mean, the Assistant Priest. He thinks I might have gotten it because of sin."

"Forget that shit. You haven't sinned any worse than anybody else," said Morton.

"How the hell do you know?" she snapped back.

"I guess I don't know. Is there something you haven't been telling me?"

Annise whipped her head away.

Gordon and Muriel returned, and the four of them started toward the pickup. As they walked Muriel strayed a distance away. Morton couldn't blame her for being absent minded these days. He went over and began to guide her back toward the others. She gave him a strangely piercing look. Next came a tap on the back of his cast. She was handing him something.

"Shhh," she said, giving him an affectionate push.

They paused under the streetlamp. In Morton's hand was the dusty bottle of Pouilly-Fuisse, the special wine from the gift shop. He was moved to a tear. He felt like kissing her.

"Thanks," he whispered.

"You're welcome," she said smiling.

"Listen, Muriel, I want you to call me tomorrow. Find a time when nobody's around. I need to know what the final decision was from the meeting."

She blinked up at him.

"At this rate I might have to steal you again," he added.

Muriel's eyes went a translucent aquamarine under the purple streetlight.

She swallowed hard. "I'll call," she said.

* * *

Chapter 38

The following morning the counselor was awakened by the ringing of his telephone. He stumbled into the livingroom and plopped into his green recliner.

"Hello," he said groggily.

"Morton, is that you?"

"Muriel?"

"Yes, it's me. I've got to be quiet," she whispered. "Most of the counselors are upstairs in one of Joseph's big Dictum Meetings. I had to sneak into the Staff Lounge to call."

"Don't get caught there. You'll get demerits or something."

"Annise will be back any second. Morton, the Arbitrators cut Joseph's therapy off with me. I just found it out. Maybe they suspect something. Do you think they suspect something?"

"Like what?" asked the counselor.

"I guess Priscilla's got pull with the Arbitrators, because they're only giving Dar/Neese three more weeks with me. Joseph wanted three months, you know."

"I know."

"I think he's more paranoid of Priscilla than he is of you."

"I'm paranoid of her too," said Morton.

"Plus, the Arbitrators told Joseph to let me come and go as I please."

"Can they do that?"

"They can do whatever they want. It's not my own Temporary Guardianship exactly. They say they want me to practice being independent. If I'm responsible for myself everybody's ass is covered. Roselawn's. Joseph's. Even the Arbitrators look good. And anyway, they know I'm not any crazier than you are."

A long pause while the counselor thought this one over.

"You're a free woman then?"

"Kind of. But you know how these things are. If I do something suspicious they'll lock me back up."

"Don't do anything rash, Muriel. Promise me you won't do anything rash."

"OK," she said. There was a momentary silence. "So when can you steal me again?" asked Muriel.

Morton sighed. "Are the police after me? What happened when I dropped you all last night?"

"From what I heard it's not kidnapping. Annise signed us out, remember? So your name's not on anything. Joseph was so mad his face looked like it had ants all over it. I think he's taking a lot of those Dexies lately."

"Stay away from him, Muriel. It's possible he's an attempted killer."

"You stay away from him, Morton. If he's a killer we don't want you to be killed."

In the old days there'd always been a certain psychological gap between them. Now, even across the telephone lines, there seemed hardly a breath of miscommunication. Proof positive, wasn't it, that the mentally ill weren't doomed to hearing gravely, dictatorial voices with no people attached? Morton was impressed.

"I'm so glad you're comprehending these things, Muriel. It takes a great burden off me. I've been feeling so tired lately. Like I'm old as the sea. Like I'm ancient," said the counselor.

"The sea might be ancient, but it is not old, Morton. It's fresh as a daisy each time somebody jumps into it."

"You're a sweet kid, Muriel. You know, in a way I'd kind of like to see you today."

There was a clamor on the other end of the line.

"Wait! I hear Joseph's elevator," said Muriel. "I've got to get off the phone. You can bet her bottom Annise is in there with him."

There came a delay, though the lines stayed open. What was she saying about Annise's bottom? And Joseph in there with it?

"Morton, is that you?" It was Annise.

"Morning, babe," said the counselor.

"Babe? Give me a break, will you? Look, I know what you did yesterday. Sneaking Muriel out and all," she said.

"Did you get in trouble?"

"Well, no. But I certainly could have."

"Joseph will hold it all against me. You shouldn't worry. I've been jerked around so much I didn't want any hitches in seeing Muriel. I didn't mean to lie."

Annise paused. "You had the right," she said finally. "The way you said it though you didn't exactly lie. You fudged. And you know what?"

"What?"

"Once I got to thinking about it I really got excited. You might not know a lot about religion, Morton, but you're almost as good as a Christian at getting at those gray areas. Frankly, I'm rather proud of you."

"You are?" said the counselor surprised.

"I certainly am. And I've been terribly cross with Joseph since I found out he fired you. It was a dirty low-down trick," she said with a hint of thrill in her voice.

"I'm glad you feel that way," said Morton.

"I don't know what it is you've got going with these schizos, but the girl was like a lamb when we got back from Venice. It was really incredible. Everybody told me what a great job I was doing. I got all the credit, only I know it wasn't me. It was you, Morty. You did it all."

"You were good with Gordon though."

"Not really. He tore the doors off the laundry room as soon as we got back." Then, very humbly she said, "I did have something to do with Sally starting to talk again."

"Sure you did," agreed Morton. "A lot of times it takes negative stimulation to get these people to perk up."

"Negative? Are you saying I'm a negative type person?"

"Of course not. You've just got your own special way of encountering sticky situations."

"I know for a fact the Fraction House thinks I'm improving. Did I tell you? They're letting Muriel come to my place for an overnight. It's all set for Thursday."

"Thursday? Isn't that our T-back night?"

"I guess it is, now that you mention it. Anyway, I'm not getting a Temporary Custody per se, but it shows Joseph has faith in me, don't you think? Isn't it great how he trusts me with her all by myself? It's almost like he's starting to see me as part of the agency."

"You and Muriel are getting to be friends then?"

"It's hard to say with these people. I'll have her Thursday. They're giving her her own Custody for that one day. Joseph said it'd be like a trial run for this apartment thing. There's a lot going on in the afternoon. Why don't you come by in the morning? June 6th is the date. Try to remember it. We can all three play Trivial Pursuit or something."

"Thanks, I'd like that," said Morton. "I'm not sure I'd mention it to Joseph."

"Joseph doesn't know I'm still seeing you. Anyway, Harvey's back in for good now. He swears he's going to work till five every day no matter what," said Annise.

"Already? I'm very concerned about him. I called his home last night but the number's been changed. I even stopped by his place but all the lights were out," said Morton.

"He doesn't look good. He's all pale and gray in the face. Joseph's still acting Director though. In fact, he's telling everybody Harvey's on his last leg around here. I've got to admit it does look that way."

"So we're set for Thursday?" said Morton. "I can't wait. We'll have a threesome."

"A threesome! God, you're kinky," she whispered excitedly.

"For Trivial Pursuit, Annise."

"Damn, too bad," she joked.

"One quick thing," added the counselor. "I didn't get to say a proper goodbye to Gordon yesterday. Is he around now? I'd like to talk to him for a minute."

"This is highly unusual, isn't it?" objected Annise. "I mean, you being severed and unbonded with him and all, in a Freudian sense, I mean."

"The injunction restricts me physically from the Fraction House. I can still talk to my friends. I'm talking to you aren't I?"

Annise thought it over. "Well, I suppose it'd be OK. Gordon thinks the world of you, Morton. You *should* say a real goodbye. I'll have him call."

"Thanks," said Morton.

~~~

When they hung up the counselor sat there trying to get his bearings. So much had happened. Yesterday he lost his job, his income. The Arbitrators were getting suspicious of Joseph. And Muriel having her own Temporary Custody? What was this about? Harvey was on his last leg, and declining fast apparently. Priscilla was doing her fancy footwork. She could be a bulldog when she wanted to. There wasn't time even for a coffee.

Morton opened his briefcase and began a meticulous perusal of his documents. He thought about shaving, but no, best to get underway immediately, head on out to the L.A. County Courthouse and figure out how to tie up these frayed ends.

~~~

In the afternoon Gordon called. Morton had just completed the long return ride from the County Courthouse.

"Anybody there with you?" asked the counselor.

A long pause. "No, only the voices," said Gordon. "But I haven't been able to make out what they're saying since Joseph moved all the television sets up to the third floor."

They'd never made small talk in the past, and this time there was no small talk either. Several minutes of important discussion transpired.

"I'm not going to say goodbye," declared Morton. "You're my friend, Gordon, and I'll be there for you as long as you need me."

"Fair enough. And the same goes for me," returned the paranoid.

"I've got a gigantic favor to ask," said the counselor. "If you don't want to do it say so and there'll be no hard feelings."

Morton could hear Gordon's breathing quicken. "Whatever you need, my friend," he said.

"It'd be tomorrow. Can you get to the main lobby at 3:15 sharp? I've been looking over your schedule. You'll be down the hall in Clay-Work. Keep an eye on the clock. Tell Wanda you have to take a leak or something. Think you can do it?"

"Lie? Sure, I can do that. A lie is utterly false, so it's bound to be a good thing."

Morton explained how necessary it was he meet with Harvey, if only for a few minutes. How far out of hand things had gotten, what with Joseph's sex shenanigans, not to mention his obvious attempts to hijack the Dar/Neese Directorship. They spoke a bit longer, working out the details. Gordon was highly interested.

"If that's the way you want it done, I can do it," he confirmed.

"Fair enough," said Morton. "See you tomorrow."

* * *

Chapter 39

The next day Morton waited until 2:30 p.m., then drove to the Fraction House. A legal injunction meant he'd be arrested the moment he set foot on the premises. Nevertheless, a private talk with Harvey was imperative.

Morton parked in the back under the overhanging trees of the Organic Therapy Garden where Joseph couldn't see his truck. He knew the Gestapo's schedule by heart. Joseph wouldn't be seeing Muriel, but he did have Sally and a few others booked for tub time. At 3:00 p.m. he'd be tied up with Sam Lorenzo, a slow, taxing case. Sam invariably strung Joseph along for an hour and a half, minimum.

Morton hurried to Odette's secret wee a.m. exit over the rusty chain-link fence, and began to make his climb. But wait, no longer was there the familiar bowing down at the top. Overnight, literally, it had been re-strung with shiny razor wire, the kind used at maximum security prisons. That Joseph was a fast operator. The counselor backed down.

Morton glanced both ways before easing to the corner of the property. High hedges blocked the view from the private residences to the south, allowing him a few moments to seek an entrance.

For years there'd been a neglected crawl hole here. This was a by-gone labor of Sally Featherman when she'd spent a full year escaping from fifteen different weak spots in the Fraction House armor. At the time, these escapes were a great perplexity, but after his recent talk with Trina Lopez, Morton knew precisely why Sally had to run away every night.

He got on his hands and knees and nosed along the base of the fence. But no, he recalled, Joseph had Sam Lorenzo and Gordon fill the old holes up, grain by grain, for their ionization therapy. The earth was packed down like concrete.

Morton returned to his truck and drove down to Vera's. He'd have to use his alternative plan.

He checked his watch. Half an hour had elapsed. It was three o'clock.

Taking care to remain safely on the public sidewalk, he hustled on foot up the hill toward the Fraction House. The trick would be finding a moment when none of the staff who might tell on him would be passing through the lobby. Stacy? Wanda? Annise? Perry Barwick? Who, really, *could* he trust?

At the front of the building the counselor jogged the long flight of Dar/Neese's concrete steps, and wedged against the wooden double doors. With one eye he peered through the thick, wire reinforced Plexiglas into the lobby. It was 3:15 exactly. No Gordon.

Morton pulled back. His heart started to pound. This was forbidden territory. It was the right thing to do maybe, but face it, he was committing a crime.

Once again he leaned to see inside. A rogue eye appeared on the opposite side of the door, enlarging in the distorted magnification of the glass. It was the Synthetic Paranoid, his pupil triply wide, like a pirate.

The counselor leapt back in terror. Gordon, meeting Morton's own wild stare, also leapt back. But they'd connected, and it only took a second for the two to gather themselves.

According to their prearranged signal, the counselor made a fist and jerked it downward in front of his face. Gordon turned and went quickly across the lobby to the fire alarm. He gave Morton a nod, then pulled the red lever firmly down.

Immediately an ear shattering clanging tore apart the afternoon calm. Gordon shot off down the hallway. Morton raced down the steps, and at full tilt traveled the half block to the north side of the building. He made a sharp right into the blind alley adjoining C-Wing, the men's dorm, and a moment later came to the steel fire exit.

Morton banged four times with the side of his hand. Approximately a minute passed while, as they'd planned, Gordon struggled from the inside with the complicated safety latches. At last the door burst open. Morton rushed in. They were concealed by the aluminum partition at the main corridor.

"I did it," called Gordon over the violent ringing.

"Thanks, buddy. You don't know what this means to me."

"It's my pleasure, Morton. I guess you know how come."

"How come?"

"Because it's phony," screamed Gordon over the clanging. "It's an absolute one hundred percent synthetic fire. I really like that concept."

"Well, uh, good. Now listen, do you remember the rest of the plan?"

Gordon nodded, but his eyes betrayed a dangerous loss of direction. Morton took him by the shoulders.

"You're running to the men's room in the lobby," Morton reminded him. "It'll take Wanda a few minutes to realize you're not outside with the others. Make sure you stay in the bathroom until Wanda comes and drags you out."

The paranoid nodded enthusiastically.

"And remember, Gordon, this is *not* a real fire. You'll be safe no matter what. If Wanda forgets and the firemen pull you out, just smile and go with them. You got it?"

"Got it."

Morton started away. Gordon jerked him back.

"The staff have probably all filed out by now," said Gordon. "Joseph might still be hanging around though. Don't go by the cafeteria and the Staff Lounge."

"Joseph's in therapy with Sam right now," returned Morton quickly. "Nobody could get Sam out of the tub in under ten minutes. If I go right now I've got a chance to slip past the Therapy Room without being seen."

"Best to cut through the courtyard and take the laundry room entrance," said Gordon. "Be careful though. Somebody busted the doors the other day. There's sharp metal hanging off them."

The two shook hands. Gordon bolted toward the lobby. Morton took off in the opposite direction, scrambling out of C-Wing, across the courtyard, through the broken doors of the laundry room and up the stairs toward Administration. He knew Joseph and Sam would be the last ones out. It was all so damn risky. Subconsciously, maybe he was hoping to meet up with the Gestapo on the stairs. Well, that'd be all right. One on one this time. They'd see who'd take the tumble.

~~~

Over the harsh ringing of the alarm Morton heard the sirens of the approaching fire trucks. He paused at the top of the steps and surveyed the length of the administration corridor. Empty.

He moved by Joseph's vacant office, the door hanging open, as usual. He needed to reach the safety of the Conference Room at the end of the hall. From there he could take the side entrance to Harvey's office. He gulped for air.

Ahead yellow light was leaking from under the Therapy Room door. He heard an ominous twisting of the designer brass handle. Morton eyed the clock at the end of the hall. It was 3:24 exactly. Joseph's OCD checking behavior kicked in every six minutes no matter what clanging and clattering happened to be going on around him. Due to this disorder he *had* to verify that no one was sneaking up on him from the hallway.

The door began to swing open. The counselor's heart leapt into his mouth. All on their own his feet accelerated, and in a split second he snapped open the door to the Conference Room and lunged inside.

After a moment Morton risked a peek outside. Sam Lorenzo was in the hallway clutching a white, gym towel around his middle. Otherwise he was naked. Sam retained the classic toe walking and hesitant baby steps of Infantile Autism, which had been his childhood diagnosis. Above the ringing and the sirens and his own loud panting Morton heard the Gestapo's fierce curses echo harshly through the asylum.

"Get *going*, goddamnit!" shouted Joseph.

Morton was appalled as the supervisor began kicking Sam's buttocks, forcing him down the hallway with hard, pounding thumps from his shiny jodhpur boots. How often did this go on, wondered the counselor? How many times had bruises been put on his friends in places no one dared look? Morton was incensed.

Before he knew what he'd done the counselor charged into the corridor.

"Go, you bastard! Go!" screeched Joseph as if he were talking to a mule.

The Gestapo thrust his fingers into Sam Lorenzo's hair and dragged him onto the stairs. By sheer luck they rounded the corner and dipped behind the cold gray tiling of the wall just as Morton would have come into view.

Stunned by his urge to retaliate, the counselor's hands began to shake, then his knees, until his entire body convulsed with a mixture of anger and fear. Had there been a silence? No, the alarms were still sounding, the deafening sirens were right outside the building, in fact.

Morton gathered himself. He could hear the commotion of the firemen storming the lower floors. He knew they'd have to open and close every door in the building looking for fire, including the closets.

Morton ducked back into the Conference Room and entered Harvey's office through the side door. Lining the walls were curiously shaped molds of bronze and pewter, New Wave sculpture, he guessed, but no closets. This was important. In addition, Harvey's desk was custom built to accommodate the doctor's sprawling three hundred pound physique, insuring a large gap underneath.

Amidst the bedlam Morton took a moment to look out the window. Below were clustered all forty clients, most of them decently dressed, along with the fifty or so staff members, including the Administrative and Maintenance people.

The staff hung out together on one side of the concrete steps, the patients on the other, like a couple of ungainly football teams. False alarms at the Fraction House were a common event, and to a person they were strumming their cheeks and tapping their feet in frustration. Even the most lost of the clients had grown weary of these nonsensical evacuations.

Apart from the group Morton spotted Gordon Theodoricus. It was as if the paranoid had telescopic vision, for at this extreme distance Morton watched as Gordon formed a circle with his thumb and forefinger and covertly flashed the A-OK sign.

Morton returned the slightest nod. What communication!

Suddenly there came a thunderous pounding in the hallway. Boots and gear. Gruff voices and doors opening and slamming closed.

"Number sixty-four. Check! Number sixty-five. Check!" they were calling out.

Morton swung Harvey's coaster chair against the windowsill and dove into the tiny square of darkness beneath the desk. He was able to fit, but barely, due to Harvey's ancient double-walled safe hiding under there with him.

"Number sixty-six!"

Harvey's office door flew open. Morton took the deepest breath of his life and tried to make himself grow small in the flimsy patch of afternoon shadow.

"Check!" cried the fireman.

The door ripped savagely closed, the cannon boom reverberating in the counselor's head as a stabbing ache. A pain, yes, only a curious emotional sort of impaling, like the way he felt when Muriel would burst into tears for no good reason.

It lasted, this ache, for most of the next hour as Morton awaited the completion of the shakedown, and the refilling of the Fraction House.

* * *

Chapter 40

Dr. Harvey Mueller entered his office like a man tired to the bone. He'd always waddled, but now he lumbered in with his head down, his left foot seeming to drag behind in a kind of palsy. Morton was on the sofa along the east wall, flanked by the uninterpretable sculptures. At first the Freudian didn't see him.

"Don't be frightened, Harvey," said the counselor quietly.

The doctor turned. Annise was right. His skin was a dangerous ashen gray.

"Morton!"

Harvey struggled to assemble the scene. Perhaps he'd been a bit out of it lately, but Morton knew he was nobody's fool.

"I realize I'm not allowed around here," said the counselor evenly. "But I have to talk to you, Harvey. I think I've found out some terrible things about Dar/Neese."

Harvey eased into his chair. His eyes tightened with suspicion.

"You're wondering if I pulled the alarm?" said Morton. "Well, I did. I had no choice. I've tried to get you at home a hundred times. I've even gone to your house. Where have you been anyway? In the hospital?"

"You've got to leave here, Allison. Don't make me call the police." He reached for the phone.

"Listen to me, Harvey. Joseph's a psychopath. I believe he's been molesting Muriel in their Therapy Sessions. He's trying to pin her rape on me, but only to deflect suspicion from himself. If the tests had been done they'd have found Joseph's semen in her, I'm sure of it."

The physician closed his eyes and began to massage slowly at his temples. "We've gone round and round on all that. Leave it alone, Morton, please."

"I can't, Harvey. This has gotten way too big. Don't you see it? Joseph's pulling the rug right out from under you. Dar/Neese used to be a decent place, but Schopen's methodically turning it vulgar."

Harvey's brow beaded with perspiration. He reached for the nitro. All at once Morton had a dramatic illumination.

"Harvey, wait! Don't swallow—"

But it was too late. The Freudian smiled. The nitro had already melted under his tongue. He sipped from his mug of cold coffee.

"I just had this flash," said Morton. "Joseph supplies you with those medicines, doesn't he?"

"Of course not. My cardiologist writes all the prescriptions. Which reminds me, in twenty minutes I'm due for my afternoon meds."

Harvey produced the two brass keys needed to open his safe.

"Pardon me a moment, Morton," said the Freudian.

With much grunting and groaning he bent beneath his desk and worked the keys in conjunction with the hand-turning dial. He gathered his personal prescription vials and organized them on the desk alongside the container of nitro.

Lasix to keep fluid off. Potassium capsules to replace the electrolyte leeched by the Lasix. Cardizem for his high blood pressure and rapid heart rate. And of course the trusty nitroglycerin pellets to blast open the heart pathways when they were in the process of clamping down and cutting off the flow, the old angina. And there were the pain pills— 'Hydromorphone,' it said on the container. God, what a lot of crutches for a guy who could barely walk.

Harvey opened his vials, removed the medications, plus a spare nitro tablet, and placed them on his desk.

"But Joseph does the inventory. I mean, he gets the boxes each week straight from the wholesale distributor. From Carney Apothecary, right? That guy Rooney brings them."

"So?"

"So what if Joseph put cyanide or something in your pills? What if he's poisoning you little by little? Didn't he give you pills right before the meeting started the other day?"

Harvey laughed. "If it was cyanide I'd have been dead a hundred times by now. Cyanide takes a person out like a bullet."

"Well, I don't know. Arsenic maybe. Something that makes you sick like you have heart disease and after a while kills you."

"You've got a creative mind, Allison. But I've had heart problems for years. These meds are pulling me back together, not hurting me."

As if in proof Harvey brought out his pipe and began to fire it up. Well, he might claim he felt good, but he looked like death warmed over. Morton felt for his own vial of capsules.

"Take a look at these, Harvey. They're tranquilizers. I've been swallowing this crap for the last ten days."

Harvey examined the label. "I didn't know you were on Librium. Has it helped?" he asked.

"Hell no, it hasn't helped. And what do you mean you didn't know? Didn't you write the script for me? It's your signature."

Harvey tapped at the vial with the end of his pipe. "These Xeroxed stickers are all pre-signed," he said. "Joseph puts them on the proper containers and fills in the client names. We've got fifty or sixty medications a day, Morton. It's a common way of keeping up with the volume."

"So in effect Joseph gave me this Librium?"

Harvey puckered his lips. "I must have signed for it somewhere along the line. I know I haven't been in touch as close as I ought to these last weeks," admitted the doctor. Harvey raised his eyebrows. "Oh, now I see what you're getting at. Relax, will you, Morton. You don't look very poisoned to me, if that's what you're thinking."

"I'm not so sure, Harvey. For tranquilizers they seem quite powerful."

"People have different tolerances. One person has a heavy effect, another virtually no effect."

Morton put his hands on his head and began to absently rub his scalp.

Harvey waved his pipe. "Nervous types tend to fabricate their own delusional realities, Morton. Best to take your medication and get off the grounds before you stumble into trouble."

The counselor walked to the Freudian's desk and placed his palms on the smooth mahogany top.

"Harvey, I'm going to be blunt with you," began Morton. "Sick things are going on around here. What would you say if I told you I just saw Joseph kicking Sam Lorenzo down the hall? Kicking him hard in the ass where nobody'll see the bruises. And that's not all. I'm pretty sure he shoved me down the steps trying to get me out of his hair. He knew I'd stand up for Muriel if I found out he was abusing her. It's possible he may have been trying to kill me."

Harvey did not alter expression. Very strange for your emotionally oriented Freudian psychiatrist.

"Did you see what happened, Harvey? You were coming down the hallway when I fell. Give it to me straight, man. Did Schopen push me?"

The physician chewed hard on the stem of his pipe. A piece of plastic chipped off and he spit it onto his desk top.

"I didn't have anything to do with Joseph firing you at the meeting, Morton," said Harvey. "I guess I know he's run a bit amuck lately."

"A bit! Christ, he's a rapist. And a thief too. Surely you're aware he's stealing your AMA articles and signing them as if he's the author."

Harvey nodded gravely. Slowly he laid down his pipe.

"And all the Dexedrine he takes. Shit, you're the one prescribes it all, Harvey."

"Dexedrine is a mood elevator," defended the doctor.

"High times, you mean. You've got to know how addicted he is by now," objected Morton.

"I know," mumbled Harvey. "I know it, Morton."

The counselor stepped back from the desk and put his hands in his pockets.

"You're an honest man, Harvey. A fair man. Or at least I always thought you were. I know you've been sick, but people are getting hurt in a big way. Somebody's got to do something."

Harvey shifted in his chair. He checked his watch. "I'm meeting with Joseph in ten minutes. Don't let him catch you here, Morton."

"I'm not taking bluffs anymore, Harvey. One way or another these things are going to be resolved. That son of a bitch raped Muriel. I *saw* him beating Sam Lorenzo. I know other things too. Like why Sally Featherman all of a sudden went echolalic. It didn't just happen, somebody drove her to it."

"Sally!" gasped the Freudian. Again he started to bead with perspiration. Morton picked up the nitro vial and handed him a tablet.

"You know more than you're saying," continued the counselor. "Stress can make a man's heart blow faster than a popped balloon. I'm deep into this now. With or without your help I'm going to get to the bottom of it. Come clean, Harvey. Help me. We'll put this place back together the way it should be. We'll make it decent again."

"I can't," said the physician.

"You have to."

"Look, Allison, do you think I let him sign my medical articles out of love? You think I don't know he's horning in on my Directorship? In a way though I think you're right. I am dying of stress. So I tend to eat more, and the heart keeps weakening. If I'd only had the courage when he tore into Sally. I protected Muriel as long as I could, but Dar/Neese will be lost altogether if this kind of thing gets out. I'm not strong like you, Morton. He's got dirt on me. I'm sorry, but my hands are tied."

The Freudian began to cough violently, checking his watch between the harsh reverberations of his flesh. The nitro had done nothing.

"Joseph will be here any minute, Morton. You've got to go."

"He's got dirt on you? What kind of dirt?"

Silence. At last the Freudian sighed deep, as if letting the steam out of his pressure-cooked hell. "Ever want to do a certain thing before you die?" he asked quietly. "Well, I'd like to go down to The Green Room with an ax and a nine millimeter Beretta and—" The physician grasped his chest.

"Christ, take it easy, Harvey!"

"When Sally went echolalic I figured out what he'd been doing. He used their Therapy Sessions to fondle her. At first it probably seemed halfway reasonable, so Sally didn't say anything. I was starting with the heart problems about then. Nobody knew, but I was feeling so sick I could hardly think. By the time he was raping her I was in and out of cardiac intensive care every week or two. But I did confront him, Morton. I want you to know that."

"What'd he say?"

"He admitted it. He laughed and told me I was in it with him from then on. See, once I knew it'd look like a cover-up to the Arbitrators Dar/Neese would go down the drain at the slightest leak. Then Muriel started doing so well, and my papers were being published... I realize it was selfish, but he had me over a barrel, Morton. He promised to quit it with Sally if I'd keep quiet. I guess I should have known he'd start up with someone else as soon as he had the chance."

The counselor shook his head. "We've got to nail him, Harvey."

The Freudian nodded. "I can't tell you how much better I feel," said Harvey. "I've bottled this up for so long. You wouldn't believe the kind of guilt that comes with hiding a lie. You'd be a hell of a therapist, Morton, you know that?"

"You by any chance a Catholic?" wondered the counselor.

"No. Why do you ask?"

"Just wondering. Look, Harvey, we have to do the right thing on this, even if it means bringing the place down."

"I could go any minute. I want to make amends before my heart cuts out. Schopen's done unspeakable things, and I've been a party to them. I agree, we've got to stop him."

"We will, Harvey. I've been to the Courthouse. I can talk to the district attorney if you're willing to testify."

Harvey mopped his brow. "I'll testify."

"I'll talk to Muriel," said Morton. "I don't know how much credibility she'd pull on the witness stand, but it's worth a try."

"They told me Sally started speaking on her own the other day. Do you think she could help us?" wondered Harvey.

"I doubt it," said Morton. "It's mainly you. I know we could get him on assault if we had a witness to the scene on the steps. Did he push me? Tell me the truth. Muriel says he put silicone or something on the floors and tried to kill me."

"He pushed you. His expression was like a murderer. This cold bland grimace. I ran down the hall, but it was too late. When you only broke your wrist I got spooked again. And then you quit. I know, there's no excuse for it."

"Will you testify he pushed me?"

"Absolutely," said Harvey. "I'm going to make the turn, Morton. It's time we put an end to his tyranny."

"Good," said the counselor. "Neither of us could pull it off alone, but together I'm sure we can take him down."

Morton stepped forward and the two men shook hands firmly.

"Now look," warned Harvey. "Joseph really is due in here when he finishes with Sam. I wasn't bluffing."

Just then they heard Joseph's voice in the hallway. "You can take the elevator down, Sam," he was saying. "If you're not in your room in fifteen minutes you'll have hell to pay."

~~~

The Gestapo's Third Reich boots began clip clopping toward Harvey's office. Morton's nostrils flared with anger. He went to the door and threw the lock. Joseph had a key, but this would delay him a few seconds.

Harvey scooped up his pills and keys, dropped them into his shirt pocket, spun his chair 180 degrees, and from a seated position jerked open the window.

"Quick, take the fire escape!" he whispered. "The alarm just rang, so if you're seen nobody will think anything. Go, Morton. And remember, I'll stand by you no matter what."

The Gestapo's hard five thump knock sounded. Morton looked to Harvey, but found the Freudian's eyes glowing wide with terror, all bloodshot and overhung with the fatty lips of his eyelids. Well, not everyone was a gunslinger, you had to accept that.

Swiftly the counselor hustled through the opening and onto the steel platform outside. Harvey frantically pulled shut the window.

Morton glanced down. He was three stories high, the iron rusty and creaking ominously under his weight. His vision blurred in the whipping wind as he saw the odd angle of the concrete steps way below. To establish balance he focused immediately on his feet, and quietly, so as not to rattle the ancient, flimsy welds, began his descent.

From inside he heard the snap of Joseph's key throwing the bolt lock.

"What the fuck's going on, Harvey?" he heard the Gestapo say. "Trying to lock me out or some shit?"

Morton backed down the fire escape. He could hear them bickering above, but soon their voices gave way to the whistling wind and the sound of the traffic below. The rails were overgrown with a patchwork of ivy, which helped conceal him from the road.

Once, when he paused to glance up, he thought he saw Joseph's head pop back inside the window. It was a long distance though, and he couldn't be sure.

* * *

Chapter 41

There was a short distance between the last rung of the fire escape and the ground. Morton made the jump, then hurried to Vera's to retrieve his truck.

As he was pulling out of the lot an ambulance roared by, siren going, lights flashing. He watched as it screeched to a halt part way up the hill, at the entrance to the Fraction House.

This wasn't unusual. Seizures were relatively common among the clients, accidental overdoses, your occasional bleeding problems when people like Odette Gunner chewed too far into their forearms. Still, Morton had a funny feeling about it. He pulled in behind the ambulance.

A small crowd began to assemble on the upper landing. What with the injunction against him Morton couldn't risk joining them. Twenty minutes went by. He shuffled his feet on the sidewalk.

Another ambulance appeared, no lights going, no siren this time. The police arrived. Casually the paramedics entered the building.

At last a stretcher came squeaking through the large double doors. Joseph had hold of one of the rails, helping to ease it down the steps. Morton was careful to remain on the public sidewalk as it bumped to a stop. The counselor angled trying to see what was up. He looked to Joseph. He looked to the group of people who were straggling down from the landing.

Morton's chest began to tighten as he realized what had happened. A long white sheet covered what was obviously Dr. Harvey Mueller's enormous three hundred pound figure, shrouding it all, his face included.

"Joseph, what's happened!" gasped Morton.

The supervisor backhanded the counselor aside. The paramedics positioned the stretcher at the rear of the ambulance. One motioned to Joseph with his clipboard, and together they stepped to the front of the ambulance.

Morton tried to think, to rationalize, but his heart pounded in his ears and nothing came but bile and venom. The counselor gripped the edges of the sheet, and like a magician at a fully set table jerked it into the wind. A swallowed gasp went up from the crowd.

Morton leaned close. "Harvey," he said low.

But Harvey wasn't pale anymore, or even gray. No, he was dead.

Morton raised his eyes to the onlookers. He recognized them all, and yet their faces were foreign. Harvey's eyelids had been fingered shut, but resolving nerve fibers were continuing to twitch in the muscles. Twitching, and now, at exactly this moment, stopping their twitching and freezing the lids eerily open at half mast, as spooky to see as death itself was spooky to stand beside.

Morton was face to face with Harvey, his hand stabilized on the Freudian's massive chest. Under his fingers the counselor felt tiny lumps in Harvey's perspiration soaked shirt. The pills—the critical heart medications! Or maybe the arsenic, worried Morton. Foul play was written all over this.

The counselor hunched close to the corpse. Deftly he reached into Harvey's shirt pocket and secretly worked out the several medications. There was something else with them. Two small brass keys.

"We'll nail him Harvey," whispered Morton to the physician's dead body. "I promise you, we *will* nail him."

It had all happened in a frenzied instant, it seemed. The fire alarm. Gordon. The good talk with Harvey. Hell, his whole life was a frenzy.

And now someone was restraining him from behind. Morton smelled Joseph's cologne and the rancid odor of old tobacco smoke on his day-old growth. A sudden pain split the counselor's side. Was it a punch?

More of a crowd was there, gasping and moaning. "A heart attack," they were mumbling. "We all saw it coming. He overworked. He was a good man though. A good man."

Morton fought for breath, then, without warning, he lurched forward and heaved a wet dressing of vomit over the Gestapo's arm and into the hot Santa Anna winds. Those nearby leapt aside as the vile spray peppered their clothes.

"Uggghhhh!" exclaimed Joseph letting loose his strangle hold, and like an autumn leaf Morton sunk to the ground from nausea.

The counselor was weak as water in the knees, semi-paralyzed with hurt and misunderstanding. He squinted through his tears and saw the sheet crumpled beside him, the shroud. He reached to tug it to him, for like a baby he wanted to tuck a hem under the corner of his chin for warmth.

But then came Joseph's hardened jodhpur boot slamming down on his wrist, the original broken wrist, crunching it into the grit and grime of the sidewalk. The agony was so intense Morton nearly passed out. After a second he heard Joseph's voice hissing in his ear.

"Looks like I'm in complete charge now, Allison. Take this as fair warning. Stay away, or the same thing could happen to you."

* * *

Chapter 42

There was little time to mourn. The need to get Muriel immediately to the Courthouse was paramount. The very next morning Morton rifled through the contents of his briefcase. If he could pull it off just right—the documents, the signatures, the official rubber stamps—well, there was a chance of gaining a little security for her future. The patient would have to appear in person though, not an easy thing to arrange.

Luckily however, Morton recalled that this was the day, Thursday, June 6th, Annise had invited him to join them for—what was it she'd suggested—an early game of Trivial Pursuit? Arrangements had already been made, but when no call came the counselor decided to drive on over.

It was around eleven when he trotted up the iron stairwell. The door was slightly ajar, so he went on in.

He paused at the kitchen, for in the middle of the living room was Annise sitting straddle-wise on a hard backed chair, her arms hanging loosely over the back. She was wearing a short pink slip. Behind her, working over the new kinked-out permanent with a big red comb, was Wanda Novice, the Social Worker.

Morton gazed uneasily at the makeshift beauty salon. Annise was majestic, it couldn't be denied—her legs split apart with the slip dipping between them in a loose U, her skin finer than satin. Wanda leaned toward the militaristic side, her hair brushed back and upward. Tight as bugrugs, these two, wondered the counselor?

"I, uh, guess I should have knocked," stammered Morton, his cheeks burning with embarrassment.

Suddenly he noticed Muriel perched stiffly on the sofa.

"Morton! You came!" she bubbled rushing to hug him. "I told them we should have called you."

The counselor felt his composure draining away. He turned and stepped into Annise's bedroom where he could be by himself for a moment. He was sitting on the edge of the bed when Annise came in.

"I know what you're thinking," said the blonde coming over to him. "You're jealous. I can see it in your eyes. Don't feel bad, it's happened before. I'm almost used to it." She was trying to be tender, but it didn't come off.

"Jealous?"

"I'm not a fool, Morton. I'm well aware Wanda's got something of a gay streak. But she's so nice. I like nice people. What's the matter with that?"

"Nothing," he agreed shuffling his feet. "Nothing at all."

Annise lit one of her new, slim black cigarettes, similar to the kind Joseph preferred.

"She's even trying to help me stop smoking," she added sipping from her mug of coffee. "And Wanda knows so much about relationships, Morton. You ought to talk to her yourself sometime."

Your Annise Chastain, lover of humanity in all its forms. Hard to criticize her for that, wasn't it?

"To be honest," she said, "I'd prefer to use you for my support system. But it seems like when I need it the most you never stroke me."

Morton reached out and softly rubbed her leg.

"Not that way, damnit! I need feedback. I need a lot of Gestalten."

"Gestalten?"

"That's right. You know, talking things out for hours and hours and getting at my issues."

"Wanda does that for you?"

"Uh huh. Let's be realistic. Sundays don't come every day. I can't run to Gary each time I get frazzled. And you're a man, Morton. You wouldn't respect a frazzled chick."

This went on. As far as confessions went, Wanda had proved she could swallow a secret with the best of them. Certainly better than that Gary dude who you could damn well bet never brought a Wiener schnitzel to full boil. And even if he had Morton was confident it'd never been served up on a steamy bed of sauerkraut where a fellow could sink his teeth into the real thing.

~~~

After their talk, Morton, a bit stunned, wandered into the livingroom and sat beside Muriel on the sofa.

"It's terrible about Harvey, Morton. People are so upset they'll hardly talk about it," said Muriel.

"I know," admitted the counselor. "I'm trying not to think of it myself."

"The mood's so black over there. I'm not sure if it's because Harvey died or because Joseph's taken over."

Wanda had the vacuum out. She was cleaning up the last snipped ends of Annise's hair. The blonde appeared with the mug of cold coffee she'd been carrying around.

"Harvey's in a better place," Annise called over. "A better place by far, you two."

"The undertakers?" wondered Muriel naïvely.

"Heaven," replied Annise firmly.

"Not heaven," said Wanda coiling the electric cord. "Nirvana is where he is. Harvey was high level. He'll coast from now on, take my word. Even when he comes back he'll be coasting."

"When's he coming back?" asked Muriel. There was no irony or sarcasm in her voice.

"Wanda thinks we have other lives," explained Annise. "We keep coming back till we get it right, don't we, Wanda?"

The Social Worker and the blonde smiled warmly at one another.

"How about you, Muriel? Do you think you've had other lives?" asked Annise.

Muriel considered it a moment. "Roselawn," she said. "But I don't remember much about it. And I guarantee you I'm never going back."

A half-second pause before Wanda and Annise burst into laughter. Morton laughed too. It was good to break the ice.

"I have to run," announced Wanda. "The Fraction House is a mess, as you can imagine. Joseph's sucking up to the families— I mean, you know, easing their minds about the Harvey thing. They're very worried. We'll do the braiding another day, OK Annise?"

"OK."

Wanda picked up her purse. "Don't forget, I'll come by for Muriel at six tonight. I've got to get her over to Cedars for her hepatitis B vaccine. There'll be a wait, probably. Everyone in L.A. county with a handicap will be in line. If we're late you'll know we went to get something to eat afterwards."

Wanda strapped on the nylon fanny pack she used as a purse. "Hug Annise goodbye for me," she said slapping playfully at Morton's midsection as she passed.

~~~

Annise entered the bathroom where she began her elaborate routine of primping before an important outing.

"What's up?" asked Morton.

"We've got a lunch date with Joseph. He's going to assess my relationship with Muriel. Film us and all so he'll have something for the Arbitrators at the next meeting."

"Lunch with Joseph? Does he know I'm coming?" asked Morton.

"You're not coming. It's going to be Muriel and me." Annise poked her head out of the bathroom. "I'm sure I told you about this. It's been set for a long time."

The counselor looked to Muriel. She shook her head minutely, almost a shudder.

"Joseph's contact with her was cut off by the Arbitrators, you know," said Morton going into the bathroom.

The tub water was running and fogging the mirror. Annise pulled her slip over her head. Underneath she was naked. Strange perhaps for your devout Catholic, but she'd never shown the first scruple about flashing her parts.

"Joseph is evil. You ought to steer clear of him," said Morton.

"Evil can be exciting," she said.

"You better be careful. If you hand Muriel over to him you could get in big trouble. Did she get her own Guardianship for today?"

Annise nodded. "Yeah, but it ends at 8:00 a.m. tomorrow morning."

"If you ask me, it's a set up for another rape," said Morton. "Think about it, Annise. If something bad happens you might even have to testify against him. It's possible you could go on trial yourself."

"Nonsense," said the blonde. "Who's going to say anything about a little lunch date?"

Morton jutted his jaw. Annise was about to step into the tub, but when she saw how hard he'd become she nervously lifted her hands to her mass of newly kinked hair. "You're saying you'd tell, aren't you?" she realized.

"Where are you going to lunch?" asked Morton.

"One of those spots on Hollywood Boulevard, I guess."

"The Green Room?"

Annise's eyes went wide. "Actually I think that is where we're going."

On the spur of the moment the counselor decided to try one of his hunches. "You better leave Muriel here," he said. "If you and Joseph take her to The Green Room again—"

Annise ripped her head in disbelief.

"Again!" she cried. "What do you mean *again*?"

Stark naked, Annise stomped into the livingroom and glared silently at Muriel. "I don't have time to bathe," she said turning and going into the bedroom.

Morton returned to the livingroom. Through the closed door he could feel her fuming as she dressed.

When she came out Annise was a veritable explosion of hair and scent. She had on a gold miniskirt with a daring slit up the side. Exactly the thing for those elevated barstools at The Green Room, mulled the counselor. She smiled her sultry everything-is-hunky-dory smile.

"I hate to admit it, but you're right, Morton," she said going to the door. "This was planned before the Arbitrators made their ruling. I can't risk my career—I mean, Muriel's welfare on a dinky lunch date. I'm going to leave her here with you after all."

"What are you going to tell Joseph?"

"I'll think of something. He's a macho type. I can wrap those kind around my little finger if I have to. All men have their price, Morton. Us girls have to know how to make the payments tantalizing enough, don't we, Muriel?"

Together they looked at Muriel. "Yes. Yes, we do," agreed the schizophrenic staring over at Morton.

"We might stop by Dar/Neese on the way back. Don't worry if I'm late," added Annise. She went to the door.

To Morton the three of them seemed stranded at far ends of the little apartment, an oblique triangle of icy miscommunication.

"I've got your number," called Muriel to Annise.

Silence. Annise's fear was palpable as it stonewalled in the hallway. "You've... You've got my number?" returned the blonde nervously.

"Yeah. I'll give you a call when you get back to the Fraction House maybe."

Annise's sigh of relief pealed through the rooms. For no, so far *none* of them had her number, not even Wanda Novice. Whatever the big secret, it was safe for another hour. A moment later she was gone.

* * *

Chapter 43

For a number of minutes Morton and Muriel sat in silence on the sofa. There seemed such a distance between them, and yet when he'd glance over at her no distance at all, just her easy, understated smile. Were everyone's days such a cracked hodgepodge of unmakable appointments and twisted left turns of emotion, wondered the counselor? Before long he'd be out roaming the city once again.

Was he really so different from Joseph and Annise, even from Wanda or Stacy Lung? After all, this crazy chase was for solace, wasn't it? For asylum. And they all deserved that, surely. Did you find it in Librium? In Dexies? How about in the Gestapo's power-mongering, or the great clueless religions?

Morton shook his head. No, the do-gooders couldn't seem to locate their feeling of peace, but neither could the criminals, no matter how much they'd stolen. Yet somehow it all got whipped together into a weird, smog-like batter, sexy as sin in its exotic newness, all of a sudden jumping out of the top of the cake as 38 D's in a string bikini. A sex asylum, that's what L.A. amounted to, and the Fraction House too for that matter.

Morton looked to Muriel. In a way she was quite the dish herself, what with that Annise Chastain figure poured into her jeans shorts. Despite his flutters the counselor knew sooner or later he'd have to come to terms with her as a full-grown woman. Morton's lips were dry. He licked them before he started to speak.

"Listen, Muriel, we need to make a quick run up to the Courthouse. Timing wise this couldn't have worked out better."

"To the Courthouse? How come?"

"To clear up a few documents. Nothing earth shattering. You know, the usual administrative business. I sign things, you sign things. It's important to do this while you're your own Temporary Guardian. Don't worry, I'm on top of it."

"I didn't worry before and you disappeared to the mountains."

"I made a mistake, Muriel. It won't happen again."

"I didn't mind you going," she returned. "Just remember to take me with you next time. I'll dress really hot and put my new perfume on. We can make a big fire in the bushes up there."

"A fire in the bushes? What are you talking about? You really haven't been acting yourself lately, Muriel."

She crossed her legs. "I tried being myself. It didn't work. From now on I've decided to be somebody completely different. Please don't look at me like that, Morton. It's not schizophrenia if I *decide* to do it. Remember what Harvey used to say? How changing personalities is good if your mind is conscious about it?"

"Harvey said that?"

"You're the one always wanted me to change. So now I'm doing it. Why don't you relax and see if you like the show?"

"The show? What show? I don't know what you're driving at, Muriel, but it's imperative we get to the Courthouse right away. Are you ready to go?"

"I'll have to bathe first," she said.

Muriel rose and stretched her arms languidly into the air. Quite a cry from the jumpy, eccentric movements he expected. In a coiling, snake-like motion she wriggled out of her shorts, then pulled off her Grateful Dead T-shirt. She ambled to the bathroom, and leaving the door open began to casually remove her underclothes. Morton looked across the hallway in confusion as with a dainty dip of her toe she tested the bath water left by Annise.

"I'm going to lay around in the tub a while. Get me out in about an hour." She kicked closed the door.

After her bath Muriel went into Annise's bedroom to dress.

"I want you to know I'm going to be a completely different woman this evening," she called out. "I've been thinking very seriously about this, so get yourself ready."

She seldom wore dresses, but this time she emerged in a beautiful blue calf length skirt. A long slit ran up the side. He noticed too how her eyelashes were darker than normal and appeared to have been curled. Really, she was decked out for a fancy French restaurant. Morton and Sassafras stood side by side, ogling her.

"Close your eyes, Morton," she said, coming up next to him. "Now smell. It's Annise's expensive perfume. *Heroin*, it's called. Don't you just love it?"

～～～

They negotiated the Courthouse paperwork with an unexpected lack of trauma. Muriel signed off on the various forms with a sleepy-eyed composure, which accorded her a tacit admiration from the masses. Composure? Well, maybe it was the revealing slit in the blue skirt. At any rate, Morton caught people staring and nodding to one another when she wasn't looking. Very interesting.

As they were pulling away, Muriel said, "We should eat something. Why don't we stop by the Taiwanese restaurant down from Vera's? I'll run in and get us carryout."

Once there Muriel insisted Morton wait outside. She'd handle the order alone. "I know what you like. Curried pork, right? Don't worry about the money. I owe you a lot more than this," she said.

Hmmm, she really *did* seem different. When she came her white high heels clattered noisily over the pavement. Inside the truck she took him by the hand.

"Do you remember that railroad bridge off Ventura Freeway?" asked Muriel. "You know, where we used to walk with Gordon and Stacy at Sepulveda Dam?"

"Yeah," said Morton.

"Let's go there, you want to? We can look at the water while we eat."

Muriel rummaged under the truck seat.

"I knew you'd forget all about this," she said coming up with the bottle of Pouilly-Fuisse she'd bought for him in Venice. "We'll have us a party."

* * *

Chapter 44

The ride along the freeway seemed futuristic and frightening, as always. At last he navigated in alongside the ancient iron railroad tracks. They parked by a dilapidated plywood shack. When they got out he saw they'd have to walk a distance along the splintered wood of the ties to reach the water.

"Can you make it in that outfit?" he asked.

"Oh, sure," said Muriel lifting off her shoes. "I'll just go barefoot."

Giving him a seductive sideways glance she reached deep under her skirt and slowly, lewdly slowly, began to roll down her stockings. It was hard to tell if this was the new Muriel, the old Muriel, or a stray, anonymous Muriel about to be released into the vast L.A. wilderness. Whichever Muriel this was, she was making it clear she was in need of special attentions.

As they made their way across the uneven ground her hips swung like a model on the runway.

She said, "You know, Morton, I sometimes think about Annise. How she really does walk the walk around the Fraction House."

This was a therapeutic sounding comment.

"How do you mean?" he asked.

"Oh, the way she shakes and shimmies and all. And she talks the talk too. I mean, with all those Valley Girl expressions she uses."

A lot of litter was blowing around. The water shone black and oily. On the horizon the sun was beginning to lower in bright purples. A low humming sound came from the nearby electric towers. At the end of the tracks lay a big square log with rusty iron bolts through it. They sat on the end and Morton opened the bottle of wine with the corkscrew he'd remembered to bring from the glove box. Muriel took a long swig directly from the bottle.

"One has to be careful about one's drinking," suggested the counselor. "It creates a false sense of euphoria, you know."

"I thought any euphoria was a false sense," said Muriel.

"Well, uh, yes, I suppose it is."

Muriel remained notably optimistic, which was a curious trait for her. Even when they began to discuss Harvey she kept a kind of upbeat, detached attitude.

"I like this distance we've been keeping from one another," she said. "Sometimes I think keeping a good distance is what lets people get really close to each other."

"In what way, Muriel?"

"In a spiritual type way. And please don't sigh like that, Morton, because you know damn well it's true."

"Spiritual? I'm not sure I know what you mean."

"Well, did you ever think how you wouldn't even be in L.A. if your wrist hadn't broken? But you're here. We're here *together*. What a wonderful coincidence. We should be grateful."

She reached for the bottle and took another long pull. Funny, since she'd never been much of a drinker.

"Certain things, Morton, are meant to be," she said opening her hands.

"Meant to be? What's that mean?"

"I don't know, but Annise always says it."

~~~

Morton furrowed his brow. They sipped at the wine and kicked their feet like a couple of kids against the pilings. They got the boxes of food out. Muriel tried the chopsticks for a couple of bites, set them aside and reached again for the wine.

"That blonde drinks a lot too, doesn't she?" she muttered under her breath.

The counselor looked over, but she hadn't turned her head. It was pleasant out there in the open, the water so glassy they could see the clouds floating in it. Every so often Muriel would reach over and stroke his back. A real stability had come over her. It was as if the locks had all been unbolted and they were flying around like doves in the soft sunlight.

"Can I ask you a question, Morton? People are saying nasty things about how Harvey died. You didn't punch him or hurt him or anything, did you? Or do something to make him have his heart attack?"

Morton tensed.

"I know you wouldn't do anything bad. But Joseph says he saw you climbing down the fire escape. And right after that they found Harvey dead."

"Joseph saw me?"

"He says he did. Something suspicious must have happened up in Harvey's office. His family wants to have him cut open and checked for crime."

"An autopsy?" said Morton.

"I guess so. I'm afraid Joseph might be trying to get you in trouble."

"There's nothing new there," said the counselor. "How do you know all this, Muriel? You haven't been hanging around with the Gestapo, have you?"

She lowered her head.

"I wish I wasn't so dirty and horrible," she said. "I hate people sometimes. It's so bad to hate. But I had to find out what was going on. I loved Harvey. And I love you, too."

"Joseph told you about the autopsy?"

She nodded.

"What'd you have to do for it? Joseph doesn't give favors away for nothing."

"I told him I'd do what he wanted in the tub one last time. I had to, even though the Arbitrators cut off his Sessions with me. It was the only way I could help you."

"In the tub! Jesus Christ, Muriel!"

"You know what he said, Morton? He said you killed Harvey. He said you snuck into the Fraction House and got in Harvey's office and scared him to death. Or shot him up with a needle or something. He doesn't want any charges against you, though. He doesn't even want Harvey cut open for crime. All he wants is me."

Morton jutted his jaw. "That son of a bitch. So he made you—"

"He wanted to. But when he tried to tell me you killed Harvey I got mad. I said, 'Morton'll kill *you*, you bastard.'"

"What happened then?"

"I squirted shampoo in his eyes and I said, 'Fuck you, Joseph Schopen,' and I ran out of there."

"You did all that for me?" Morton was deeply moved.

"The other times it was my fault," said Muriel. "I let him get away with it. They say a woman can't be held down and have it done to her if she really doesn't want it. This time I really didn't want it."

"Don't be too hard on yourself, Muriel. You've always done your best. All a person can expect in this life is to do their best and let the rest of it go."

"You give me too much credit," she said looking away. "You do it, though. Like not taking a lot of crap off Joseph and Priscilla and them. And with Annise—always watching out for her even when you don't work there anymore. I can be devious. But you're connected to the core, Morton. To the spiritual universe, not to some dopey Catholic religion."

"What do you mean, Catholic?"

"Well, you know, all their dumb beads and saints, and the way they don't use birth control and make the man do all the work in bed."

She caught his eye for a quick instant, then waved her hand. "But that's neither here nor there," she went on. "It's me I've got to think about. I'm the one who has to quit being so hateful and numb to people's feelings like the old Muriel sometimes was."

"But you were never hateful or numb," objected Morton. "You're talking like somebody totally alien to who you've always been."

A sharp silence.

She said, "Somebody like Annise, you mean?"

In a way, Muriel was right. Annise *was* alien to herself. He'd been influenced by her ability to grasp his melancholy, but everyone, really, had their extra sensory perceptions. By degrees he'd become alert to his fear that the blonde might be akin to Roxanne and The Green Room gang, all dolled up with eye jobs, nose jobs, cheek jobs, chin jobs. Making their great offer of purebred sex and unlimited lust to the unwary male. Overwhelming him with first infatuation, with satisfaction and gratefulness because it'd been *given* to him, a bestowal of the finest blonde crotch straight from the heart. But from then on, as everyone knew except the poor sucker himself, he'd have to pay through the nose, for the surgery had been plastic, not authentic flesh and blood like what your addled Muriel Gonska types offered. A lot of times, pondered the counselor, it was easier to see the reflection of the great sphere through a debased crack or blemish, like your schizophrenics did. So women of large caliber, though with eccentricities or even madness helped a guy see truth more than the bubble blonde types, though they might have bigger hooters.

"I've been watching you press the place where your cast used to be," said Muriel low. "You're upset, aren't you? It's probably due to that sleazy bitch. I know you, Morton. You're hurting yourself because of her. I wish there was something I could do to make you feel better."

Muriel downed the last of the Pouilly-Fuisse and flung the bottle into the distance. It clanked metallicly across the gravel without breaking.

"You're absolutely right, Morton. I told you before, from now on I'm going to be a new person," she said, a hint of slur in her voice. "And I want you to be the very first to see me this way."

The silky blue skirt, probably a loaner from Annise, peeled seductively back as Muriel clamored to her feet. She reached out her hand to help him up.

"A new person?" said the counselor dusting off.

"Uh huh. There's secrets in me, Morton. And below them, there's more secrets." They stood there facing each other. "You're smiling. You don't believe me," she said.

"Change is tough, Muriel. "You might be underestimating it."

"In everyone you see, Morton, there's a new person living right underneath the old one. It's not every day these things are actually exposed."

She wore a thin Orlon top, obviously without a bra. Exposed was right. Her eyes flashed in the twilight. She started back toward the truck, then abruptly stopped and cocked a leg sideways onto the railroad track. The skirt rode high on the horizon. A sight to see there among the rust and the shacks as the early minutes of daylight saving time pulled in toward darkness.

Morton picked up on the routine. It was a blatant seduction, and not too shabbily done either. In fact, he was rather touched at how quickly she'd mastered the classic moves.

"Come, Morton," called Muriel curling her fingers. God, but she could be a vixen!

The counselor hesitated.

Muriel put her hands on her hips, another uncommon trait. "Come *on*, for Christsake," she repeated. "There's something in Annise's room I have to show you before she gets back."

"What?"

"You'll see when we get there. But believe me, it could be very serious to do with our future. Annise may have her spies," noted Muriel slyly. "But I've got the key to her box."

Morton raised his eyebrows.

"Now let's get going," she said wheeling and striding out between the silverish tracks.

* * *

Chapter 45

Back at Annise's place they nibbled more out of the boxes of Chinese food.

"Taiwanese, Morton," corrected Muriel. "It's Taiwanese food."

They put the leftovers in the refrigerator beside Wanda's stores of spirulina and carrot juice, and under the packet of hamburger Morton had taken to bringing over for Sassafras. Muriel got Annise's gallon jug of white wine from under the sink, poured a milk glass full and handed it to the counselor.

"You better drink up," she said. "I think you're going to need a bracer for this."

She led him into the bedroom. As always, the calendar and the tray of colored pencils caught his eye. Morton had known from the start Annise had a lot of, well, 'friends' was the word she used, but the calendar with all its codes and notations to keep them straight brought it home in a kind of naked way.

"I want you to know I'm not a snoop, Morton," said Muriel.

She opened the tiny kid leather purse she'd been carrying and handed him a key. Morton recognized it as the one to Annise's locking box.

"Wanda and Annise were in here all morning ooohing and aaahing over something," she told him. "Then they went down to Matthew's Place—you know, the little religious cafe. I came in to change clothes was all. I didn't want to see any of that. They left it all strewn out on the bed."

"Her sex toys, you mean?"

"Yeah, the toys. But something else too very scary. I'm only saying I found the key in the bathroom. Annise must have left it there. I guess I put it in my pocket. I had to. I knew this was something you needed to see. Here, take another drink."

She passed him the glass. Then she got the box out and they sat on the bed much like he and Annise had done so many times. Muriel crossed her legs, the slit in the skirt ascending just shy of the secret auburn garden as one by one she began to remove the items. The negligee. The horses head whip. The ball bearings.

As she leaned to the task Morton could see her breasts lolling bare under the drooping neck line. The pistol appeared. He pushed her hand away and removed it himself. A fierce little thing. Pure death snuggled in close beside the weirdly curved vibrator and the square packet of bonds. Despite himself the counselor felt the fire.

At last Muriel lifted out a folder. On the front Annise had written, *My Confessions*. Inside were the pages from her laser printer.

Hmmm. So she hadn't been joking about inputting her sins each Saturday night. Morton had an ugly premonition. He looked up at the calendar with the abundance of penciled in initials. A bolt of fear shot through him. He found his Librium vial and quickly washed one down with a giant gulp of wine.

"I'll go get us another drink," said Muriel, and she left with the glass.

~~~

Morton swallowed his pride and began to read *My Confessions*. After a minute he knew it was more than pride he'd have to swallow, it was vomit. J.S.? Yes, that was Joel Sincowitz, all right, as she'd said. Only they'd had intercourse three times last week. H.H.? Hudson Harkness. Morton didn't know him. They'd done it twice. The counselor could hardly believe the schedule she'd been keeping. R.S. was there—that was Rodney Stonesipher, the ex-boyfriend. L.S. too. Lance Stonesipher, the brother.

Bitterly he read on. The details were terse but graphic. She was filthy, truly filthy, and seeking it out in this compulsive, spread-eagle way. Friends? Well, they might have been intimate, but they couldn't have been very close, since not a one, excepting Morton himself, had been allotted more than an hour of her precious time.

A wooziness swept over him, a looseness call it, yes, a sort of high, vulgar looseness. Sometimes that happened when your heart sunk without your permission and all of a sudden you didn't know which way to turn.

~~~

Muriel came in and handed him the fresh glass of wine. He took a long drink and immediately felt the effects.

"I'm sorry, Morton. I know how much this hurts you," said Muriel. She stroked his shoulders.

The counselor's head slumped. Damn, but that new Librium was strong! She cupped his cheeks and tenderly pulled his face to her breast.

Morton turned sluggishly through the rest of the pages. He couldn't get over the sheer quantity of men. She was juggling six or eight of these so called 'friends' every week, and new initials were continually showing up on the calendar.

"Look here," he said. "She's got Joseph Schopen down. Jesus Christ, Muriel, she told me she'd never have anything to do with Joseph."

Morton flopped sideways onto the bed. His eyes watered with exhaustion. He was hopelessly sleepy. He reached for the pillow, but by accident dragged some of the scented toys toward his midsection. He sensed a curious arousal. Sex in any form, even of the vilest, most taboo varieties had the potential to get a fellow going. Why *was* that?

"It's all right, Morton. It's all right," he heard Muriel saying.

She was so close he could feel her breath tickle his ear as she comforted him. He shifted and saw Annise's lovely risqué mouth. No, no, it was *Muriel's* mouth, but lovely and risqué nonetheless. He was half loaded, caught in an underhanded daisy chain of arousal, Annise having screwed all those guys and yet holding back like some lily white virgin on Morton himself. The toys. The intense kissing and the awkward penetration of hands where organs should have been. Was it truly the sharp air of crime which made life so stimulating? Doing the wrong thing didn't work, but maybe if you did it with *zeal*— Apparently you had to be hesitant and gung ho *simultaneously.*

Was this Annise's view? On the one side you had your guilt ridden Catholicism, and on the other your Librium and hot rum toddies, he guessed. Either way there was a multiplicity of nymphomania and long armed lechery mucking around the asylum.

"Morton, roll this way," Muriel was saying.

She rippled her shoulders and scooted closer beside him. He felt her recline passively on the bed, though she'd never been the passive sort before.

He struggled to an elbow to see her. Lazily she lifted her fingers through her hair and beckoned him toward her. She made her eyelids flutter. She was different, yes, he thought. In fact, there was hardly a thing about any of it he remembered from the old Muriel. He felt her pulling him toward her. A slow, loving embrace, the skirt lost high on the hips. No longer could he deny it. She was sexy and real.

"We can do whatever we want, Morton," she whispered. "I'm my own Guardian today, remember? Everything's strictly kosher, like you always want it."

A moment passed. "I know what I'm up for doing," she said, her mouth parting ever so slightly.

She eased the counselor onto her. Their lips met in a sultry, naïve kiss, not the criminal heat he'd expected. She wasn't crazy by a long shot. To be honest, he'd known this for quite some time. Romance that hadn't begun as a fantasy wasn't really romance, was it? Or maybe it amounted to the *only* real romance. Hell, what did he know?

After a couple minutes Muriel tapped his arm.

"Hey, Morton—"

"Yes?" He opened his eyes.

"I don't think it's working."

"It's not?"

"I don't think so."

"What do you think the problem is?" he asked.

"I don't know. I guess... I guess I'm not sure who I am today."

"You're not sure?"

"I want you to want me. I'm trying to change, I really am." She slapped her hands on the mattress in frustration.

"I know you are, Muriel."

"I want to be a different person. A totally different person so you'll want me."

"But who, for Christsake? Who in the world could you try to be if not yourself?" objected Morton.

A moment of silence passed.

"Annise Chastain," she muttered. "I want to be like that Annise bitch so you'll want me."

"Oh, Muriel! Listen, baby, if it's any consolation, I want you to know you're doing a damn good job." He hugged her around the neck.

She started sobbing. A like moaning and weeping all mixed together. It got so turbulent the counselor considered popping another Librium to keep the anxiety down.

Suddenly a noise came from the other room. They froze.

"It must be Annise!" exclaimed Muriel.

A second later she'd stowed the locking box and was into the hallway, her clothes smoothed better than if she'd had all afternoon to do it. She opened the front door.

"Hello, sweetie," said a voice. It was Wanda.

"I'm all set to go for my hepatitis shot," volunteered Muriel.

There was a tiny crack in the bedroom door. From the bed Morton watched as Wanda stepped inside. "Annise here?" she asked.

"No."

Wanda nodded. By now she was aware of the blonde's habits.

"Morton's sleeping," said Muriel. "Annise will be back soon. We can go on to Cedars if you want."

"OK," said Wanda. "Is that what you're wearing?"

Muriel kicked her leg naughtily out the slit in the blue skirt. The counselor cringed at her audacity.

"Isn't it all right?" she asked, her voice going to a sexy tinkle.

"Whew whee!" ogled Wanda. "Sure, you can go in that. No problem. God, I'd be proud to be seen with a chick— I mean, with a lovely woman like you."

Morton peeped into the hallway as Wanda opened the door and like a butler held it there. Muriel said, "Wait here, Wanda. I'll be right back."

Muriel returned to the bedroom for her shoes. The counselor looked up. She leaned and winked at him. Then she strode away, Wanda Novice still holding the door for her.

That Muriel Gonska, he reflected putting his hands behind his head. She wasn't so blind to working those slippery gray areas herself, was she?

* * *

Chapter 46

Annise returned a couple hours after dark. Morton was on the sofa with the lights out. Without comment she flipped the switch on, entered the kitchen and looked under the sink. "Want a glass of wine?" she asked.

"Uh huh," he muttered.

"I guess Muriel went for her hepatitis shot."

Annise came with the glass of wine, leaned and kissed him on the forehead. He could smell the fragrance on her hair as it washed across his chest, the ultra-pricey *Heroin* mingled with—yes, it was unmistakable—the Gestapo's acidic *Paca Roma* cologne. She wasn't disheveled. No, he'd never catch her out of uniform.

"Why does she need those shots anyway?" asked Morton.

"Because half the people at Roselawn are infected with it. You know that as well as I do," said Annise.

"Roselawn? My God, are they really going to send her back to that place?"

"It looks like it," she said. "But I'm not sure of all the details."

"You should be, hanging out with the Gestapo all the time."

Annise eyed him. She got up and put a CD on. They sat there strangely subdued with this like whistling bagpipe music floating in the background. There seemed everything worth saying, a mountain to communicate, yet all they did was cross their legs and drink, the blurry silence eating into the mood like those locusts out of the Bible. A solitude of the heart it was, at least for Morton.

"I suppose Muriel will be back before long," he said.

"I doubt it. There's a big conference tonight. Wanda said Muriel would probably bolt if we told her about it. Sandra Dar herself is going to attend for once. And two or three board members."

"Really? Why didn't you tell me? What's going on over there?"

Annise shrugged. "She might come later. And anyway, you're done with that place. Can't you try to forget it for a while?"

"I can't forget it," said Morton. "Everybody says she does better when she's seeing me. And now this with Harvey. I don't know if you're aware of it, but Joseph's all over her."

"So what? She's pretty," said Annise. "She's going to have to face these things in the real world."

"Face what? Rape? Nobody deserves that. I mean, don't you care just a little bit about her, Annise?"

"Of course I do," she insisted snapping her glass down. "But what about me, Morton? Can't you see what a wreck *I'm* becoming? They're working me to death. There's always a thousand things going on in my life, and nobody at all to talk to. These last couple of days I've even seen lines around my eyes. See here? See all these little lines?"

She seemed awfully testy. Was it that time of the month? Or maybe she was concerned about the tumor. She'd promised to see a doctor, but each time he asked about it she hedged. She turned the music off.

"But, Annise," began Morton, "if you all didn't tell Muriel— I mean, it's Wanda's obligation as the Social Worker to be truthful—"

"To hell with Wanda Novice. Don't you know what she is, Morton?" Annise wheeled around. "She's a fucking lesbian! Everybody at the Fraction House knows it too. And do you know what she did this morning? She came right up behind me and adjusted my bra straps. She said they were twisted and she unhooked them and re-hooked them and everything. Can you believe it?"

"You're a sexy girl, Annise. Wanda sees that too."

"I am not! Here," she said. "Get me another drink. I mean, will you *please* get me another one?"

Morton was waking up to her devices. She employed the distraction method. Go to bed with Joseph, throw up the smoke screen of Wanda or some other nonsensical lines around the eyes issue. Once you were wise to the clues the plot wasn't so hard to see. He went to get her a glass of wine.

"You need another one too," said Annise coming into the kitchen.

"Just for the record, it's not *Nah*vice," said Morton. "It's *No*vice. The way you say it it's like she's a greenhorn or something. She's not, Annise. She's very skilled."

"I know what *novice* means," she said glaring at him. "It means she's not experienced. You don't have to explain everything to me just because you went to fancy Johns Hopkins."

Johns Hopkins? Morton never said that. Hopkins was the school Joseph had the crooked diploma factory print up for his fake degree.

Annise left and returned with a dictionary. "Newly acquainted," she growled thumping the book. "Exactly what I said."

She turned and stomped into the bedroom. Morton shuffled in after her. She was removing shirts from her chest of drawers, unfolding them, folding them up again and stuffing them back in the drawers.

"I've tried to give you hints," she fired. "I've tried to let you know how much it irritates me. But you keep on doing it."

"Doing what?"

She pulled out a sweater, unfolded it, folded it back and jammed it into the drawer.

"Everything, Morton. Just everything."

The counselor gulped his wine. "Listen, I want to talk about Joseph. I want to talk about the calendar and a lot of other things."

"You're off the wall, Morton. You better take one of those Libriums and pull yourself together."

She stormed out of the bedroom. Without a second thought the counselor popped the pill into his mouth.

In the living room Annise began to look over her collection of the Maccabees and her Irish picture books. Interpreting her was similar to the way people described reading the Bible. It could mean anything either of them wanted it to. This was a problem.

"Did you know?" said Annise breaking the silence. "Wanda's been in Confrontational Therapy for six months now. You didn't? Maybe it's Transactional Therapy, I forget. She's got ODD—Oppositional/Defiant Disorder. Anyway, her therapy is very productive. Wanda says screaming hateful stuff at each other is the only way she keeps from flying off the handle the rest of the week." She paused thoughtfully. "I was wondering if that sort of thing would help us?"

"We already have it, don't we?"

Annise squinted at him. "At least *I'm* seeing a therapist. I'm trying to get it worked out. You're not doing anything."

"A therapist? Really? Who?"

"By the way, Harvey's viewing is tomorrow," said Annise changing the subject. "Are you going? The funeral will be a day or two later, I guess."

"I thought his family wanted an autopsy. If ever an autopsy was warranted, this is the time."

"I don't know why you'd be so hot on it, the way all the gossip is. Harvey's family thinks there could have been foul play. I mean, a bunch of people saw you sneaking down the fire escape. Joseph included," said Annise.

"So?"

"So an autopsy might incriminate you."

"*Me*! What do you take me for, Annise?"

"I'm not taking you for anything. I'm talking about the law. You can screw around with justice, but you can't screw around with absolute circumstantial evidence. At least not if the autopsy shows something up. Quit staring at me. Joseph's going to cover for you. You should be grateful, Morton. First he said he saw you run down the fire escape. Now he's saying he didn't see you. What could be more decent of him than that?"

"The Gestapo's covering for me?"

"He's concerned about you, Morton. I don't know why you can't see it."

"I'm after the truth, that's why. Joseph doesn't want Harvey cut open because he'd be found riddled with poison. It's like when sperm was inside Muriel. If they'd have checked her they'd have found Joseph Schopen in there. And if they'd check Harvey they'd find him in Harvey too. Not me. I didn't do anything to anybody."

"Can you prove that?"

Morton gritted his teeth. In a sudden moment of clarity he realized that no, he couldn't prove it.

"I'm no murderer, Annise. But when it comes to somebody like Joseph I might be willing to change my tune."

Annise gasped. A twinkle of excitement shone in her eye.

Tense, temperamental minutes passed. The critical subject *was* going to be addressed. This was the time for it, but perhaps not the place. Morton suggested they go out to dinner.

Annise hesitated.

"Don't worry, I'll pay," said the counselor brusquely. He was getting a bit peeved with her scenes lately.

"OK. But I'll have to wash my hair," she said.

"It looks clean to me."

"It's filthy, Morton. And I'm all out of creme rinse. Would you do me an itty bitty favor?" she asked turning soft. "Would you run down to the corner and get some?"

She found a piece of paper and wrote '*Cloister Creme Rinse.*'

"Thanks so much, Morton. Danny's Market. You can't miss it." She stepped back and waved goodbye, though he was standing right there in front of her.

At the checkout counter Morton had a hard time believing how much it cost.

"Nine dollars for creme rinse? Is this really possible?" he asked the checkout girl.

"Oh, yeah, it's possible," returned the girl. "*Cloister's* the silkiest of them all. It's like if you put Teflon on your hair. No matter how you move it falls back perfect. It's worth the money."

"Well, OK, then," mumbled the counselor.

~~~

Back at the apartment he climbed the stairwell and turned the knob. It didn't open. He'd gotten used to rapping and going on in. This time though the door was locked. He could hear her padding around, lighting a cigarette probably, taking a few extra seconds to put her slippers on. Finally she came.

"Why is the door locked?"

"What?"

"The door, Annise. I left it open so I could get back in."

"I was about to hop in the tub, Morton. I always lock up when I bathe, you know that. Did you get the creme rinse?" She looked into the bag. "Yes, this is it. Come *in*, will you?"

Annise's bubble bath foamed absurdly over the rim. Morton folded close the toilet lid and sat down as she lowered gingerly into the steaming water.

"Remember the talk we had about fidelity, Annise?"

"Sure, I remember."

"You said you absolutely believed in it."

"So?"

"So do you?"

"Of course I do. Christ, we've been through all this, haven't we?" She shifted under the bubbles.

"You left the key to your box out. It was on the sink with your makeup."

"My key?" Annise became very still.

"I couldn't wait any longer. I had to know for sure what all those initials on your calendar meant."

Annise was stone faced. "You didn't trust me?"

"You're always with Joseph. You smell like Joseph half the time. I saw your Confessions, Annise. I know it's not only Joseph. It's Lance. It's Joel. It's—" Morton felt suddenly ill.

"Did you hear what Rodney said that day in Venice?" he asked her. "He told me not to end up like road kill on pretty Beaver Boulevard the way he did. What'd he mean, Annise?" Morton took a swig of wine.

She hung her head. "Where's my key now?" she said.

Morton dug it out of his pocket and handed it to her.

"You think I'm horrible, don't you?"

The counselor was silent.

"Let me tell you something, Morton. I don't even like those guys. I know they lie to me. But they're such shitheads they can't even make it *sound* true. Don't you see? That's why I don't bother with a relationship."

"But you keep going to them, Annise."

"They're not real though. They're fabrications. They're fantasy. Christ, do you think anybody in their right mind could do such things?"

"Not real?"

"Not in my mind's eye. That's where a person lives. I wanted to be a virgin with you though. It's what a person *intends*, not what they actually sneak around and do. I've been keeping you on a pedestal, Morton, can't you see this?"

"But what about our relationship?"

"Toys aren't for real when you're a grownup. Those people are only for one reason. It doesn't have anything to do with a relationship. They're incapable of relationships. I'm doing what I have to, Morton. Us Catholics are always about to blow apart with passion. It's kind of like being terribly angry and out of control. You can't take it all out on one person. Everybody in the grocery store gets a piece of your mind."

"Doing what you have to? Damnit, Annise, you're risking everything. You're risking your life. Bad men are out there. Bad diseases too."

"I wouldn't jeopardize you, Morton."

"But you are jeopardizing me. I read those Confessions. I saw how long the list is."

"I'm safe though. I swear I am. Nobody gets a chance at me without protection. You know how scared I am to die. I go every month for the test. Let me show you the paper."

She surged out of the tub, and leaving a movie set trail of foam headed for the locking box.

Morton followed. She was shaking she was so nervous dumping the lurid contents across the rug. Frantically she searched for the paper.

"Here it is. See? This is last week. 'HIV negative. Other STDs negative.'"

"What are STDs?"

Annise wagged her head at his naïveté. "Sexually transmitted diseases," she whispered going red.

"But why, Annise? Why act like a... a..." He couldn't bring himself to say it.

"I do it out of love, Morton. It's not for my own satisfaction at all."

"Love?"

"You might not believe this, but I swear on a thousand Bibles it's true. It's the Trickle Down Theory, like they have in economics. If you give love to one person, though they may not love you again or call you back for a week or two, or even ever, that love still goes to the next person they meet, and the next, and so on. So in the big picture you're adding more and more love to world."

"You mean love or sex?" asked Morton.

"Love. Think about it a minute. Don't you have a warm feeling somewhere in your heart for the times you've been laid?" Annise cringed at the dirty word. Morton shrugged.

"Admit it. You do, don't you?"

This was the thing about Annise. Bold, yet in her way modest and shy. She came at a topic from every direction at once, which was an asset, wasn't it? A quality to be desired in a woman, right? Still, there was no getting around her personal venue of pornography.

"This isn't the point," he objected. "The point is you deceived me. And frankly I have trouble respecting people who deceive other people. All that crap about protection. You're always trying to make sure I don't use any protection."

"I have to use the rhythm method with someone I want a relationship with. For us Catholics it has to be birth control without exactly being birth control, you know what I mean? Shit, Morton, you're the only decent thing in this godforsaken city. I know I can be a bitch sometimes. I need to stop that. I need to stop everything keeping away your respect for me."

"But why me, Annise, when you've got half of L.A. county on the string? And I know they all like you."

She gave a heavy sigh. "That's exactly the problem. *You're* the kind of person I need respect from, Morton. Can't you understand? I want you to want me because you *don't* like me. You don't even like my type. Of course the others are going to want me, but only because I don't want any of them."

"But Rodney really likes you, Annise."

"Joseph," she corrected glaring absently at the calendar.

"But Joseph really likes you."

"It makes me feel bad when people like me, Morton. I don't deserve to be liked."

The counselor began to see deeper psychological issues at work here.

"Don't talk that way, Annise," he said.

"And the more they like me the worse I feel. Right there's the hitch with Joseph, if you really want to know. And it's why I'm so attracted to you."

"Why?" he asked.

"I told you, because you're not interested in me. Deep inside I know that's exactly what I deserve for being so underhanded about things."

"So all this with the men and the calendar is going to stop?"

"If you say so."

"Joseph included? And anyway, what about adultery? I mean, fornication. That's what you've been doing."

"Look," she said fanning out her Confessions on the bedspread. "This is my salvation. Gary—I mean, you know, the Assistant Priest, has seen every single week from top to bottom. When a Catholic gets absolved, Morton, she starts all over again totally unbesmirched. Totally immaculate, like a baby."

The counselor furrowed his brow. Annise was coiled in a sheath of slowly bursting bubbles and glistening droplets. A sight to see there on the rug with the little Buddha looking over her shoulder, the little Madonna rather. His torment seemed small and dim, a weak light through a long narrow tunnel. It flit through his head that the recent Librium might be coming on, easing the pain of the confrontation. He sipped harder at the wine.

Such was your modern Catholicism, he reckoned. Well, he was doing his best to understand it.

He noticed her pausing to caress the gun as she began to clean up the mess. She flashed him her patented ultra-feminine smile. It had only one story behind it, and they both knew how it read.

* * *

Chapter 47

Annise left suddenly for the bathroom, not an abnormal trait for the female.

Morton felt dizzy and overheated. He took his shirt off. He undid his belt. The barrel of the pistol, he could see, was sticking up around a new packet of stocks. The room began to spin. Annise appeared.

"Getting naked again?" she said. "I was hoping we could be more modest this time."

Modest? She opened the closet and shifted the coat hangers. She mumbled something about a gown he didn't quite hear.

"Are we going to bed?" he wondered.

"I'm really on fire. Do you mind if we go out to eat later?"

She left again for the bathroom. Morton struggled up and started looking through the closet. Modesty, he kept thinking. When in doubt do the most religious thing, right? Which was cover up with fig leaves your, uh... your...

Nothing in there seemed very suitable though. He noticed a baggy maroon gown. That might do.

Another sip from the wine glass. Everything becoming foggy and unreal. Then, in the next instant mysteriously lucid, as crystallized and tangible as a diamond chandelier. He crawled under the covers and waited for her.

~~~

Annise returned, opened the closet and swung the hangers back and forth.

"Where's my red gown?" she asked. She checked behind the chair. She bent over and looked under the bed.

"Morton, where's my red gown? I saw it a minute ago."

He shifted uneasily in the covers. "I, uh, might have made a mistake, Annise," he said low.

"Why? What have you done with it?"

"Well, I guess I'm wearing it," he said shyly.

"Oh, Morton, you can't be!"

Cautiously he lowered the blanket. They could see lace around the wrists and at the hem. The neckline plunged far down.

"My God!" she cried. "That's ridiculous! For Christsake, take that thing off!"

"But why?" he objected.

"Because, it's stupid. It's not like you to do a thing like this."

Morton got to his feet, peeled it off and handed it to her. Underneath he was nude.

"I thought you didn't like me without my clothes," he reminded her returning to the bed.

"I don't. But I'm certainly not going to make love to a transvestite either."

~~~

She didn't seem to hold it against him though. Of course, she was naked herself. Not even wearing the little gold anklet with the cross on it. Her hair remained wet and tangled.

Before they started she spent a lot of energy checking over the dates on her calendar. She went to the bed and hoisted a leg over him. She reached up and pulled the cord twice on the green paper lantern she'd gotten in Taiwan. It dimmed and swayed gently above as they began to make love.

"Don't you think we should use protection?" whispered Morton.

"Birth control?" she asked.

"Well, yeah."

"I... I have to use rhythm with somebody I love," she said meekly.

He heard what he thought was a flutter in her voice, but at the time didn't make anything of it.

"You... You love me?"

She smiled and looked away.

He hadn't been aware of what a healthy lust could do to a Catholic once they finally caved in to the drive. More like molten lava when it came at you than mere licks of fire. At last the steam of her breath and her buttocks and her pert high breasts doing the thinking for them.

Over her shoulder, however, he couldn't miss the impact of that enormous calendar. Yet in a strange way it added a seamy eroticism to the mood. Other men, he pondered? And miserable Joseph only a few hours ago? Joseph Schopen, the murderer. And here they were doing this thing which could give life, should it accidentally take.

Pregnancy? He'd never really thought of it, though Annise had mentioned it on a number of occasions. What kind of wife would she make, anyway? She wanted a little Morton, she'd said. An infant in swaddling clothes to nurse in the way a woman was meant to. So she'd said.

They were really getting stoked up, when out of nowhere she grasped his hips and held him very still.

"Morton! Stop!" she said.

He slowed.

"I'm sorry. I'm so sorry," she panted.

"No, Annise. Don't be sorry. Everything's all forgiven now," said Morton.

"I can't follow through with this. I'm doing something horrible to you. Something really terribly horrible. And what's worse is you don't even know it."

"Please, Annise. It's all going so perfectly," pleaded the counselor.

She was poised over him, eyes taut as marbles. "I can't," she said. "I just can't."

By degrees, though, he realized they weren't going precisely by the rules. Because in the dead center of this burning anointment of the flesh she maneuvered herself around backwise and ripped her head toward him.

"I want you to say something for me," she squeaked as they resumed. "I want you to tell me I've been a bad girl. I need to be punished, Morton. Tell me you're making me. Please do it. Say, 'I'm making you do this, you bitch.'"

The counselor opened his mouth, but he simply couldn't say it for her. There was bizarre, and then there was *bizarre*. She whipped her head around.

"Say it, goddamnit!" she cried. "Say, 'I'm making you, you miserable bitch!'" Her eyes were hot and red as she squinted at him over her shoulder. They frightened him.

"I'm making you, you miserable bitch," he whispered weakly.

It worked at first. But soon came this drying inner sag. Her head rotated again. "Spank me, Morton. I'll never get over this unless you help me. I've got to be spanked and it has to be totally real." He hesitated. "It's either the hand or the pistol. Take your pick."

"The pistol?"

"I have to be forced. This needs to be like a rape or else there won't be the first bit of therapeutic effect. Rape may be the worst thing that can happen to a person, but if you've been really bad it's the sweetest feeling punishment." A smile of inner turmoil came at him over her shoulder. "You know what they say. 'Happiness is a warm gun.' Now quit wimping around and do this for me."

"It'll be painful, Annise."

"Sometimes pain can be perfect," she returned. "Rocket fuel hot. Pink welts and a few tears can do wonders for a wench."

"It can?"

"Sure. It's a documented fact Carmelite nuns whip each other in the inner sanctum. Look, God wouldn't have the balls to make spankings hurt so hot unless there was something super fine about it. He's not in this for his health, you know."

Morton heard a threatening quality in her voice. Was she about to panic?

"Do it!" she hissed. "Do it right now!"

In the spirit of the moment he halfheartedly swatted her across the buttocks.

"Talk to me," she insisted. "Tell me you're making me. And mean it!"

The counselor struggled to find his role. When she looked back again he peeled up his lips in a vague attempt to bare his teeth, "I told you," he said reluctantly. "I'm making you. Now turn back around and do it."

"Say, 'You miserable bitch.' I have to hear you tell me."

"You... You miserable bitch," he muttered weakly.

Luckily that last seemed to do it. The crazy game played right and true, even if it went against your grain and had to sting your palm in the process.

Her arms flew apart and downward like wings. She clutched at the covers. At last the body freed up and thrusting every which way. He heard her groaning out words she'd never in a million years have uttered. And this, she cries hurling back her head. And this is my *cunt*!

There was more, and not necessarily the tenderest things he'd ever heard either. Her voice spiked and irascible, like glowing charcoal, like one of those demon-possessed actors in the movies. She was talking about her father, it seemed. Or maybe it was *the* Father, he wasn't sure.

Soon he felt it building in her. Her arms swept close to her body. She screeched out the name of Jesus and his mother, and others Morton wasn't too familiar with, then dropped flat onto the mattress.

A terrible thing? A violent thing? No, of course not. It was a performance of beauty and wonder. In sympathy with her exhaustion he arched along her torso like one of those pictures of clocks melting in the limbs of trees.

As the counselor was learning regarding women, it wasn't always over when it was over. Annise seemed lost in the fury of her own release.

Morton made an effort to continue, but he was over heated and began to cough. It was one of those little tickling spasms in the back of the throat he was prone to. He tried to stifle it, but it wouldn't hold. Sometimes these things happened, and always, it seemed, at the most inopportune moment. He made an effort to cough with his mouth shut, to sort of swallow the spasm the way you might choke back a sneeze. His body, he knew, was jerking around strangely, yet there was nothing to do about it. It occurred to him that Annise might interpret this as, well, more excitement say than what he was actually experiencing. His heaving motion was accidentally mimicking climax.

Sure enough, her eyes bolted open. He felt her deliver a weird twist, as if to pull free. Then, rethinking it he assumed, she reached awkwardly around, snatched him by the hips and drew him powerfully to her. For many seconds she held him there.

Morton surged again with a cough, trying desperately to turn his head away. A cough though, that's all it was.

~~~

After a minute Annise kicked out of the covers and rushed to the calendar. She stared intently across the rows of weeks. At last she picked up one of the colored pencils and made a notation in the margin.

"Jesus Christ Almighty!" she cried placing a group of fingers on her forehead.

She made the sign of the cross, then turned and gazed at him. Lovingly almost, it felt. She rushed to the base of the bed, feverishly gripping the rail. She beckoned him to her and started hugging him.

"Thank you, Morton! Thank you! Thank you! Thank you!" she exclaimed. "You've given me the greatest gift one person could give another."

The counselor didn't try to psychoanalyze it. Hell, everybody from Joseph Schopen to Sigmund Freud had failed at that.

"You're welcome, Annise," he said simply. "You're very welcome, my friend."

* * *

Chapter 48

The moments passed. Finally the day returned—the night, rather. At last they were sensing what had been done, and that they were there together, a couple.

After her initial enthusiasm the mood flattened as if a steam roller had cruised through. Annise sat on the edge of the bed, slightly slumped, then stretched onto her stomach and stayed there for the longest time, her head turned toward the wall.

The counselor stroked fondly down her shoulders in an effort to caress her back to herself. Before long he came to the troubling place at the crease of the buttocks, the weird little mound under the skin. He felt carefully, anatomically so to speak, and by her uneasiness he knew she was aware of his probes. A mass was there, no doubt about it this time. He thought he heard something. Yes, tiny, subdued sounds were coming from deep in the pillow.

Gently he tried to turn her, but she resisted. Her glass of wine was on the night table. She reached over and downed the rest of it.

"Please don't be upset. Nothing's wrong, Annise," said Morton.

"Nothing's wrong?" she echoed lifting up kind of woodenly.

Annise snatched the red gown off the floor and slipped it on. She went to the vanity and lit a cigarette.

"What'd I do with my drink?" she asked looking around. She grasped herself at the temples. "My God!" she moaned. "What have I done, Morton? What have I done, what have I done?"

There was no consoling her. She launched into a barrage of words, a torrent of accusations and criticisms the counselor could only partially put together. The ugliest of things had happened, she said. A sickening thing. A hellish thing. She lifted her rosary off the mirror and every few seconds recited one of the beads. There was a real evil in all this, she told him. An infestation of evil. You always knew it too, because the guilt wouldn't wash off and you fucking stayed dirty.

"No, Annise. It was beautiful. It was perfect. Next time will be better, you'll see."

"Next time! Don't you realize what has taken place here? Don't you even know why—" She gritted her teeth. "Why I've got this cancer?"

Morton tried to touch her but she jerked away.

"This entire business is useless," she said. "Pathetic and useless and evil. I really wish you'd go."

"Go? What do you mean?"

"I mean one of us here is a whore. I'm not blind, Morton. You think I don't know you're out to get all you can from me? I see you eyeballing my stocks. You're like all the rest. You want a pretty piece to show off on your mantle. I've got a beautiful soul, mister, and it's obvious you don't give the first shit about it."

Morton found his clothes and began to dress.

"And the craziest thing is you don't even *care* about money," she went on. "You're like those street people who take what they can and bolt under another bridge for the night. Now my body's all screwed up. Christ, you'd make a person pay soul *and* wallet if you could take them for it."

Morton knew he needed to keep quiet, but this was too much.

"It sounds like you're talking about yourself, Annise, not me," he said boring into her. "Where's the money for Danny's Market? For a hundred errands I've done? And even when you fuck you do it anonymously, and afterwards take that back too. Then have it all back, sweetheart. I give every last bit of it back to you."

He made a motion like he was handing her something. A cold second went by.

"It wasn't me," she said low.

"What?"

She looked up from under her eyelashes. "It wasn't me, Morton. It couldn't have been me."

"What are you talking about?"

"I... I didn't have a choice," she muttered. She ran her fingers nervously through her hair. "I didn't want to. You made me do it. You did. You knew I never wanted to right from the start." She lifted her head. "You even said I had to do it. You said, 'I make you, I make you,' didn't you?"

"You told me to," said Morton.

She sighed. "A man isn't supposed to do everything a woman tells him to. Everybody knows that."

"They do?"

"What kind of a world do you think we'd have if men did everything women said?"

"A sexy world?" ventured the counselor.

"An insane world. A violent world. If you had any idea how many Catholic girls need to be spanked, and how many kids end up getting spanked because their husbands won't—" She halted. "Ah, hell, forget it. Plus, you called me—" A shiver racked her body. "You called me a miserable bitch."

"No, Annise, this is all wrong."

Morton reached out to comfort her. She slapped hard at his hand.

"You're the batterer," said Annise. "A person doesn't do anything they don't want to do. And we both know damn well what you just did."

"What'd I do?"

"You... you forced me. If that's not the definition of rape I don't know what is."

"Rape? You're saying... You're saying *I*—"

It took several moments before he understood what she was telling him. Even then it was difficult to believe. Her stare was carnivorous and hard, and at last he did understand. The nightmare came blowing like a fire storm across his forehead.

The counselor shot to his feet. This startled Annise. She recoiled into the vanity. Tiny decanters of scents and lotions tumbling recklessly off. Liquids draining into the carpet. The fumes rising and mixing with the lingering cigarette smoke.

Morton was shivering, inside and out. He was about to say something hurtful, but decided not to.

He finished dressing, not once looking her way.

Then he turned and went through the door, slamming it behind him so hard it flew straight through the jamb and into the bedroom side, where it dangled limply on its hinges.

He walked to the front of the apartment. Sassafras trotted at his heels. He was about to slam that door too, but instead paused, and said, "You're a good girl, Sassafras. I love you so much."

He petted her small, silky head, then eased out into the dark L.A. night.

* * *

Chapter 49

Outside it was cool and windy. Sometimes Morton could smell the sea in the air, but not this time. He walked past Matthew's Place, the little religious cafe. He passed The Rusty Fisherman, a new lounge Annise had shown him. Although it was a bleak, moonless night the jumping headlights of the automobiles and the brilliant L.A. streetlamps made it seem like high noon.

The counselor returned to his truck and drove to Vera's Russian Diner. He bought a newspaper from the machine and opened it on the counter.

God, but desperate people were out there, he read. Shooting each other with automatic weapons. Losing arms and legs. Going on kidney machines. Over here hearts blowing out from too much fat in the diet, said page two; over there starving to death from the rice famine, said page three. California, he saw on page five, was second only to New Jersey in one significant feature—pollution. Interesting? Or was this dangerous information he'd be better off not hearing about?

He came to an article on cancer. At first a shaky chill for Annise ran through him. Yet these things were printed all the time. They listed the statistics. One in three was bound to come down with it. Which meant either Muriel, Annise, or Morton himself...

He asked Vera for two glasses of water and a cup of black coffee.

"Men who drink much water drink much alcohol first," noted Vera. "This is not like you, Morton."

She waddled away. That Vera. Legs like tractor wheels and arms like tree trunks, but as honest and decent as they came.

Morton pushed the paper aside. He noticed an attractive black haired woman several stools down. What, he wondered, might be at the base of this pretty one's spine? It was late. Morton smiled. She smiled back. Something of the old L.A. run and hide between the legs of a new person was stretching between them.

Sexual relevance! Awesome how a mere shadow of a vibe could lift a person's despair, though the card might never be played.

~~~

Annise was distraught. More, she was haunted by the repercussions of her own behavior. It was a moral axiom, wasn't it, that people wouldn't do a bad thing if they honestly knew it was bad? After all, she was a people person. Not so much a lover of nature as a lover of humankind, of the multitudes, of men and women and babies. She was like the overbred Persian cat racing around the back alley. The nine lives? Well, they had nothing to do with avoiding death. They were simply doing different activities each day with different people and being thoroughly absorbed in each life, all nine of them sometimes, including, Morton had to accept it, Joseph Schopen's life. Risky business, to be sure. Unsafe in more ways than one. Who knew what horrendous messages those ladies in The Green Room kept hidden in their Dirt Devil vacuum cleaners? She swore she was safe though.

Vera came to refill his coffee. "This blonde girl. She drink alcohol?" she asked.

The counselor shook his head adamantly. It was a lie maybe, but a white lie. Best to temper gossip with a side order of discretion.

Vera wagged her head in response. "I do not believe," she grumbled.

Annise, Morton felt sure he'd intuited, was not purposely malicious. He recalled one of their early training days. She'd been trying so hard, yet Harvey had to bring her in for a talking to.

"He told me I was twisting people's minds. You have to remember, Morton, those minds *came* twisted. I was only twisting them back where they belonged."

It wasn't that Annise didn't take criticism, rather she simply didn't hear it. She wanted no obstacles getting in the way of her joys. Even when she was sad she found a way to turn it around and call it happy. "Sometimes I'm so optimistic it worries me," she'd said. She could tell you hard things too, but she didn't always mean them the way they came out. A fellow had to listen carefully for the underlying tenderness. Like the time she said, "I like your looks this way, you know, with your beard grown out a week or so, all scruffy and rugged."

"You mean when I'm ugly?"

"Well, yes. It puts me at ease to be around somebody inferior."

And of course she harbored other qualities which were downright endearing. The night in the Cuban bar, for instance, when she'd looked over at him with such innocence. "I don't see how married people manage to get to work on time," she remarked.

"Why wouldn't they?"

"It seems to me they'd get wrapped up in making love every morning. And I'm hardly ever on time to begin with," she said smiling.

"Every morning?" wondered Morton nervously. "Would you make love *every* morning, Annise?"

A look of dismay came over her. "Well... Yes." Her voice had lifted an extra octave.

No, he decided, it wasn't too late. She said she'd stop it with the other men. With Joseph too, hadn't she? Fairness, that was the thing. Fidelity too, for that matter. He slapped the counter. No one should be beyond putting a measure of humility into their life.

Yes, by God, go back to her. Straighten this misconstrued crap out. That was the respectable thing to do.

* * *

Chapter 50

Morton parked in front of Annise's apartment. He didn't go directly up, but instead spent a long while walking the nearby streets, breathing the crisp night air. He waited until his head rang clear and sober. He wanted nothing in the way this time.

When he finally mounted the stairwell and checked his watch he was alarmed to find it close to 2:00 a.m. He'd been away for hours.

The lights were off. She'd gone to bed. As a last hope he twisted the knob. She'd locked it, naturally. He twisted it the other way, and click, the latch tripped. What a stroke of luck!

The hinge creaked as he stepped onto the carpet. An odor of spilled perfume was all through the place, but now it somehow smelled rich, lusty even. The shades were drawn tight. He had to feel his way down the hallway.

In the living room he caught a scary glimmer from the wall mirror. It startled him. But no, it was his own shadowy reflection.

He heard a kind of breathing sound, and sensed a small motion on the sofa. He didn't blame her, he wouldn't have slept in the bedroom either. Too much hell had broken loose in there.

Cautiously the counselor tiptoed to the edge of the sofa. He knelt and placed his hand on her shoulder. Gently. So very gently as he himself would have preferred it under the same circumstances, he touched. She shifted. There was a tiny childlike moan as he felt her coming around.

"Hi," he whispered.

"Hi..."

"I decided to come back."

"Uh huh."

"I'm sorry about the way I was before. I know I can be erratic sometimes."

"I understand. It's OK."

Her voice grainy and unfamiliar from sleep. Her breath wonderfully clean smelling, not the slightest hint of tobacco. Morton put his hands on her arms and began to massage.

"I don't ever want to hurt you," he said.

"I know you don't."

"I want to help you. I'm trying to help you."

His hands found her breasts. Were massaging there. Massaging...

Incredible the suppleness of sleep, how the body changed into a different body, a nighttime body that began to receive and not repel.

"I'm back to my old self now," she said very low.

Her old self? Damn, but those multiple personalities could run around in most anybody.

"I'm so glad," returned Morton.

In the pitch blackness they had no way to meet eyes and get the guilt and terror she was sure to put on this in her waking hours. Of this which was really the most natural of events.

He felt her ease more fully onto her back. As he touched farther he found she was wearing a slip, one longer than he was used to. How right he'd been to walk, to think, to reconsider. To not abandon this person, who now, as he angled gently into position, was opening so fairly to him. In his caresses he noticed how her hair was so much softer than usual. She must have spent hours brushing the kinks out of the new permanent.

And now their bodies beginning to move in these minute cat bite strokes, so delicate and understated they were almost not moving. Yet feeling inside the far away places they lived in and the people they could so easily become if only they'd let themselves.

"You're beautiful," he said.

A moment passed.

"So are you," she whispered back.

Things were suddenly so good every part of her body became the same importance to him. She held the beauty of the world in her eyes, and he couldn't remember having seen the beauty of the world. But it was there. In the little glints of her eyes. At last he was sensing it.

The rush of excitement began to peel down his spine. The darkness was so black it was bright. He could actually feel it glowing under his eyelids. Then there was a noise. Something she'd mumbled?

As he squeezed open his eyes he realized the light had come on. Must have been— Must have been *switched* on!

He looked over his shoulder. There, by the counter, in her red gown, hair still fully kinked like before, stood Annise. Her mouth was so open he could see the white stuff coating her tongue. Her eyes were like springs they were so bugged out.

Morton rolled his head downward, and gazing up at him, her face brightly illuminated by the ceiling light, was sweet little Muriel Gonska, the schizophrenic.

Shocking moments passed. Morton's heart somersaulted as he glanced back and forth between the two women. Without knowing it he'd jumped off a cliff higher than the third floor of the Fraction House.

In the inelegant midst of it all—he couldn't help noticing— Muriel's hands continued to clutch tight as vices in the small of his back, refusing to let loose.

* * *

Chapter 51

The next morning Morton rose, swallowed a Librium, and left for the hectic freeway drive out to the Shearer-Kaplan Laboratories in Glendale. This was in the so called think tank quadrant of the county where large, low lying hangars honeycombed with antiseptic offices sprawled out over the desert acreage.

The receptionist eyed him nervously, but sent out a page for Trina Lopez over the intercom. If they were going to cut Harvey open for crime—an autopsy rather, Morton would have to move fast. Verify poison in Harvey's pills. Verify poison in Harvey's body. And there you had it, the Gestapo convicted!

"Trina's a wonderful woman," said Morton to the girl. "We used to be partners. I mean, you know, at work I'm saying. Do you know her well?" He sat down. He was more and more out of himself these days, though he couldn't put together why.

Trina appeared. "Morton!"

She wasn't wearing her nurses cap, but the rest of her outfit was the same, including her thick coke bottle glasses. He was glad for that. Not everything changed like the wind.

She led the counselor to her office. Morton gazed around at the calculators, the folders, the line of half full beakers and nearby Bunsen burners.

"I am a research analyst. I make many friends here, Morton. We are trying to fix medicines better for people," explained Trina.

"That's why I've come," said Morton. "Did you hear about Harvey?"

"Harvey should quit that place. He is too good to try to live in such a hell."

"In a way he did quit. He died, Trina. It looks like he had a heart attack in his office."

"He... He died?" Trina breathed deep.

The counselor went on to explain the big meeting scene, his firing and what not, the shove at the top of the steps, and finally his suspicions about Harvey's death.

"Horrible things are going on around there, Trina. Sometimes I think I'm losing touch. I'd just finished talking with Harvey when it happened."

"You do not look yourself, Morton. Do you stop shaving now? And your hair so long and falling everywhere. Look there."

She pointed him toward the mirror.

"Your eyes are bloodshot and your pupils so little, my friend. And your voice is slow. You have not been drinking, maybe?"

That Trina. Bolt straight to the point without regard for your goofy frailties. It was refreshing, really.

"No, I haven't been drinking. Trina, I think Joseph had something to do with Harvey's death. I heard the family's considering an autopsy, but Joseph's fighting it. I need your help."

Morton produced a small envelope. Out of it he funneled the five pills he'd slipped from the Director's shirt pocket onto Trina Lopez's desk.

"I think one of these is poison," said the counselor. "Or maybe all of them are poison. I believe the Gestapo's been packing the capsules with something to make Harvey sick. Can you have these tested for me, Trina? See what's really in them?"

"Certainly," she said. "But you look sick too, Morton. Have you been taking something?"

Morton brought out his Librium vial.

"Here," he said, handing her the container. "It'd be a good idea to test these too, I guess. I know they're not poison though. They make me feel a thousand times better. In fact, they're so good I can't seem to quit taking them."

"Hmmm," said Trina searching the counselor's eyes.

"I think Joseph's a murderer. I told Harvey I'd catch him no matter what. And by God I'm going to."

"I believe you. I fear Joseph may have been tampering with the client meds for years. I have always had suspicions why he started leaving his office door open all the time."

"Yes?" said Morton scratching his head.

"Is it not obvious? He is protected in case any of the medications turn up wrong. He leaves them out on his desk. He can say someone entered and switched them."

"Like me," said Morton. "He knows I was with Harvey right before he died. He could say I had access to Harvey's medicines. He could frame me. He could say I put the poison in—"

"But if he does not want an autopsy he would not be trying to frame you, would he?"

Morton felt so limber he envisioned doing the splits and popping right back up for a quickie fistfight with the Gestapo. His morals were intact, in their way, yet a kind of unreality swept over him, a looseness of emotion bordering on indifference. He proceeded languidly through his consultation with Trina.

"How long since Harvey passed away?" asked Trina.

"Two days. He died on Wednesday."

"I cannot promise, but I will try to have tests done over the weekend. We need to know soon. We must stop this badness."

"Monday? They might bury him by then."

"Sometimes, if it has to be done, the law will exhume a body. Do not despair, my friend."

"One more favor," said Morton as he started to leave. "I need a blood test. Or urine, or whatever it is."

"All right," said Trina. "What do we test for?"

"HIV and STDs."

"HIV! Morton! Certainly you are not shooting drugs." Again she studied his eye carriage.

"Of course not. I've had a couple of dates lately. I mean, with friends, only I'm not sure they're..." He trailed off.

The research analyst was quiet.

"It's really not so odd, Trina. Hanging out with friends and all. A lot of people have certain acquaintances they see. I mean, we're not necessarily going to marry these people, we're just, you know, engaging them in a very regular loving way. Don't you agree? Because the human being is a person needs to give love out, Trina. Anyway, will you call me when you find out about all this?"

"I will call."

"Thank you," said Morton. He reached for the vial of Librium.

"Oh, no you don't. I'm keeping these," countered Trina Lopez quickly plucking the container off her desk.

"You're keeping them?" The counselor weakened inside.

Trina blinked with a sudden change of mind. "You are right, Morton. You must keep some. To stop taking them all at once might be dangerous. I do not know what is in these, but I have an idea it is much more potent than little Libriums."

Trina removed most of the pills, then handed him the vial.

"Harder than Librium? Like poison, you're saying?"

"Whatever it is," said Trina, "you're addicted to it."

* * *

'L.A. 2000:' Sex Asylum

Chapter 52

When Morton returned to his apartment he found an envelope in the mailbox marked with Dar/Neese's fancy calligraphy. Inside was a form letter with the underlined places typed in. He read it there at the curbside.

> *We at <u>Dar/Neese</u> have learned how traumatic the moment of Fraction House termination can be for our clients.*
>
> *Under the reigning Los Angeles County Ordinance, it is <u>Muriel Elaine Gonska's</u> right to request a Designated Morale Supporter to be present at the time of her closure.*
>
> *It is <u>Muriel Gonska's</u> wish that one <u>Morton K. Allison</u> be named her Official Morale Supporter.*
>
> *Therefore we at <u>Dar/Neese</u> ask for the honor of your attendance, <u>Mr. Allison</u>, at her upcoming Termination Meeting, scheduled for <u>June 25th</u> of this year.*

Joseph's Schopen's signature was scrawled so harshly at the bottom it could have come from one of the bunker stages of Adolph Hitler. Beside it was the word 'Director,' which had been Harvey's title.

Early in the history of the Fraction House Sandra Dar noticed how upset her clients became when they were about to be transferred out. To reduce stress she laid down a by-law allowing the clients to invite a so called Morale Supporter to their Termination Meeting.

As the months passed Harvey began to notice that the clients were selecting along the lines of high powered attorneys, independent psychiatrists, even other schizophrenics. By the time Dar/Neese picked up on the error experts in the field had already declared it a sensitive, client-oriented innovation. A powerful self-help system all halfway houses ought to offer.

Within months the fat cat bureaucrats declared it a county ordinance. So, desiring to keep their funding, not to mention their good name, Dar/Neese found themselves stuck with—well, in this case, Morton.

The counselor heard his phone ringing. He hurried inside.

"Allison?"

"Yeah?"

"It's Joseph."

Silence.

"Look, the two of us are making fools of ourselves," said the Gestapo. "You want to help Muriel. I know you don't believe me, but I want to help her too."

"By raping her?" said Morton. "For your information, I know about Sally too. Your days are numbered, Schopen."

"You're a lot of shit," said Joseph. "There's no evidence of anything anywhere I've been, and you know it."

Morton gripped the receiver so hard he heard the plastic stressing.

"You're making this hard on me," continued the Gestapo. "I'm trying to reconcile with you, Allison. I can explain everything if you'll let me."

Morton didn't answer.

"I've got videotapes. They're of Muriel," stuttered Joseph. "I want you to see how—stay calm now—I want you to see how provocative she can be. And, ummm..." Joseph appeared to hesitate, "There's another woman, er, interacting with her, if you get what I mean. Someone you know quite well, I'm afraid. Once you take a look at these tapes I think you'll agree we should put them in Harvey's casket for safekeeping. Otherwise—"

"Another woman?"

"That's right."

"I don't know what you're getting at Schopen, but sex isn't against the law."

"I'm glad to hear you agree with me, Allison. On the other hand, if the Arbitrators see this tape Muriel goes straight to Roselawn. It's not only sex. There's drug use."

"Drugs!"

"Quit acting so shocked. Bring your ass up here and talk to me about it. We need to get this mix up resolved before the Termination Meeting. You come clean with me and I'll come clean with you, I swear it."

Silence.

"It's in Muriel's best interest," said Joseph.

Morton sighed. "All right," he said.

"Good. Show up tomorrow at nine, we'll make things right. Oh, and Morton, tomorrow is Saturday. We're making it casual day and wearing our worst outfits."

"We are?"

"Come in your jeans and those ignorant suspenders you always wear. You'll fit right in."

The counselor had a thought. The injunction against him was still in effect. Could this be a trap? If he was arrested, they might be able to block him from attending Muriel's Termination Meeting. His mind raced. He'd need a decoy.

"Uh, how about ten, Joseph?" he said. "I'll wear my railroad hat. It's casual to the max."

"Ten it is!" boomed the Gestapo.

Before they hung up, Morton could have sworn he heard Joseph clapping his hands together with glee across the lines.

~~~

The same day, an hour before the cafeteria opened for supper, Morton dialed the Staff Lounge. Stacy Lung and Wanda Novice would likely be hiding out there with their brown bag health food, seeking a few minutes of solace. Stacy answered.

"Stacy, Gordon called me earlier, but I was out. He said he'd be in the lounge."

"He's not here, Morton."

"He must have forgotten. Can you run get him?"

This was a shade off from absolute honesty, but your investigators sometimes had to wade around in those mucky borderline areas lawyers used to get at the bigger truths.

Stacy balked. Typical of her.

"I'm afraid he'll hold it against somebody if he doesn't get my call," pressed the counselor. "Last time he lost it he tore the doors off the laundry room, remember? Joseph was *very* pissed."

A few minutes later Gordon was on the phone.

"Don't talk, Gordon. Listen to me. I've got a big favor to ask you."

"I loved the fire," said Gordon.

"Shhh. This is top secret. You're scheduled for an hour free time tomorrow between nine and ten, aren't you?"

"Yes."

"What I want you to do is put on a pair of jeans and those red suspenders I gave you last Christmas. Then meet me at Vera's at nine. Think you can pull it off?"

"Sure. I'm not restricted anymore."

"I'll explain the rest in the morning. But believe me, Gordon, this is going to be so phony we'll both end up stronger men for it. By the way, you're, uh, not afraid to go to jail, are you?"

"Jail? Did I do something wrong?"

"No, of course you didn't."

"Great! Then I'd love to go!"

The counselor was touched. That Gordon. His love of the artificial was more sincere than your born again Christian's prayers to the Holy Ghost. Quite a fellow, the paranoid.

"You're a gem, Gordon. A real gem," said Morton.

"Thanks," said Gordon. "Muriel's here."

"What?"

"Muriel's here. You want to talk to her?"

"Sure."

"Hi, Morton."

"Hi, baby. I mean, not baby. Christ—"

"It's OK about the other night on the sofa, Morton. Annise knows you thought I was her," said Muriel.

"Thank the Lord!"

"You should thank me. I'm the one had to explain it all to her."

"Thank you, Muriel."

"You're welcome. And Morton—"

"Yes?"

"I want you to know you were *very* good."

The counselor smiled through the lines. "So were you, young lady. So were you."

Morton could hardly believe he was saying these things. He felt intoxicated and at the same time antsy. He patted his pockets for the Librium.

"I have to go. Stacy wants us for supper," said Muriel.

"Wait. I have to ask you something. This is very important. It could affect the outcome of your Termination Meeting."

"Yes?"

"Joseph says he has videotape. He says— He says you and another woman... And you were taking drugs or something. I thought you might be loaded when I found you curled up on my rug. Is any of this true?"

She didn't answer.

"Muriel?"

"Yes?"

"Is any of it true?"

A long pause. "Yes," she said.

Morton heard the receiver drop to the floor. A moment later someone hung it up.

* * *

Chapter 53

The next morning the counselor put on his black dress pants and his nylon baseball jacket with 'DODGERS' stitched across the back. Then he met Gordon for breakfast at Vera's Russian Diner.

They had a nice time, joking with Vera, talking about the old days when Gordon first arrived at the Fraction House. Harvey and Joseph had him pinned down as was one of those schizos who heard voices, and then acted out what he thought the voices were telling him.

"You better rape that woman," he'd be overheard mumbling to himself. Or, "Shoot this man. Shoot him now or *you're* the one who'll die."

As it turned out though, and as Harvey and Joseph determined after they'd given him serious sedation, Gordon had been overhearing Sam Lorenzo's TV set playing the afternoon soap operas. He'd been listening through the walls and mumbling the words so he could figure out the storyline. The bosses, it seemed, would have felt a little remorse. On the contrary they counted themselves super fortunate to have diagnosed the paranoid so early, because otherwise they'd have lost him and all his funds when he went into an independent apartment, which was protocol for people who were only borderline crazy like Gordon. No, better to keep him at Dar/Neese where he could improve at a rate which allowed the Gestapo to shuffle Gordon's funding as he saw fit. Once you opened your eyes, pondered the counselor, the conspiracy wasn't so tricky to put together.

Morton had brought his alligator-skin briefcase to Vera's. "I want you to carry this, Gordon," he said. "It'll be phonier than sin. I'll get it back when the fallout blows over."

"Fallout? Is the bomb coming too?"

"It's just a phrase, Gordon. I didn't mean it literally."

Gordon undid the latch. "It's empty," he said.

"I know. I left my document collection back at the apartment. This is simply a matter of falsifying one thing for another."

"I can dig it," said Gordon investigating like a cat the inner pockets.

Morton rose.

"What's this?" asked the synthetic. He'd found a plastic loop with two brass keys attached.

Morton took a look. "I don't know," he said. "Drop them back in. Remember what they say in the program—when the keys are ready the lock will appear."

"What program's that?" asked Gordon.

~~~

When it was time the two men walked up the hill toward the Fraction House. Due to the injunction Morton paused a distance away from the entrance.

"You look good," said the counselor. "The jeans. The suspenders. Here, put this on." Morton handed the paranoid his striped railroad cap. "Beautiful," he said adjusting it. "You look just like me when I get paranoid."

Gordon smiled wide. We all had our quirky ways of getting happiness. One man's grin was another's scowl. Freedom, decided the counselor, amounted to how well you pursued your fetishes.

"Good luck, my friend," said Morton.

~~~

Gordon looked up and down the street. Then he checked the sky above him, just in case.

At last the paranoid mounted the steps. As Morton expected, when he reached the landing two uniformed policemen surged through the double doors. According to plan, Gordon spun and darted away. He was quick on his feet, and he managed to turn into the back alleyway before the officers could catch up.

Morton watched from the opposite sidewalk as they gripped the paranoid hard at the biceps and began to guide him farther up the street where they'd stashed their cruiser. Morton saw the rolled injunction papers carried like a baton in one of the officer's hands.

The counselor strained to see upward along the outside of the building. And yes, there was Joseph Schopen glaring down from Harvey's office like a hunchbacked generalisimo on his kingly balcony, seedy voyeur to the end. Morton's suspicions were confirmed. It *had* been a trap. The police would let Gordon go, of course. But had Morton himself taken the bait serious jail time would have been involved.

Three floors away the counselor could see the supervisor's grotesque smile—check that—the new *Director's* grotesque smile. Harvey was dead. As far as your crafty coup d'etats went, this was a bloody one, and it was likely to get bloodier still.

The police car moved into the distance. Morton began a side to side wave to the Gestapo. Joseph's head poked farther out the window. It took a minute or so, but by degrees the Gestapo recognized him.

The counselor waited until he could see the toothy, cigarette-yellowed smile disappear. Morton pointed his finger and brought his thumb down, as if he were firing a gun, a derringer maybe, like the kind Annise owned. It was a long way up, but Joseph saw clear as a bell what he meant.

The counselor turned and headed back to Vera's for his truck.

~~~

Morton wasn't home for ten minutes when the phone rang.

"For your information, Allison, Harvey was finished off an hour ago."

"What do you mean, finished off?"

"Cremated," said Joseph. "Burned to a crisp. His blood stream is nothing but cold ashes now."

Silence.

"Let's see, by supper time we'll be scattering him in the Organic Therapy Garden," said Joseph.

"He's been cremated?"

"Your smartass evidence just went up in smoke," said the Gestapo clicking down the phone.

* * *

Chapter 54

Trina Lopez always came through. On Monday morning she telephoned to say that the tests were quite complicated. They were going to take longer than expected.

"It won't make any difference if you find the poison," said Morton sadly. "They burned Harvey up on Saturday."

"Cremated?"

"I'm afraid so. I guess Joseph convinced the family or something."

"We must think of Muriel," returned the RN. "We must do what is right. I will contact you as soon as the results are back."

Gordon called, thrilled about his phony arrest. "Joseph wanted to break my neck, Morton. But he said he was going to break yours instead. Watch out for him."

"I'll watch out."

"By the way, about your briefcase."

"Yes?"

"I mailed it off. I took it to the post office all by myself."

"Thanks, I appreciate your efforts," said Morton.

"I didn't trust any of the nuts working here to give it to you."

"Good thinking, Gordon. You're a man after my own heart."

"And you're a man after mine, Morton Allison. Something's been bothering me," said Gordon heavily. "Maybe you could give me satisfaction on it."

"I'll try," returned the counselor cautiously.

"Those two keys keep rattling and rattling around. I have to know, Morton. Did the lock ever appear?"

The counselor searched for a therapeutic answer. "Not so far," he said. "But the shooting match isn't over yet."

He heard Gordon sucking his lips. "The shooting match?" said the paranoid nervously. "I didn't know we were in a *shooting* match."

"Well, we are. And the bullets are starting to fly. So keep your head down."

"Don't worry, Morton. My head's been down for thirty-seven years. It's not likely to come up at the sound of a couple of gun shots."

~~~

Two weeks went by.

Annise didn't go out of her way to avoid the counselor during this period. She really did work a great deal. He would phone with high hopes. Her answer: "I'm sorry, Morton, I can't today. Wanda needs me something terrible. You know how bad a shambles the Fraction House is right now."

Ever since they'd discovered the cancer, or whatever it was, Annise had been struggling to cope. She'd developed a sort of compulsion to reach back at odd times and test if the thing was still there. When it was, well, problems. This stimulated much friendly advice around the Fraction House—ala southern California style—on how to get cured. Macrobiotic dieting. Laetrile treatments. Psychokinesis to retard cell growth. Wanda, she told him, said if she could *see* the damn thing she was certain she could help. Annise was mixed up. It was hard to bandage a wild animal, no matter how gentle you tried to be.

Well, all right. He had those loose ends to wrap up at the Courthouse. Fortunately he had his Librium caps, so he could calm his nerves when he had to. Addicted? No way. Just because he liked the feeling didn't mean it wasn't a legitimate prescription, did it?

The following Monday the call came from Trina Lopez.

"When is Muriel's Termination Meeting?" she asked.

"Tomorrow."

"You must come to me immediately, Morton. I have found bad information."

"Bad? What do you mean bad?"

"I mean like I said. You had better come right away."

At Shearer-Kaplan Trina Lopez escorted Morton briskly into her office. "Shut the door. It will lock by itself," she said.

Morton saw the series of tiny plastic Ziplocs, each with a single pill inside. Trina angled her head at him. "You did not shave again," she noticed.

The finicky RN gathered her papers. "All right, Morton. You must listen closely. First, these Libriums. They are not Libriums at all. The outside looks like them, but the capsules are filled with Dilaudid."

"Dilaudid! That's a poison, isn't it?"

"It is a very serious narcotic. And badly addictive. More addictive even than morphine. How much have you taken?"

Morton scratched his head. "I used maybe fifteen out of the first bottle. Then Annise changed them out for a fresh vial. A hundred in there, I guess."

"Annise gave you these?"

The counselor wondered how much the Dilaudid might be affecting his troublesome sexual staying power with the blonde. It was a shot below the belt. He found himself unnaturally angry.

"I didn't end up taking all of the first batch. They were too strong at the beginning," he said.

"Sí, I think they were, amigo. The first ones must have been a smaller dose, so you would not become nauseous. This built your resistance. Next came a powerful amount to hook you."

"Hook me? But why would Annise— No, she can't be that evil, Trina."

"Morton, these so called Libriums have double the prescribed dose of Dilaudid inside them. Someone wants you doped up on narcotics. From the looks of you they are succeeding."

"I'm... I'm not aggressive like I used to be, am I?"

"You are very smart, my friend. Perhaps you are only slower smart right now."

"Joseph is trying to kill me, Trina. Annise would never— I mean, I don't think she would—" Morton thought hard. "But Dilaudid wouldn't kill me, even if it was double the dose, would it?"

"It would make you like drunk. Worse than drunk. Stupid perhaps. Then unordinary things happen."

"I don't know. It seems like the Gestapo could do better if he wanted me out of the way."

"This is what I must tell you," interrupted Trina. "We tested Harvey's medicines. There was only powdered sugar in the Cardizem capsules, for his high blood pressure. And in the potassium capsules, sugar. The Lasix was in a tablet form—it was made of cornstarch."

"Jesus Christ," groaned the counselor.

"I am saying there was no medicine in any of these pills. His nitroglycerin was a tablet also. It was sugar, only mixed with a tiny bit of cayenne pepper like you can buy at the grocery store. This was to mimic the stinging effect real nitro has under the tongue."

"And his pain pills?"

"They too were empty, Morton. I mean, the tablet was made of plain sugar. This is what we found."

"So Harvey wasn't poisoned after all?"

"Not with these pills. The medicines had all been removed. But if he wasn't getting his medications his blood pressure would stay high. He would retain water. He would experience much pain. Heart problems are unstable and hard to treat. An overweight man—I am saying a very obese man like Harvey could easily die from not getting his medicines." Trina blinked. "I was there to make sure of these things."

"Forget the guilt, Trina. Joseph is the killer. He's the one responsible for all this."

Trina picked up one of the Ziplocs. "In this tablet, Morton, we found residue of hydromorphone. It has been replaced with sugar, but traces were there."

"Yeah, that was his pain pill. What's hydromorphone anyway?" asked Morton.

"Dilaudid," said Trina. "They are the same medicine."

"Hydromorphone is Dilaudid? I saw that on Joseph's desk a few weeks ago. I saw it again in Harvey's office right before he died. I remember he complained about the nitro getting old. He must have noticed it wasn't doing anything for him. Dilaudid, huh?" pondered the counselor. "Is that a legitimate med, Trina? Narcotics for a heart problem?"

"Well, it is not illegal. Sometimes this is done for extreme pain. Usually only in the hospital. But Harvey must have had terrible angina. He could have prescribed it for himself, or else his cardiologist."

"Joseph suggested it," said Morton. "I heard them arguing one day. Joseph acted like he wanted to keep Harvey alive and ease his pain."

"Yes?"

"I'm saying Joseph has tampered with the drugs from start to finish. He put sugar in Harvey's pills so he'd get sick and have a heart attack. That's why it took him so many months to die. And he used Harvey's real Dilaudid to fill my Librium caps with narcotics. *Double* the narcotics. He wants me messed up. And it's working. I'm definitely messed up. I'm not sure why he wants me loaded, but I'll find out."

Trina shook her head.

"Everybody knows Joseph has that fancy chemistry lab in his basement," said Morton. "I'm sure he's quite professional at his quack science. You can bet your ass he concocted all these fake meds."

"I kept the paperwork on the tests," said Trina. "I can put it in my safe if you want. It would not be much proof though. Anybody could have made those pills."

"Yeah," agreed Morton. "And Joseph always sweeps up after himself. I'm sure he's destroyed anything incriminating."

"I fear you are right, amigo."

"Tomorrow is Muriel's Termination Meeting," said Morton. "I have to get her out of there before I do anything else. I'll take the tampered pills and the test results with me. They might help. By the way, Trina, a letter came from the Fraction House. I'm her Designated Morale Supporter, so I'll be in there mixing it up with those bastards."

"Be careful, Morton." He turned to go. "Wait. I have something for you," said Trina. She handed him a small vial of light green capsules.

"Librium?" Morton was astonished.

"Yes. A doctor friend of mine prescribed them. You must take these, Morton. You will be sick from Dilaudid withdrawal if you do not. You will not think straight."

The counselor was rubbed the wrong way. Trina in on the conspiracy too? Take drugs to counteract the drugs you've already taken? But it really wasn't so uncommon, was it? Internal medicine could correct as easily as distort. And Trina had never steered him wrong.

"I implore you, Morton. Take these or else you will go crazy."

"All right."

She handed him an invoice sheet from the laboratory. "Results of your blood work," she said.

Interestingly enough, it resembled the yellow form in Annise's locking box. 'HIV Negative. Other STDs Negative,' he read. The counselor sighed deep.

"Let me ask you something, Trina. Without an autopsy on Harvey there's no way to prove he didn't have those meds on board, is there?"

Trina shook her head. She said, "Even if they had done an autopsy we could not prove Joseph gave him empty pills. Joseph would say Harvey did not take his medicines."

"That son of a bitch," said Morton.

Buck Buchanan

"That bastardo," said Trina Lopez, then immediately turned red.

* * *

Chapter 55

Monday night before the meeting Morton got his alligator-skin briefcase down. He was into the second stack of forms when he came across the raffle tickets. They'd be perfect.

The next morning he went to his bedroom closet and decided on his bold purple blazer and the striped, seersucker pants. These would be a good distraction for the kind of hocus-pocus he was looking to pull off. He didn't have to go by the Courthouse today. All that had been seen to.

As he pulled up to the Fraction House he spotted Joseph at the top of the steps, his arms folded militantly. No worry, the injunction was powerless now due to the counselor's special designation of Morale Supporter. Morton mounted the steps confidently.

Over to the left was Priscilla Daddio. Her black hair was in a bun, but it was a loose bun and she kept stuffing it back up with her long, thin fingers. Annise was by the railing, her permanent losing its flashy billow by now. Wanda was beside her. Muriel lingered a distance away, almost in the bushes. She was wearing her conservative tweed skirt and stockings. Two men in navy blue suits, the State Arbitrators, were waiting by the double doors. They would make the ultimate decision regarding Muriel's future.

As Morton reached the landing Wojeck and Emily Gonska came up behind him. They stopped and shook hands. Wojeck certainly looked the part of a rapist. Big, ugly, pock-faced. He was a silent, lumbering type, which seemed at odds with his hotshot, monied career in gene splicing. Remarkable the talents people had. Wojeck was your one in a thousand perpetrators Morton felt was genuinely repentant, and over the years the two had developed a pretty good rapport. Muriel wasn't likely to forgive him, but at least the hell and high water had subsided.

"I'd like to thank you for everything you've done, Morton," said Wojeck patting the counselor on the shoulder. "I understand you've been under the gun around here lately. I want you to know I don't believe anything Joseph says. Not the first word. And believe me, he's saying rotten stuff. We owe everything to you. And so does Muriel."

Emily, the short, redheaded mother, said, "To be honest, if it wasn't for you, Morton, me and Wojeck wouldn't even come to these shitass meetings, would we, Wojeck?"

That Emily, roundly floozed in the garish L.A. style of foam shoulder pads and rouge red makeup. And not your highest life linguist either, one noticed.

Wojeck nudged Morton aside. "I just keep wishing somebody decent would marry the girl up. She's a good age for that, you know. But shit, me and Emily don't hardly know anybody decent, except for you."

They chatted a minute. When Morton saw the opportunity he opened his alligator-skin briefcase. Playing the charlatan had never been his forte. On the other hand, leaving the blind to lead the blind might cause them both to tumble into the ditch.

"Listen, Wojeck, I've got these raffle tickets. They're for a wonderful cause." Morton took a minute to describe the details. This was an important exercise. Do not short shrift it, he told himself.

Priscilla Daddio, who got paranoid when people started signing things, trotted over. She examined the raffle proposal.

"A Teenage Pregnancy Campaign?" she said suspiciously. "Is Morton really into this?"

The counselor gave a big up and down nod.

As it turned out Priscilla agreed Teenage Pregnancy was a weighty cause. When Morton mentioned the opportunity to win a spanking new Cadillac, Priscilla passed him a dollar, then jotted her name and address at the bottom of the intricate, folded over raffle proposal.

It was a harried group this morning, and the raffle idea eased the tension a bit. Morton approached each of them and carefully laid out the campaign.

"Only a dollar?" asked Annise.

Her eyes lit up, and he remembered the special corner of her heart reserved for wagering. Wanda came over. The two conferred. They seemed cool and withdrawn this morning, so unlike them. Morton flashed to the shady collusions of the first meeting. Could that be happening again? After a moment they smiled and bought four tickets each.

Morton went to Muriel. He was worried about the upcoming meeting, and spooky feelings were in him as he stepped close to her. For several minutes they stood there whispering. Finally Muriel said, "I'd like to buy some, but I don't have any money."

"You don't have any money?" repeated Morton loud enough for the others to hear.

Muriel shook her head despondently.

Joseph eased over. "I couldn't help overhearing," he said. "I wish we could all see this as a time for reconciliation." The Gestapo shuffled his feet self-consciously, then reached for his wallet. "Let me pay for Muriel's tickets."

Morton flipped quickly to the proper pages.

"Good God boy, where'd you get those pants!" exclaimed Joseph. "And that jacket. Purple?"

"She wants three, Joseph," said the counselor showing Muriel where to put her name.

Morton slapped his forehead. "Wait, I just thought of something. You can't sign for yourself, Muriel. Dar/Neese has your Guardianship right now."

Muriel looked confusedly around. In her three-year old voice she said, "Would you sign for me, Joseph?"

The Gestapo took the pen and began to write. "Here too," said Morton pointing. "And once right here."

Joseph, a bit downcast himself it seemed, forked over the money. "By the way, I know there wasn't any medicine in Harvey's pills," whispered Morton passing the Gestapo his stubs.

"You wha—"

Joseph's eyes grew queerly dilated.

"You're dead meat, Allison," replied the Director. "And after today your girls are *my* meat." Joseph nodded to the two women, Annise and Muriel. "In fact, they've been my meat since day one. Remind me to show you the video. Once you see it, your view on life will change."

A hundred replies went through Morton's head, but he said nothing.

* * *

Chapter 56

The Conference Room had been completely rearranged. No longer was it plush and rich feeling with Harvey's decorations, but cold and austere, like the new lantern jawed Director himself.

Since Morton was Muriel's Morale Supporter they were required to sit together on the sofa. The tape machine was running of course, but in addition a specially appointed stenographer had been retained to get everything down. This was going to be the real thing.

Joseph brought the meeting to order.

"We're going to hear important testimony from a special witness who will throw incriminating light on one of Muriel's caseworkers," he said.

Annise began to squirm. Morton felt for her. She could end up in real jeopardy if the Arbitrators found out about that sexy night of mistaken identity, what with she being the supervisory counselor and all.

A chair was placed in the center of the circle. Joseph motioned for Annise to sit in it.

At first it was difficult to tell where the questioning was headed, until Morton heard the phrase, "Mr. Allison's bizarre style of counseling." He could hardly believe it! And yet by degrees he realized Annise was getting into the ugly ways he'd done Muriel damage. So here we go again, he thought. What was this, the Fraction House trying one final time to prove Joseph innocent and Morton guilty? And how could Annise buy into it?

Muriel and Morton stared at each other in disbelief as Annise recounted the time he'd given Muriel the spicy bean burrito in the midst of a new bout of bowel problems, along with the ruckus the next morning when the housekeeper called in sick and Joseph had to pick up her bedclothes.

"There was a *gigantic* stink about it," said the blonde, and they all laughed.

Annise continued. She related a conversation with Muriel concerning the day Morton came in depressed.

"What she said he said was, 'I had an argument with a hot blonde last night. I feel like I've got a big fat bone in my heart today.' So what I'm saying is Muriel told me she stared at his crotch because she didn't understand what he was trying to say by that bone business. Muriel's face turned beet red. She said, 'A bone in his heart, Annise? Do you think that's really where he meant he had it?'"

Joseph intervened. "This represents our point entirely," he said. "Sexual innuendo. Misapplied psychology. Dangerous male/female interactions."

The Arbitrators leaned forward. In the midst of her assault Annise flashed Morton a wink, as if it were all a barrel of good clean monkey business. Well, they'd had their earth shattering talk a few days ago, the one that pillaged his whole world picture. It wasn't a customary thing to have a bombshell the size of the San Bernardino mountain range dropped into your lap. As she continued Morton remembered back to last Friday when Annise had telephoned him.

"I want you to come right over here and get on top of me," she'd said. "I know how it upsets you because I hardly ever let you have the top. But everything is about to change. You're the man, Morton. You should have the top sometimes."

"I should?"

"I'm really and truly a changed person. Not the way you think either. Come over here," she urged. "But one thing, I insist you leave the minute you finish."

"The minute I finish? Wow, what a gas! You've certainly got creativity, Annise."

He went over. And there *was* a different feel to it. She smiled up at him all the while. Very strange. Afterwards he started to dress.

"What are you doing? Aren't you going to stay?" she asked.

"You said I had to go home the minute I finished."

"Goddamn you, Morton. You know I didn't mean that."

"You didn't?"

"Of course not."

He saw her cheeks fire up. "Has anybody ever told you how insensitive you can be? You have a way of making a person feel stone cold dead inside."

She seemed quite upset. He pulled her close and rubbed the place between her eyes.

"I wish you wouldn't listen to me when I'm wrong. It hurts a woman when a man believes everything she says."

"I didn't mean it, Annise."

"You did though. You listened the way you listen to all the terrible things I say."

A tear came into one eye. She lifted the corner of the bedspread and wiped at it.

"I wasn't going to tell you before," she said. "But I have something exceedingly important to say. I've decided to go ahead and say it too, whether you want to hear it or not." Her eyes cleared. They had a curiously fresh, hopeful look now. "You're going to find out sooner or later anyway. So I might as well go ahead and tell you. The fact of the matter is... Well, I'm... I'm..."

"Yes, Annise?"

"Pregnant, Morton," she whispered. "I'm pregnant as a dog and I'm going to have your beautiful beautiful baby. What do you think of that?" she asked grinning.

* * *

Chapter 57

Annise came to the end of her talk.

"Things I've said might make Morton here—I mean, Mr. Allison—look bad. But I want everyone to know he can be very good sometimes too," she concluded.

She gave the counselor a timid smile, rose, and took a seat next to Joseph.

A period of feet shuffling elapsed. The Gestapo produced what appeared to be a plastic cup of lemonade along with a handful of papers.

"Our investigations have turned up proof of Mr. Allison's wickedness— Ummm, misconduct rather," Joseph flapped the forms. "These are the results of Allison's Employment Urinalysis. Let the record show narcotic drugs were found in the man's bloodstream. This is very condemning, because hard drugs were also found in Miss Gonska when she was examined at Cedars-Sinai. After he raped her, that is."

"Drugs!" exclaimed Annise. "What drugs?"

Was she honestly shocked? Wojeck turned his head back and forth between Joseph and Morton.

"Dilaudid," hissed Joseph. "One of the grossest street pharmaceuticals out there. Obviously none of this was prescribed for her. Or for him. We've checked." Joseph scowled at the counselor. "She'd been doped. And Allison is the individual who doped her. There's no question about it now."

This was one Morton couldn't have seen coming. Too sly. Too deep in the conspiracy corner of things.

He gripped his briefcase. The results of Trina's Librium tests were inside, along with Harvey's doctored meds. But the Arbitrators weren't the police. And sugar pills weren't proof of anything, especially not with the evidence burned to a crisp at Harvey's cremation. The Librium? Well, when you got right down to it anyone could have spiked it. Morton himself could have spiked it and had it tested. Like Trina said, the Gestapo always left his office door open. He had an out at every turn, literally.

Suddenly the counselor sensed the trembling in his hands. Dilaudid withdrawal, just like he'd been warned. Secretly he swallowed one of Trina's prescription Libriums.

"Dar/Neese has no blame in this charade," declared Joseph. "The escape. The rape. The drug use. It's all on Allison's shoulders. The Fraction House has been innocent from the very start. The patient had setbacks, and we've acted to correct those. Gentlemen," he said to the Arbitrators. "Miss Daddio. Roselawn has no right to Muriel. We at Dar/Neese feel her therapist should be immediately reinstated so he can get back to—so the work can go forward, shall we say."

A hush so loud it echoed through the room. Joseph set the urine cup aside, and with one button undone at the top of his white satin shirt grinned his somnolent lady killer grin across the circle at Muriel. She looked back at him in terror.

Muriel gripped Morton's hand. She was feeling abnormally cold all of a sudden. Joseph always worried the parents might make a play for Guardianship. He was about to call on Emily, but she started first.

"Excuse me, Mr. Mueller. I mean, Mr. Schopen. But me and Wojeck gotta be someplace at ten-thirty," she said. "And frankly we ain't too familiar with this psycho stuff you're talking about."

"Excellent," said Joseph. "I mean, this would be a good time to hear from the parents. We'll hurry the meeting along. You go right ahead, Emily. The parents' input is crucial."

"Years ago me and Wojeck bought out in the suburbs," began Emily. "It's not like it used to be, Mr. Schopen. The city keeps 'enroaching' and 'enroaching' till me and Wojeck can't hardly breathe even in Burbank, can we Wojeck? I'm only thinking of Muriel. You know, what would be best for her."

"Certainly," said Joseph. "Certainly you are."

"Like I say, it's all different now," Emily went on. "God knows I'd give Muriel my heart and soul if I could, wouldn't I, honey?" She peeked quickly at Muriel. "But, lately they been building houses in between the houses already been there. And later on they put other houses in between *them*." She clasped her hands. "I'm only saying the place has got so 'clusterphobic' it's like an asylum out there. We can take her though, if you want. We're dying to have our little girl back, aren't we, Wojeck?"

"Very much so," agreed Wojeck. "Except—"

"Not only that," persisted Emily. "But every summer they put a 'band' on water for two or three months, so Muriel wouldn't be able to have her little 'mulsh' garden like she used to. And of course Wojeck's got his 'hyenal' hernia now, so I wouldn't be able to cook her the spaghetti she liked so much."

Amazing, mulled the counselor, how a sexy, clearheaded little thing like Muriel could emerge from those two.

Emily, of course, was defining a common problem with the parents of nuts, which was treating the child like an infant after they'd grown up. Harvey used to say this was due to the parents themselves wanting to remain infantile. He had a point there.

Emily finished. Fortunately the parents didn't want her. Good. The Arbitrators piped up with their brownnosing, thanking Emily far too warmly for her honest input.

"One final point," broke in Priscilla. "Dr. Daddio sees that after this recent date of June 6th the patient appears to have miraculously stabilized. Can this really be true?" She tapped her pen skeptically.

"Annise?" said Joseph.

"I'm afraid so," agreed the blonde. "She's been totally sane ever since the two of them—" She glanced at Morton. "I mean, since the night Muriel spent at my place. Or, you know, since that date rather. I wrote it all down in the files, Priscilla." Annise writhed at the boldness of her deception.

"But wouldn't Dr. Mueller— Oh, excuse Priscilla. Dr. Schopen," she continued, "consider it somewhat abnormal for Muriel to suddenly behave normally, when Muriel has always behaved *ab*normally in the past?"

One of Joseph's new Dictums was that smoking wasn't permitted in the Conference Room, but now he pulled out the thin black cigarette he kept stashed behind his ear and lit it anyway. He took several nervous drags. He produced his razor knife and began his Obsessive/Compulsive habit of thumbing the blade in and out of its aluminum housing.

"Such extreme shifts are evidence of a deepening mental illness," declared Priscilla to the Arbitrators. "By rights this patient belongs at Roselawn. Nobody gets totally sane overnight. Priscilla herself can verify this."

The stress level, even for the professionals, was palpable. Muriel stiffened as the cruder points came forth. Every so often she would slip her fingers across the cushion and Morton could feel her icy, nerve racked touch along the back of his hand. It struck him how big a day this was for her, the biggest of her life, probably.

~~~

A lull came. Wanda got her organic spruce bark chewing gum out. She handed pieces down to Annise and Joseph. Periodically Morton and Muriel would accidentally brush knees, and each time it seemed Annise's eyes were locked on them.

"May I say something, Joseph?" asked the counselor.

"Of course, Morton. Of course you may. The Morale Supporter is entitled to make any comment he or she chooses to our Arbitrators. Please, be my guest."

That Joseph Schopen, maximum suck up if there ever was one.

Morton opened his briefcase and flipped past the raffle forms.

"I feel we've missed a couple of points, is all." He uncapped his pen. "I have here a copy of Muriel's original Guardianship Release Statement. Remember, Joseph? This was in the batch you dumped into the wastecan a few weeks ago. It released the

Fraction House from liability so she could move into the apartment on her own."

"So?" said Joseph nasally.

"There's an important place here on, ummm, page three it looks like, where they're asking for a psychiatric classification of the patient. According to the Guardianship Release Statement," continued Morton, "I see Muriel was classified by Harvey—Dr. Mueller, that is—who was the consulting psychiatrist, as mentally competent. Isn't this right?"

"Mentally competent?" muttered Joseph.

"So it says here."

Priscilla put a hand on her hip.

"May I have a look?" asked Joseph quickly.

Morton passed a copy around the circle.

The Gestapo crushed his cigarette out. "We're in the process of reviewing all this," he replied. "We simply haven't had a chance to downgrade it yet. Obviously things have changed since then."

"But aren't these forms still valid, Joseph? I mean, nothing was done to overturn them, was there?"

"Technically, they probably are," he mumbled. "But we're not as stupid as you—" Joseph glanced at the stenographer. "Look, Allison, I admire your research. But as usual, you're way out of bounds."

"I am?"

"You're forgetting entirely about the most critical document of all. As you know, there's something called a G-F form. And it can only be validated through a complicated procedure at the Los Angeles County Courthouse. The patient herself would have to have signed it. It would need notarizing. And it could only be valid if she were her own Guardian at the time of the signing. I made sure this was never—I mean, this simply wasn't done."

"But if it had been done—"

"It wasn't, Morton. Even if it had it wouldn't be legal unless the Director himself, meaning me, had signed the attendant Sanity Verification forms in... in..." Joseph hesitated.

"In triplicate?" said the counselor.

Slowly Morton removed the three pages Joseph signed an hour earlier under the guise of the Teenage Pregnancy Campaign.

Dead silence.

The counselor angled the forms so they could all get a good look.

"As you can see, Muriel's notarized signature is on all three of these G-F papers," continued Morton. "And Joseph Schopen, the current Dar/Neese Director, has signed in the appropriate places. Plus, they've been properly dated and rubber stamped and all that important crap that goes along with it." Morton glanced at Annise Chastain. "This *is* your signature, isn't it, Joseph?"

"No, it's not my signature! I mean, it's my signature, certainly it is, only I was tricked. You all saw it. I signed for a raffle, nothing more!" cried the Gestapo.

Morton jutted his jaw. Whatever the Gestapo's complaint, a signature was still a signature. There was no carbon dating on a Bic pen. A ripple of satisfaction eddied through the counselor. At last the beguiler himself had been beguiled.

Much agitation. Emily Gonska jerked at the flange of hair near her ears. Wojeck's eyes were hard on the Gestapo.

Quickly Morton turned to Muriel. "For the record, Miss Gonska," he said. "Did you autograph these forms of your own free will? I mean, without coercion or connivery or any kind of sneaky business? And knowing full well what they were?"

The stenographer tapped away.

"Oh, yes!" bubbled Muriel. "Yes, I did!"

The counselor pulled the patient to her feet. "As of this moment you are your own Legal Guardian, young lady. This means all your funds are yours to do with as you please. Roselawn can't get their grubby hands on you now." He glared at Priscilla. "And neither can Dar/Neese. Congratulations, baby!" He hugged her around the neck.

Joseph's eyes had gone hazy. Over Muriel's shoulder Morton saw the hint of legalese trying to rise in them. It was all sinking in. And no, there wasn't a damn thing the big mouth Director could do about it.

"Why you son of a bitch!" lisped the Gestapo.

Joseph sprung to his feet. His arm was still in the strap of his designer satchel. It snapped away from his shoulder as he lunged across the circle. Annise's witness chair was in the way. The Gestapo kicked the feet out and sent it flying in the direction of Priscilla Daddio. Full force he came at Morton.

He was inches away when Wojeck Gonska lashed out with a forearm that caught Joseph at the throat.

The Gestapo wheezed for breath as Wojeck bent him backwards. Everything went dangerously silent. The rest of them, including the Arbitrators, remained frozen in their seats, gripping the leather arm rests like startled astronauts.

"Honey, I want you to go with Morton now," grunted Wojeck to Muriel. He tightened his grip. Joseph began to change from white to blue.

The counselor tugged at Muriel's arm.

"Go on," pressed the father evenly. "I don't want to have to hurt this here man, do I Emily?"

At first Muriel's legs wouldn't work. Morton had to half drag her down the hallway and onto the stairs. Then they did work, and the two of them raced out the front doors and down the concrete steps to Morton's pickup. It was like a dance it all happened so fast, a lurched over jerk your partner tango all the way out to the road.

In the car Muriel threw her arms around Morton. She kissed him many times across the side of the face.

"Where are we going?" she asked as they zoomed away.

The counselor power shifted through the gears, laying rubber like a teenager in second and third.

"Home, my friend," he said smiling over at her. "We're finally going home."

* * *

Chapter 58

As Morton drove across town, he noticed the teddy bear, Little Morton, beside Muriel on the seat. She must have smuggled him into the meeting. She always said she'd never leave him behind. Morton looked over. He saw a tear rolling down her cheek.

"What's the matter?" he asked. "Aren't you happy about this, Muriel?"

A moment passed. "Yes," she said. "I'm happy."

"Good. Very good." He patted her shoulder.

"It's just my eye keeps crying," she said rubbing away the tear.

"No, baby," he consoled. "It's not your eye. It's you. *You're* crying inside yourself. At a time like this it's probably an appropriate thing to do."

"You're funny sometimes, Morton," she said wagging her head back and forth like in the old days.

"I am?"

"Yes. Look here." She pried her eyelid up. "See? I got sand in it running down the steps and water's coming out now."

Hmmm, she was right. Her eye really was crying. How was he always misinterpreting these things?

~~~

They stopped in front of a small stucco building. It was the apartment Joseph had rented for her in Culver City.

"This place?" said Muriel.

"The landlady gave me the key yesterday. Everything is all taken care of," explained Morton.

He led her up the short sidewalk and opened the door. A fold out sofa bed was against the far wall. A small Formica table was in the kitchenette area. The floors were bare. Morton let go of Muriel's hand. She gave a long, heavy sigh.

"Are you all right?" he asked.

"Yes. Sometimes I just don't breathe for a minute or two," she answered.

Morton showed her around. He opened and closed drawers. He pointed to the fuse box. He pulled apart the curtains.

"You've got to try to make it your own special place, Muriel," he told her. "Decorate it any way you want. Put pictures on the walls. Bright colors are the best."

Morton got his wallet out and laid some cash on the table. "We'll even things up later," he said.

Long moments passed.

"The important thing right now is your freedom," he went on. "Shops are all around here. The landlady lives three houses down. There's a coffee shop right up the street. OK?"

He touched her cheek. He petted the top of her head. A full minute must have gone by.

"OK, Muriel?" he asked again. "Isn't this OK with you?"

She looked slowly up.

"OK, Morton," she said. "It's OK."

~~~

The counselor spent the following day up at the Courthouse setting Muriel's papers in order. The day after he was at the Fraction House packing and loading her clothes and personal effects.

To his surprise Annise was a great help in guiding him in and out the back doors so he could avoid Joseph. And this after condemning him so in the meeting.

"I'm sorry about the stuff I said the other day," she explained right off. "The Arbitrators found it in the Anecdotals. They came to me directly, Morton. They told me I had to say those things or else I could be brought up for review or something. Like an inquisition. I was trying to do a good thing. I really was. I didn't know you were handling the legal stuff for her."

"It wasn't all that bad, Annise."

"I'm going to make it up to you. I promise."

She was wearing a pair of crisp new Levi's, fitted tight as peppermint tea in an iced down pitcher. As they were making hurried trips to the truck she caught him in the rear hallway and dove into his arms, then reached into her back pocket and pulled out a flattened piece of paper.

"Look, it's the results of my pregnancy test!"

Morton followed her red fingernail down the page.

"Right here. See?" she said. "Absolutely unmistakably positive! You're really something, Morty, you know that?"

"Yeah, I know."

"There's something else. I've been waiting for a chance to tell you this," she whispered excitedly. "I loved it the way you were so strong with those people the other day. I saw how you manhandled that horrible Joseph."

"Wasn't it Muriel's father who did that?" recalled Morton.

"Oh, no! It was you. And you know something?" she said squeezing him.

"What?"

"I'm just terribly terribly pleased with myself."

"You are?"

"Uh huh. A woman has an intuition about these things. I must have known how wonderfully good you were from the very beginning. Otherwise I wouldn't be carrying your child right now, would I?"

"I guess not."

"Look at it this way, a guy like Joseph would never in a million years pay up for a baby. Or a wife either for that matter. That's something to think about."

"A wife?" The counselor jutted his jaw.

Annise clutched him again. She stepped backward until she'd pinned herself against the wall.

"My God," she uttered breathlessly. "You feel so fucking powerful!"

She thrust her mouth over his with one the hottest kisses he'd felt since he'd mistaken Muriel for her on the sofa.

* * *

'L.A. 2000:' Sex Asylum

Chapter 59

So Muriel had two full days to adjust to her independence. In the interim Morton telephoned her a couple of times. Naturally. That was only courteous.

On Thursday he drove over with her belongings, as well as with all the legal forms and whatnot. As her own Guardian she'd need access to these things.

He started to go straight in, but he thought—no, better knock, better do it in a very normalized way right from the start. Show a little decent respect for the girl's privacy, that's what was required here. He tapped lightly.

"No need to knock, Morton. I always leave it open for you," she called.

~~~

The first thing he noticed was the walls. Not noticed exactly—got bombarded with was more like it. Five or six paint cans were lined along the baseboard. Different size brushes were spread out over the floor on newspapers.

From top to bottom the room was a miraculous panorama of color, all drawn on by hand. It was strikingly artistic. On the wall to the left was a giant cactus, only with human arms and legs. To the right were snow capped mountains descending into a lush green pasture. An enormous silver river meandered into the corner and swept upward across the ceiling. Leaping out of the river were huge yellow fish with what looked like mascara laden eyes. It was incredibly moving. Morton set down the box of documents he was carrying.

"My God, Muriel, what have you done here?" he asked her.

She looked over. Very serene really. "I put pictures on the walls. Like you told me," she said.

"Would you, ummm, call this abstraction?" he wondered.

"No, it's all real."

Buck Buchanan

He looked closer. Those fish eyes were the same shape and color as Annise Chastain's, no mistaking it. The mascara had been drawn on with the blonde's meticulous attention to detail. People and their talents—such hidden treasures! And yes, it was real all right.

~~~

Muriel was like an oriental philosopher the way she remained so placid and easy about the transition, which was a great comfort to him.

Occasionally he'd spend the night at her place, setting Little Morton aside to open the fold out sofa. Muriel slept in the bedroom.

One morning he awakened to noises of her puttering around the kitchen. She was making oatmeal, a new skill for her.

"Add a dash of salt when you start stirring," he called.

"OK," she said.

Later they sat down to eat. Something was obviously wrong. They quit chewing.

"How much salt did you put in here anyway?" he asked looking over at her.

"Only one dish," she replied. "Like you told me."

On the counter he saw the plastic salad bowl she'd used for the measuring. Hmmm. The counselor could see important issues beginning to unfold.

Over the weeks Morton discovered how much training his client really needed. Today they were going to the supermarket. He would show her how to stand in lines, how to weigh fruit. Muriel was so excited she accidentally pulled her socks over the cuffs of her slacks as she was dressing. He pointed it out to her, in a tender way though.

It was an extremely hot day. They came out of the grocery store with four overstuffed bags. Cans of soup. The soft drinks. A turkey. Several jars of asparagus, which he felt would be good for the kidneys. The fierce L.A. smog lay over the parking lot like cellophane melted over a chocolate cake. Morton got into the truck and turned the ignition. The battery ground for several seconds, then died.

Muriel helped him fiddle with the wires, but finally they had to balance the groceries in their arms and head on over to the bus stop.

"My severance money from the Fraction House should have come weeks ago," said Morton as they walked. "It'll probably be there today."

"I hope it never comes," said Muriel.

"Why do you say that?"

"Because you'll leave for Arizona."

"Oregon."

"I mean Oregon. And I'll never see you again."

Morton jutted his jaw.

"My Social Security check comes in a couple of days," volunteered Muriel. "We'll get you a new battery then."

The wait for the bus was unbearably long. At last it arrived. They lingered while the mass of troubled looking people clambered on.

A group of heavyset Mexican ladies rushed up. He pulled Muriel aside to let them board.

As counselor and client started timidly up the short steps the doors ripped closed.

"Sorry, folks," said the driver through the glass. "Full up here."

It pulled away. They returned to the grocery store and Morton explained how to swipe one of the loose carts at the far end of the parking lot. They began pushing it, a miserable, sweaty piece of labor humping the thing up and down over the curbs. At one point a small dog rushed them. Its hackles were up. Teeth bared. They had to run two full blocks to get away, each with a hand on the side of the cart. Perspiration was rolling off them.

"So, baby, how do you like being free?" panted Morton when they shuffled up to her apartment.

Over the next couple of weeks a weird kind of rhythm began to develop. Annise's tumor continued to enlarge. Not to anything grotesque, but as the days passed they couldn't help noticing the changes. At the same time a strange heat was taking her over. It caught Morton by surprise, for the things they'd begun to engage in were more like scenes out of the Swedish magazines than the way a couple of red blooded Americans might behave.

In addition, Annise was seeing a lot of Wanda these days, which separated their time to where he could get over to Culver City and fulfill a few of his obligations to Muriel.

Muriel, on the other hand, was busy acclimating to her new emancipation. She told him how reporters from one of the local TV stations had been out to interview her.

"Joseph set it up," she said. "He's been dropping in on me, Morton."

At the mention of the Gestapo the counselor's heart pounded. He'd been searching for a way to underpin his evidence, a blueprint for confirming the man's guilt. There wasn't much point in going to the police. He'd talked it over with Trina Lopez, and the bottom line was a heart attack wasn't a murder unless you had unmitigated proof. You couldn't just shoot the jerk like in the movies. Too bad.

"The Fraction House has been handling your affairs for years, Muriel. I suppose he's going to be around," replied Morton.

"He doesn't have to be here. He brings his camera like he's taping his documentary. I'm afraid of him, Morton. He says things. He calls me his... his..."

"His what?"

Muriel's neck blanched red. "His cunt," she said.

"Oh, Muriel—"

"The thing Joseph wanted most in the world was to take over Harvey's job and be a doctor," she said. "Then he wanted Annise, but only because you wanted her. And he hates you. Now the thing he wants most in the world is me. I know it. I can tell from the ugly way he stares. He's going to make me—"

"What did he do, Muriel? Has he been molesting you? I want to know. When was he here anyway?"

She shook her head. She was unwilling to tell him the specifics for fear of some violent confrontation. It was time to get over that.

"The smarter you get the more Joseph wants you," said Morton. "It's a power trip for him. He gets a sick thrill when he manipulates a smart person."

"Maybe not smarter. Maybe harder to get than his other women," said Muriel looking shyly up.

A number of battles were flying all at the same time. The counselor scratched his beard. Yes, it was a beard now, not a growth.

"He's going to get you, Morton," said Muriel. "Every time he comes over here and I refuse he says, 'I'm going to kill that son of a bitch.' He means you. He thinks we're, you know, lovers."

"He killed Harvey," said Morton.

Muriel was unruffled. Well, decided the counselor, if you knew a man was rotten to the core the particulars of his rottenness wouldn't be much of a revelation.

"Joseph told me you think Harvey's pills were changed. Like maybe somebody messed with them. Joseph doesn't believe it. He says Harvey dropped dead like a lot of fat people do."

"The Gestapo substituted empty pills for Harvey's heart meds, Muriel. That's why he died. Harvey was weak and Joseph took away his medication."

"Joseph always gets what he wants, Morton. He got Sally and nobody could stop it."

"You knew about Sally?"

Muriel nodded. "It was before you came. I told Harvey. That's all I could do, Morton."

"I'd have stopped it if I'd known," declared the counselor tensing.

Muriel sighed. "He doesn't even talk about Annise anymore," she said. "She used to be his number one—well, 'cunt' is the word he uses. Not now though. Now that I'm free it's me. I know exactly what he's after, Morton. It's no good to keep a person prisoner in a prison. It's only filthy for him if he locks them up in the real world. It has to be total manipulation for him to be happy. He's still screwing her, but that doesn't mean he cares about doing it."

"Oh, no, he's not. Annise swears it's over."

Muriel started crying. Morton pulled her to him.

"I wish I could be like Annise," she sniffed. "I wish I could make believe there was a God and have him be in my image like normal people do. It's hard to live in a miserable state of despairs like this."

"Affairs," corrected the counselor.

"Affairs?" said Muriel excitedly.

"That's the line, is what I'm saying. We all want peace of mind. I know I'd give anything for it."

"Mind?" said Muriel. "Are you sure that's what you'd like a piece of?" She looked at him hard.

Ah, your recovering schizophrenic's vivid imagination. It was truly a thing to behold.

* * *

Chapter 60

Morton continued to see Annise, but always at her discretion. She was like a shower with stripped out knobs, hot and cold both in the same blast, and if you tried to adjust the temperature you'd get all of one or the other. This might have had to do with the tumor. She kept saying she'd have it looked at, but never did. Overall though the picture was improving. Yes, improving... He had to get things straight with her, that was all.

The counselor's apartment was looking sparse. Muriel's place had been only partly furnished, and over the weeks he'd transferred much of his furniture to help her out: his recliner, the coffee table, the dishes, the tomato and green pepper plants he'd nursed were placed in the small backyard behind Muriel's bedroom. Subsequently he had to sit on his livingroom floor when he used the telephone. He laid the receiver between his legs and dialed Annise.

"Oh, Morton, I wish you'd have called earlier! Wanda was here this afternoon, and all we needed was one more person to play Twister with us," she answered excitedly.

"I don't know how to play Twister," said Morton.

"Wanda could teach you. She's got incredible patience."

"Well, uh—"

"You were so right, Morton. That name Novice does not fit her one bit. She's moving up at the Fraction House too. She took over Joseph's old office. He's in Harvey's now you know."

"So did you get the doctor's appointment?" asked Morton.

Silence. Odd shuffling sounds. He had a feeling she was checking over the calendar.

"Why don't you come on over," she said. "Aphie sent me this present right out of the blue. You're really going to like it, Morton. It's a skirt." Her voice went deep and sexy. "And don't tell anybody, but it's *ultra*-mini."

Buck Buchanan

Their conversation ended. Thoughtfully the counselor scratched his chin, then took the bull by the horns. There was the physician's referral outlet he'd been in touch with earlier. He'd need to get back with them. After that he sprung for the long distance call to Maryland. Important information he'd been seeking could at last be verified with a simple phone call.

~~~

When he arrived at Annise's he found her fully done up. Eyelashes pre-curled. Hair brushed to a high glistening sheen. He couldn't remember when she'd been ready so far in advance. She'd already showered, and the skirt— Well, suffice to say you needed to press your stopwatch that instant to keep it from striking midnight. That Aphie had taste like nobody's business.

A staggering woman, this Annise Chastain, thought the counselor as he went into the kitchen. A person so close to the throbbing volcano of L.A. culture she was practically afire herself without knowing it. Morton wished he'd brought along a gift. A little silver earring or something.

"So how's mistress Muriel these days?" she asked coming up beside him.

Morton jerked his head around. Yes, she was smiling.

"Oh, fine," he said smiling back. "She's fine, Annise. You should see the paint job she did on the walls."

"No, thanks," returned Annise as she lit a cigarette and pulled the ash tray over. "I'm around so much nuttiness at work. Did I tell you? They paired Gordon with Sally Featherman, and unloaded them both on me. I hope you won't take offense, Morton, but I'd prefer to keep my distance from Muriel."

"Oh, I won't take offense, Annise. I really won't," he assured her quickly.

Morton got a pot out and put a hot dog on to boil.

"I really do admire you though for standing by her," said Annise. "It's not everybody who would put themselves out like you have." Annise turned him from the stove and hugged him.

She kissed him deeply. "And actually spending nights with her!" She backed up and stared proudly at him. "Christ, Morton, that's so selfless."

"Aw, no it's not, Annise."

"Oh, yes it is. In fact, it's the very reason I wanted to get all dolled up for you. Didn't you notice?" She held her arms out and spun around in a full circle. "I wanted to show you what a truly fine man deserves. It took Wanda and me all day to do it up like this."

"You and Wanda?" he muttered.

"Women don't usually get along with each other. But after a girl understands men, women start looking a lot better," said Annise. "As friends, I mean."

"Friends?" The counselor's brow furrowed.

"Wanda knows about men too by the way. You ought to ask her advice, Morton. I mean, if you don't understand your relationship don't you think you could use advice?"

"Like what kind of advice?"

"Well, like sex for instance."

"Sex? What does Wanda say about that?"

"According to Wanda, even if you put your finger on the clit every single day, only once a year will every move, every itsy bitsy touch, be perfect. If you don't understand this, all it says about you is you're not a woman."

"So what did she tell you to do about the tumor?"

"Wanda doesn't tell me what to do, Morton. She suggests, nothing more."

"What did she suggest?"

"She knows a very capable woman mid-wife she wants me to see."

"For a tumor on your butt? That's absurd. You need to see a doctor."

"Wanda is a very enlightened person, Morton. She doesn't truck with doctors."

"She doesn't?"

Annise came to him again. He was overwhelmed by the way she was letting her hands roam so freely. By the way she would switch from a kiss to grasping his head and rolling it between her breasts. He'd never encountered such aggression from her. For a fleeting second it crossed his mind that dallying half naked with Wanda Novice all afternoon could have elevated her to this.

As they heated up Morton struggled to meet the occasion. Wanted her? Yes, yes, he did. On the other hand, there was a timid flutter in his midsection, a wave of fear, it felt like. She had taken him into her hands. Maintain! he told himself. Maintain!

But it was no use. When she realized the problem it was like a rip in fine silk the way he felt her ego tear.

"Oh, Morton!" she cried drawing back. "It's not happening."

"Don't stop, Annise. It'll be all right," he answered.

"But you don't want me," she said looking innocently up. "You can't hide it. I've got the answer right here in my hand and I can see perfectly well you don't want me."

"I do though, baby. I'm just off guard or something."

She pulled away and turned to the mirror over the kitchen sink. "I'm a dog," she said. "An ugly selfish dog like Sassafras, aren't I? That's why you don't want me."

Sassafras heard her name and trotted into the kitchen.

"I think Sassafras is gorgeous," said the counselor.

He tried to turn Annise toward him but she held firm.

"I know what I'm saying, Morton," she interrupted. "Wanda even knows it. It's no wonder you're not excited. And as far as Wanda goes—shit, I don't even think a woman would want a life with me."

"What are you talking about, Annise?"

"I'm only now beginning to understand this," she told him. "I've always been ugly. I've known it from the start too. People pretended I wasn't. I pretend it myself. Like I did around Trina and Stacy and them."

"No, Annise. Listen to me. You're beautiful. You're so beautiful you stun people."

"No," she said becoming stern. "You're treating me like a child, Morton. I am *not* a child."

"But, Annise—"

"Don't you think I know all this is phony?" she said opening her arms and showing herself. Her unhaltered, perfectly formed breasts were clearly visible through the flimsy blouse. Her precise female hips were cocked sensuously under the ultraminiskirt.

"I'll tell you what's real though," she said reaching behind. "This thing." She grasped hard and gave a sharp squeal at the pain.

"It's enormous. And it's getting bigger every minute. Wanda and I had a good long look at it today."

"You and Wanda did?"

"It's like I'm a goddamn leper," she said bitterly.

"Stop it, Annise. I'm telling you, you're beautiful. This is a God's honest fact of evolution. You *are* beautiful. Why the hell don't you believe me?"

"You've never told me," she said.

"I haven't?"

"Never. Not once in all this time."

"Well, I guess I'm trying to understate it. It's so obvious I'm afraid if I say anything it'll be like a joke or something," he defended.

"So now I'm a joke," she said sneering. "You know what Gordon told me the other day? And you realize how intelligent those people can be when they want to."

"What'd he say?"

"Well, he found out about the tumor and all, and he came up and said it was the most wonderful thing he'd ever heard. He said now I'd never get cancer and die a horrible death looking like an old witch in some roach infested hospital. He said—" She choked back her tears. "He said he was glad it was me who got cancer too. Because... Because I'm the most synthetic person he'd ever met."

"He was complimenting you, Annise. That's Gordon's way."

"You know what else he said? He goes, 'Your father is rich, blondey. If anything messes up during the surgery, he can pay for it all. Funerals are terribly expensive these days.'"

She climbed onto the swivel stool and hung her head in her hands. Morton rotated the chair toward him.

"This is exactly the point, Annise. You've got to see a doctor. You must have the thing fixed so you don't go that way. Especially with the baby coming."

"Little Toni, you mean? Did I tell you? We're calling her Toni. I didn't? Well, boy or girl, we're calling her Toni Chastain—I mean, uh, Toni Allis—" Annise trailed off. In terms of anticipations this was going a bit far.

"Listen," she said taking him by the shoulders. "I want to go up to The Shamrock. They've got a really good band tonight. And I'm all dressed and everything. Take me, will you please?"

"But, Annise—"

"I absolutely promise we'll have the hottest round ever when we get back home. OK?" She slumped her shoulders. "Why not, if I'm going to die anyway?"

"Die? What's dying have to do with this?"

"You need to remember, Morton, the Devil always gets his due. I've thought this over a lot, and there's a very good chance you and me are precisely what God owes him," she returned with a sinister slitting of the eyes.

"That's crazy, Annise. Somebody we know might need death, but it's certainly not you."

"Who do you mean?" she asked tilting her head.

"Joseph," said Morton. "He's the killer. He's the one messes in everybody's business."

"Joseph is Joseph's business. There's a line about that in the Bible too if you've ever read it. If God wants Joseph, Morton, he'll put the gun in somebody's hand. And he'll shoot it too. The messenger only carries the message. God loads all the ammo."

"Does God go to jail for it?" asked Morton.

"Christ, you demand a lot. He'll go to jail *with* you, if that's what you're wondering."

"All right," said Morton. "You win. I've got something important to tell you, but let's go up The Shamrock first. I think I need to get you in the mood for it."

Silence. A rolling of the shoulders. A twisting of the legs.

"You know I can't stand a secret. Come on now, out with it."

"Does Aphie know about the tumor, Annise? Do your parents know?"

"Nobody knows. Just you and me and Wanda."

"And everybody at the Fraction House," suggested the counselor.

"Not everybody."

"What about Gary? I mean, your Assistant Priest."

"That's confidential," replied Annise.

Morton thought back. "But he knows about it, doesn't he?"

"No, he doesn't know. Even if he heard it through Confession he's not allowed to know what he heard in an earthly sense. He has to forget he knows it right after I tell him. It's all right though. Gary is *very* sympathetic. And it's not impossible the thing could go away by itself, you think?"

"Listen, Annise, I went ahead and did something maybe I shouldn't have done. You're going to be upset with me for this, but I found a doctor who can handle the type of problem you have. I used Dar/Neese's physician's referral service, you know, so your insurance would kick in. I went ahead and made an appointment for you."

A sharp quiet fell over them. Morton waited.

"You... You made an appointment for me?"

"Yes. I had to. In fact, it's set for tomorrow morning. You're off aren't you?"

"With a doctor?" she muttered weakly.

"Right. A surgeon."

She lunged forward. The counselor feared a blow and tried to protect himself.

"Oh, Morton! This is the best thing I've heard in my entire life!" she cried. She threw her arms around him. "Don't you know it's what I've been waiting for all this time? Not consciously," she added quickly. "I never knew it consciously until this minute. My God, what a genius you are! My mother always handled these things when I was growing up. I guess I never got, you know, mature that way."

~~~

Next was The Shamrock. They didn't however make that. Instead they had the good hot round she'd mentioned right there. Right then, in fact, as she sat awkwardly on the high swivel stool. She was really a torrid piece of abandon these days. And who'd deny what a powerful asset the ultra-mini aspect of her skirt was?

Suddenly she palmed his chest. "Wait. I just thought of something. You'll drive me there, won't you? I'll need somebody with me."

He said, "Yes, baby, yes. I'm going to drive you. Of course I'm going to drive you."

The actual moments were short. Her skin changed like a movie screen. Red to deep yellow. Moist to cold. The shifts were so quick and extreme he worried something more dangerous than lust might be underlying them. Not a demon exactly. And certainly exorcism wouldn't be needed if he was it. But maybe something else that haunted her and hurt her inside, and reversed everything to where it became—well, good. Or bad maybe. At any rate, whatever the ultimate consequence it was exactly correlative to this they were in now. And once started there was no interfering with the convulsive hip slamming joy. At least he didn't think so until she unexpectedly drew him to her and held him fiercely there, one of her techniques he was finding.

"Sometimes, I even think I love you," she whispered hotly. "But I don't. Because if I did I wouldn't feel so sick and sweaty like this."

Back to it. The perfume winding into her own rising odor and filling the kitchen. The hot dog had thickened to three times its size and was bubbling up out of the pot behind them. And just like that it was over. All melted and crystallized and seared so hot you didn't dare touch it. A streak of lightning strained into a dish of butter!

"God," said Annise slowly opening her eyes. "What a fuck!"

* * *

Chapter 61

Morton spent the night. The next morning, before the appointment with the surgeon, Annise moved quickly through the rooms, bumping into things, then wheeling around to stare angrily at them. She rubbed her forehead. She lit cigarettes, but immediately stubbed them out.

The counselor followed her into the kitchen. "Let me help," he said sleepily. "Would you like cereal or something?"

Her hands fell to her sides. "You know perfectly well I'm not allowed to eat anything."

"That's usually before surgery, Annise, not for an examination."

The doctor's office was near Cedars-Sinai Medical Center, in the West Hollywood area. On the drive they heard a radio report saying a lumber treatment plant south of the city had caught fire. Preservatives used in the wood were producing a cloud of what the Disc Jockey called, "slightly carcinogenic fumes." They were beginning to blow toward L.A. proper. Gordon, reflected the counselor, would be standing out in front of the Fraction House about now, breathing deeply.

Annise reached over and gripped Morton's hand. "Oh my God!" she said, her eyes wide. A minute later he saw she had bowed her head. She was praying.

They took the elevator to the fifth floor of the Medical Arts Complex. When they came to the office door Annise stood there flabbergasted. The brass plate read, E.A. WEINSTEIN, M.D.— PROCTOLOGY/SURGERY.

"Proctology! Shit, Morton, this man cuts assholes!" cried Annise snatching a bunch of hair.

Despite himself, the counselor couldn't help a tiny snicker.

In the waiting room several people were sitting on one or the other buttock, their faces screwed up in silent but obviously immense agony. Morton and Annise pulled close on the sofa. Under his eyelashes he could see them secretly staring at her.

What on God's green earth, they were wondering, could bring such a magnificent blonde in *here*? Then, faces all sour and tormented, they'd look slowly over to him.

Annise's name was called. While Morton waited one man, a very obese fellow, shifted clumsily on his seat. When he did this the vinyl cushion gave out a strange popping noise. He'd been one of the gawkers.

"Oh my!" Morton exclaimed thrusting his hand to his mouth.

The others lifted their noses and glared over at the man. Embarrassed, he rolled his shoulders from side to side, which caused more popping from beneath.

"Sorry," he muttered. "Sorry about that."

They wagged their heads in disgust.

Morton took the opportunity to step into the hallway to the pay phone. Five minutes leaning there against the wall while it rang. Hmmm. He was antsy. His breath came in shaky gasps. He remembered the withdrawal concept and fished out one of the real Libriums.

As he was about to hang up, Muriel answered.

"Jesus Christ, girl, why aren't you getting the phone?" he said.

Silence.

"Muriel?"

"Yeah?"

"Why didn't you answer?"

"No reason. Are you coming to visit?"

"Well—" He glanced over his shoulder. "To be honest, it doesn't look like I'm going to get there today. A lot's been happening. If you've got a minute I'll tell you."

"I usually have all the minutes in the world, Morton," she said monotonally. "But right now I don't have any of them."

"Look, I had to go to this appointment with Annise—"

"To be honest, Morton, I'd rather not hear about it," she interjected.

"But, Muriel, I wanted you to know—"

"I really don't want to discuss this," she repeated. "I've learned how much it upsets me and I'm not going to do it anymore."

Jealousy? It felt kind of good to the counselor. How come Annise never showed any? Through the lines Morton recognized a male voice in the background.

"What's that I hear?" he asked quickly. "Is Joseph there again?"

A grotesque silence was transmitted fully formed into his receiver.

"Muriel?"

"I'm here," she said low.

"What's going on? Are you in danger?"

"Not yet," she muttered.

"You can't talk though, can you?"

"No, I can't."

"Do you think he's going to hurt you?"

"I'm never sure. He took me shopping. I've got new clothes. I'm going to start dressing like the rest of the girls in L.A. If anybody knows about female fashion it'd be Joseph."

"I'll be right over. Don't go with him. I'll protect you, Muriel. I promise I will."

"No. You can't come now!" In a super quiet whisper she said, "He'll kill you, Morton. Stay away from here. I mean it."

The front door of the doctor's office opened.

"Mr. Chastain?"

It was the receptionist. Morton cupped the phone.

"Your wife is finished now. She was asking for you," she said.

"My wife? Uh, yes. OK, I'll be right in."

He turned back to the telephone. "Now listen, Muriel—" he started, but there was only the dial tone.

Inside, Annise was at the nurses' window. She waved him over.

"It's a cyst all right," she said a little loud. "He's scheduled me for surgery. They're going to do it at the Surgery Center across from Cedars-Sinai."

"Is it dangerous? I mean, is it cancer?" asked Morton.

"I don't know," she said filling out a form. "He said hair causes it. I must have eaten too much hair or something."

"Hair?"

"He told me the only thing left was prayer. Prayer to the Almighty," she said solemnly.

"The doctor told you that?"

She looked him in the eyes, nodded several times, then turned back to her writing.

~~~

On the way home Annise got her cigarette case out and lit one. A few minutes into the ride she said, "You know, Morton, when a person gets a bad illness they start thinking a hell of a lot about things. Would you mind if I shared something personal with you?" She twisted her hair.

"Absolutely not. I would welcome something personal, Annise."

"Sometimes I feel like you and I have gotten so friendly it's almost like we irritate each other. Do you ever feel that way?"

Morton tightened. "What about the rest of the times?" he asked. "What about the times we're not so friendly? Are they any better?"

"You mean when I feel cold?"

"I guess so," he muttered hesitantly.

"Well, it's always like I'm never doing what I want. Now that I think of it, when I'm feeling cold it's in a way the hottest of all." She gave a quiver. "I mean like so hot it makes me almost nauseous. Do you know what I'm saying?" She looked quickly over at him.

Morton shook his head. "No, I don't think I do."

"Sometimes it amazes me how ignorant you are of sin and degradation and all. You don't seem to have the first idea of why evil is such a horrible thrill."

"I don't?"

"No," she said. "Because if you did you'd show respect for how miserable a person can be when they start to feel really good inside. And quit making faces. All this has been in Scripture right from the beginning."

Annise's mascara had run dark under her eyes. She rummaged in her purse and came up with the plastic makeup case and eyelash curler. For a fleeting instant it crossed the counselor's mind that she might have looked... Not to him... *Never* to him... But to herself, well, maybe a little bit cheap.

"What about your heart, Annise?" he asked her. "What about your feelings? Aren't feelings what really changes the future for people?"

"Feelings don't change anything, Morton. Fate is what changes the future. I've told you a hundred times."

They came down San Vicente Boulevard and turned left onto Wilshire. She pulled the rear-view mirror around and began to fix her makeup. She tossed her earrings onto the dashboard. All at once she lifted her hands to her face.

"Life gets so black sometimes," she said looking rigidly ahead. "Cancer. Pregnancy. The fruitcakes at the Fraction House. It makes you feel like even God can't stop it he's so far away. Aren't any moments just themselves, Morton? That are pure and real so you can live like a human in between? I mean, aren't there *any* like that?" She tugged at her bra straps in irritation. "Everything is always something else," she lamented. "Always either yesterday—which I feel terrible about by the way—or tomorrow when I may not even be alive. But never, *never* just today."

She was tired. Unexpectedly she lowered her head to his lap. A beautiful head, rich and fragrant and healthy. As they were coming into her neighborhood she slowly rose up.

"Morton, I hope you know I didn't mean any of the stuff I said before. I really didn't. Not what I said about you or about God. Will... Will you forgive me?"

"Sure," he waved.

"You really will? You'll really forgive me?"

"Yes," he said. "I forgive you, Annise."

"Jesus Christ! What a fucking saint you are. In all my life I don't think I've ever met anyone as saintly as you!"

Morton turned the engine off, but neither of them moved to get out. She was leaning against the window now, her makeup case still between her legs.

"You're aware of the problem though, aren't you?" she went on.

"What problem?"

"You hating me. Admit it, Morton. You do, don't you? Hate me, I mean?"

"Of course not, Annise. Why would you say such a thing?"

"Because I hate myself. I've always hated myself. This is no secret, Morton. We all feel like that."

"We do?"

"Uh huh. Only now it's going to be even worse. Don't get me wrong, I understand how ugly I am, but if they're going to cut me— And you know damn well they're going to have to." She bit her lip. "Don't you see? Ugliness is one thing, but I'll be—" She lowered her eyes. "Maimed. That scar is going to be there forever, Morty."

"Not badly maimed," he objected reaching out.

She turned the mirror to scrutinize her makeup, then slapped it back his way.

The radio had been on low. In the newly subdued atmosphere they heard the Disc Jockey talking. Annise spun the volume knob. "The nasty toxic cloud has moved west, friends. It's heading out over the ocean," said the voice.

Over the fine countenance of Annise Chastain came a look of blasted out wonder. With the speed of a trigonometry conversion her eyes unclouded and returned to their indigenous riveting green. She began to smile. Her lips formed the defining pout of your magnificent L.A. blonde. She gave the counselor a frisky push on the shoulder.

"See," she said. "I told you so."

* * *

Chapter 62

Annise went ahead inside. Morton lingered in the truck. "I'll be up in a second," he said.

For the longest time he remained in the silent ticking vehicle, the heat rising visibly off the hood. He kept running over Harvey's definition of insanity, which was doing the same idiotic thing over and over and expecting different results. He was touched with a bit of that, no question. But wasn't it also doing a lot of *different* crazed things *one* time?

When he was younger the counselor believed love was having a woman in his brain and thinking about her all the day long. Seizing on her with pure abandon so the two of you remained wrapped in a gauzy, umbilical bubble of joy. Obviously the woman had to be doing this too. But the fact of the matter was nobody stayed with you all the time, not even in your brain. Except— Well, except you. Yourself. Your soul. Really, love amounted to respecting your own fractured personality enough that you wouldn't need to fixate on the other person and place her on some vaulted pedestal. But of course you had to respect her on an equal level in order not to sweat where she'd head off to when you weren't around.

Love. Christ, when you boiled it down it wasn't much more than having a hot date waiting at home and trying like wild to forget she was hot, while in a detached way going about your own daily business.

Independence! Yes, that was it. No. *D*ependence. That's what love was. Because in a bizarre psycho-sexual way you were compelled to get her editorial opinion. Her ability to make you compromise and quit being lackadaisical about important issues like childbearing and job quitting and whatnot. Right? Was this not right?

Morton scratched his head and moved on up the stairwell.

Buck Buchanan

A fear shot through him. Joseph was at Muriel's! Jesus, how deep you could drown in these things. He had to go there immediately.

* * *

Chapter 63

Immediately? No. This with Annise was too important to slough off. He hurried up the stairwell and turned the knob. Amazingly, the door opened. Was she finally catching on? As he clicked it shut he overheard Annise whispering to someone. She'd carried the telephone into the bedroom.

"OK," she said low. "See you in a bit."

It was close to noon. Morton went to the kitchen and began to prepare hot tea.

"Oh, you're here," said Annise joining him in the kitchen. "Never mind that stuff. I want the gin."

He made her a tonic on ice. No gin, she being pregnant. She wouldn't notice. They went into the bedroom. With her fingertips she touched him along the arms. She reached out and began to caress his face. Warmly. Looking deeply at him. She pulled closer and slipped her arms over his shoulders.

"But, Annise, I want to know the diagnosis. It can't really be hair, can it?" persisted the counselor.

In response she lowered her head and fished for a cigarette.

"I'm thinking of something. Did you ask if they can do surgery to a pregnant person?" said Morton.

"He told me it'll be under a local. You know, numb the area they're going to work on. They don't need a test for pregnancy like in real surgery."

"Are you certain of that?" pursued the counselor.

"Look, Morton, I'm not going to be telling some yo-yo doctor I'm knocked up. It's none of his business. Particularly if I'm not quite married yet."

"What do you mean yet?"

On they talked, her warmth gradually increasing, her lips glowing redder and more supple with each sip from her drink. Ah, the placebo effect, better than real gin sometimes. Every few minutes she would draw his face dramatically to hers.

"Do you think this is what being in love is like?" she asked softly.

Morton started to answer, but she placed her fingers over his lips. The air filled with gravity.

"Make me another?" she asked holding up her glass.

"All right." He went to the kitchen.

"Remember Harvey always saying how horrible loneliness is for an adult?" she asked when he returned. "How it's best for a person to be lonely when they're a kid, like I was? Because later, when you get older, you're happy with any friend who'll have you."

"I think Harvey had a few problems," suggested Morton.

Annise twisted her hair. "I wonder about Muriel sometimes. Do you think she's happy? No," she added quickly. "She couldn't be. Muriel doesn't have a friend either."

"It took Harvey a lot of time in therapy to get over his issues," said Morton.

"I've got a therapist. Not Gary, I mean, the Assistant Priest. He's not considered a qualified head doctor."

Morton nodded to the calendar. "I've seen the new J.S.'s up there. They don't stand for Joel Sincowitz, do they, Annise?"

She lowered her head.

"It's Joseph Schopen, isn't it? Jesus Christ, Annise, how could you?"

"He's trying to help me, Morton. He's tried to help me all along."

"How? By regressing you in the tub? Get serious, will you?"

There came a knock at the door.

"My goodness!" cried the blonde running to open up. "Will you look who's here? It's Wanda! I wouldn't have expected this in a million years. Would you, Morton?"

~~~

The two women went into the bedroom. The counselor listened from the kitchen as Annise attempted to describe the cyst. Naturally Wanda was skeptical. "Hair?" she said. "I don't think I've heard of that."

Morton scratched his beard. The situation was slipping out of control. Here she'd been advised to go under the knife, yet hadn't found time to tell her parents. Hadn't mentioned it to Aphie. Didn't seem to know the first thing about the risk ratios. Maybe, like she said, the Lord God had a handle on it. In the meantime though, Morton found the number and dialed the doctor's office. He talked softly from over by the stereo where they wouldn't hear.

"My apologies for troubling you," he said. "Perhaps you can help me. It's regarding, ummm, Mrs. Chastain," he said reluctantly.

"Oh, yes. The lovely young lady we saw earlier today," replied the nurse.

"Right. She's a bit confused about the diagnosis."

The nurse was very cordial. It wasn't at all unusual to misunderstand these things, she told him. "Will you hold? I'll get the file," she said.

She came back and ran it down for him. A polyneidal cyst, it was called. Small hairs, she clarified, tended to grow inward from a dimple on the coccyx.

"It's virtually harmless, Mr. Chastain. It's much like an ingrown toenail. They're almost always benign. You really shouldn't worry."

"I shouldn't?"

"Oh, no," confirmed the nurse. "We see this all the time."

~~~

Wanda couldn't stay long. She'd managed to shoot over on her lunch break. When they emerged from the bedroom Morton noticed the Social Worker carrying Joseph's small Sharp camcorder. Hmmm, what kind of films might *these* be, wondered the counselor?

"I heard you took over the Gestapo's office," said Morton.

Wanda's jaw tensed. "There's nothing the matter with that. They made me the new Clinical Supervisor. I had to have an office."

"I suppose so." Morton felt listless, as if a depression were taking him over.

"Joseph's in Harvey's office now," said Annise. "He redesigned the whole third floor you know."

"I know," said Morton.

The two women hugged, backed off, hugged again.

"I'll be chanting for you, Annise," said Wanda. "We'll get up to Venice soon and go rollerblading."

Morton walked Wanda down to her car.

"Annise is going to be all right," he said low. "I called the doctor's office."

"She's very upset, Morton."

"I understand. They explained the entire thing to me, though."

The two of them leaned against Wanda's mid-size Buick, a family car really, as he told her the details.

"I didn't want you to worry. I realize you care about her," said Morton.

"Thanks, that was nice of you," said Wanda. Her eyes were damp. "Candidly, Morton, it goes against my grain to say this to the opposite sex, but you really are a good man."

The new supervisor leaned and kissed the ex-counselor on the cheek. It was the right thing, and Morton felt good about it. She entered her car and drove off.

~~~

When he returned to the bedroom Morton was set on his heels at the sight greeting him. Annise had fallen fast asleep, one foot hanging limply off the bed. In addition, she was stark naked. Whew! What a welcome, ruminated the counselor with a smile.

He noticed the locking box, historically an indication of things to come. It was open and kicked sideways in the bunched up bedspread and haphazard array of pillows. Some of the rarer items had spilled out around the lid. It briefly crossed his mind that the toys, even sex itself might be an intricate blocking mechanism, a Garden of Eden hideout from the wolf's teeth of hard-core truth. Sassafras came in wagging her tail. She started to hop onto the bed.

"No, girl," whispered Morton easing her down.

Poor dog, always at the wrong place at the wrong time.

Morton took a moment to replace Annise's IRA and the set of small chrome handcuffs, petite but functional, obviously styled for a female wrist. He scooped up the shiny brass cartridges he'd unloaded from the *Smith & Wesson* derringer that time and dropped them into the Winchester box beside the horse's head whip.

He came across a medication vial, hidden partly under the covers. It was his old Librium prescription, the original one Annise had swapped out in Venice. Librium? No, wait, it wasn't Librium at all. He knew this now. Dilaudid is what it was. Christ, had she taken it?

He checked the cap. It was on tight. He put his ear to her face and listened to her breathing. He gingerly lifted her wrist and counted her pulse rate. Normal. A lot steadier than his own, in fact.

The counselor heaved a sigh of relief. Gently he raised her leg back onto the bed. She didn't stir. What an exhaustion it all was for her, he thought. Sin. Degradation. The sudden shock of forgiveness, only to be followed by a chronic renewal of despair. Even more disturbing were those secrets in the middle of her bright blonde pie which possibly weren't but could be considered lies, depending on your interpretation. And if they survived as lies they were lingering nastily overdue, up for payment so to speak, and dragging down her heart like a couple of cement overshoes. Honestly though, he couldn't blame Annise for her fatigue. Life in metropolitan L.A. was enough to make the Pope himself a little jaded in the joints.

As Morton was putting the box away his eyes roamed to the calendar. All those initials—struck through now, yes, thanks to their agreement. Nevertheless, they attested to a heavyweight sensuality. The more sex a person engaged in did tend to make them sexier in your head. And there, printed in red on the day in question, were the words 'Little Toni.'

A rush of warmth passed over him, followed by a jolting chill. Maybe it wouldn't be so bad to have a baby with a beautiful woman. A lovable slutiness steamed up from the golden sweep of her hair as it coursed in wisps across her arms and off her hips, an aura of angelic submission she never exhibited, at least to him, in her waking hours.

Morton fixed the pillow. He got a blanket from the closet and fluffed it over her. Something hard was under the sheet. He lifted it. In her hand was the pistol, the derringer, its gleaming trigger guard ringed her forefinger like a Third World wedding band.

"Oh, no," murmured the counselor.

Immediately he recalled their early talk about the rapist, about suicide. He took the thing away and finished tucking her in.

As a test, to check if she was pretending to be asleep, for he knew she was capable of faking, he whispered, "Muriel and I care for you, Annise. Don't worry, we won't let you die in some roach infested hospital."

She remained still.

He turned the radio on low, left a pleasant note on the coffee table, and drove quickly to Muriel's.

* * *

Chapter 64

When he turned into the Culver City area Morton noticed a foul odor coming from the engine, like burned oil. He kept sniffing for the source, until finally, leaning over the steering wheel, he realized it was his own odor, a heavy male stench rising from beneath his arms. It was the smell of stress.

He was in the process of squirting breath freshener under there as a quick fix when he saw this person walking along. Female. Early twenties, it looked like. He slowed. And very saucy too what with those tight aqua-marine shorts and the hair stringing down from an old-timey hippie hat.

He glanced up the street toward Muriel's apartment. No, the Gestapo's car wasn't there, thank God.

He crept along, kind of craning his neck at the girl, when he realized what he was doing. Good Lord, he thought, what kind of a lecher are you? Sincerity? Hah! In L.A. *all* the roads were Beaver Boulevard. Even he had to laugh at what a farce it was.

Just then the girl looked up. Hair tumbled around her cheeks under the funky looking hat. In a flash their eyes met. He looked harder. By God if it wasn't Muriel! Sweet little—

Morton zoomed across the traffic and stopped the opposite way along the curb, a highly illegal maneuver. Had her hair really lightened so much these last weeks? He rolled down the window.

"Oh, hello, Morton," she said.

He eyed her. She had on a very skimpy halter-top. Her sandals were laced far up the ankles. Things flowing jelly-like and curving out suggestively in various directions.

"Where, uh... Where did you get those clothes?" he said.

Shyly she looked herself over. "I told you. Joseph bought them for me. Don't you like them?"

"Well, I suppose—"

"I see other girls dressed this way. I think I'm finally getting normalized, Morton. Into the mainstream and all like Harvey always wanted. Aren't you proud of me?"

"Did Joseph leave?" asked the counselor glancing around.

"Yes. He had a woman from the TV station with him. They're going to do a piece on me."

"Great."

"Not really. It's to make him look good so he'll keep getting my father's money."

Morton stared up the road. "They interviewed you? In that outfit?"

"Why not?" said Muriel.

Moments of quiet. She glared at the traffic.

"Where are you going?" he asked. "Up to the market? I can drive you if you want."

"I'm going to see my friends," she said.

"Friends?" An irrational notion caught him. Might these be the Annise Chastain brand of friends?

"I'll be late if I don't go on," said Muriel. She started to walk.

Morton clamored out and strode along beside her. When they came to the bus stop Muriel sat on the bench and crossed her legs.

"Look, Morton, the only friends I have are at the Fraction House. I'm going over there to visit them." There was a feather of irritation in her voice.

"To the Fraction House?"

"I told Joseph I wouldn't ride with him. I'm going by myself."

A loud roaring sound approached. It was the bus. The doors swung open.

"Muriel, this isn't fair! I came to protect you," he called as she stepped up.

"Maybe you need to protect your blonde," she said stonily.

Muriel boarded and moved through the aisle, hat cocked all weird.

The counselor started to enter behind her. He slapped his pockets for change. Nothing. His truck was a block down the road. Still running probably.

"Stay away from that goddamn Gestapo!" he called as a shroud of black, greasy smoke surged out the engine grates. It swirled around him like in one of those 18th Century gunpowder wars.

When it at last cleared he saw her face pressed against the glass of the rear window, much like the long ago night she'd been swooped away by the ambulance.

The bus chugged heavily into the distance. He waved to her through the closed windows.

She waved weakly back, and was gone.

* * *

Chapter 65

Morton parked in back and used the key Muriel insisted he keep on his ring to enter the rear of the apartment.

For several minutes he stood in the doorway. It seemed so cold in there. So unfurnished, even with his donated recliner and sofa. Hadn't he noticed this before? For the first time he realized he'd never been alone in this place. What was it he'd told Muriel about people who weren't comfortable alone with themselves? Shit, hard to remember the things you once declared you'd never forget.

Morton noticed a short stack of pamphlets on the kitchen counter. Muriel's silver hairpin was on top of them. He lifted the small piece of jewelry and turned it in his fingers. It felt warm, like a rabbit's foot, like a souvenir you'd save to caress when she wasn't around. He slipped it into his pocket. He'd present it to her later, put it in her hair himself maybe, the way you'd do for a good friend.

He began to absently leaf through the pamphlets. Pictures of northern Oregon, looked like, and mailed directly to Muriel's address. Brochures from the Chamber of Commerce apparently. Hmmm, what was this about?

He wandered into the small concrete backyard. His plants were gleaming in their boxes. Well, her plants now, as it was working out. Tomatoes had formed, large and green and smelling of the rich mulched soil.

He returned to the kitchen and looked in the refrigerator for the jug of iced tea he knew she kept there. It seemed barer than he remembered. God, how fast things changed these days. And what was this strange square bottle hidden in the side door? A fifth of Rumple Minze peppermint schnapps, 100 proof, active ingredient for the Gestapo's trademark Snakebite. How had a desperado like Joseph Schopen gotten so mixed up in his life?

Morton got the bottle and a glass and sat at the table. His wrist started to ache. It hadn't felt like this in months. He began to press into the bone. Pain. What a sweet, funny feeling. In his heart, the counselor sagged. Psychologically a person could plummet into a stupor as bad as the drugged up physical kinds. Ultimately there was no avoiding the abyss. So much to be resolved, but what exactly did you do? He felt like he'd been thrashing around in some chlorinated L.A. quicksand, chest high and rising toward his throat. The Pasadena variety, he wondered? Or was this simply one of those dreams where you're caught naked in public and desperately embarrassed, because, God forbid, you were trying to keep afloat without the bright spandex bathing suit everyone else was wearing.

He drank the schnapps. Hot. Fierce. Like an animal. This was the first time, he kept thinking, the very first time he'd been here alone.

A perpetual turbulence assailed him these days. He worried about everybody uniformly. Maybe Annise was right. Maybe there weren't any moments that existed all on their own, pure and free where you could lie back and feel like a human. Maybe it really was all black, like she'd said.

He took the bottle and sat cross-legged on the cold livingroom floor. He was wearing his Dodgers baseball jacket. A lot of people wore jackets in L.A. A clank resounded against the glass, and he felt a heaviness in his pocket. It was Annise's derringer, which he'd hastily appropriated back in her bedroom.

Did it matter really how much time was passing? It might have been hours. He didn't know. Sitting there switching the gun from hand to hand. Thinking things over.

He remembered the famous argument with Annise about the word novice—how you pronounced it. She thought he was being uppity due to confusing his schooling with the long years Joseph made up about going to Johns Hopkins.

"You think you're so damn smart," she'd snapped. "You act like you're God. I bet you do think you're God sometimes."

He smiled. "Yes, I do. Now come over here and give God a little kiss." He puckered his lips.

Buck Buchanan

"Jesus Christ! You really do think that!" she exclaimed grasping her forehead in dismay.

But if there was one thing Morton understood, it was that he was *not* God. And when you looked hard you saw Annise Chastain was not necessarily your working stiff's guardian angel either.

He was thinking of Sassafras with her nervous, paranoid eyes, how she was constantly interrupting their lovemaking. Morton persisted in edging her away with the side of his foot, but the inevitable growl came.

"She makes you feel so guilty," said Annise.

The blonde fell out of the mood. The counselor went to the kitchen, and through the cracked door saw Annise secretly using her teeth to peel back a hangnail on her finger. She entered the kitchen and squeezed the tip. A drop of blood pulsed up.

"Ouch, Morton. Look what Sassafras has done," she said.

Annise glared at the menacing beagle.

"Oh you bad dog!" she scolded slapping at Sassafras with the dish towel. "You bad bad dog!"

Surely this was not the proper way. Things were going to have to change. He needed out of the soul-sucking desert quicksand, out of the opulent, kidney shaped swimming pools of ultra-suburbia and into the gentle salts of the ocean, of the Pacific, into the minerals and the mellow organic ores of human nature he knew were out there somewhere. How though, huh? How?

It was getting dark. So barren in there. Except for the walls of course. The closet door had been left open and he could make out something staring down at him from the upper shelf. It was Little Morton, Muriel's doll. But Little Morton always stayed on the sofa, like a pillow.

The wrist throbbed. He cocked and aimed the gun. *Sacred* Little Morton, he wondered? The one she would never under any circumstances leave behind? Wherever in this horrible hateful world she went or was sent to or found herself crazy in she would never, she told him, never leave Little Morton behind.

In addition, a gray wad of his stuffing was hanging out from the seam along the side of his head. Was this the way she took care of her friends?

Let it go, just let it go. Realistically, the foremost thing was Annise anyway. Yes, definitely Annise. He eased the hammer down. It wasn't loaded, he'd seen to that during their first eccentric session with the locking box.

"All right, Annise," he said out loud. "Time to take a long hard look at... at..." He hesitated. The doll's glass eyes had begun to glow a supernatural red in the new darkness. "A long look at little Toni?" he wondered. "At little Toni Chastain? Er, Allison, rather? My... My daughter?"

Such thought processes!

~~~

The counselor rubbed the pistol hard against his temple. The steel was cool. Firm. He cocked it for practice, and once again eased down the hammer. He changed hands and rubbed the barrel against his opposite jaw. Like a small epiphany it occurred to him this was probably what Annise meant when she talked about turning the other cheek, making sure you were able to take the abuse evenhandedly from either side.

It was then he heard the high whining foreign engine out front, which he knew to be Joseph's poorly sculpted gold-colored Jaguar.

Morton scrambled to his feet and peered through the front curtains. Twilight had receded to a dark gray. The Jaguar's windows were shaded with a deep titanium tint, yet he was positive he saw the Gestapo draped lewdly over his passenger.

This would be Joseph's way. Everything clouded and indistinct, but the morose pawing and thrill seeking going on nonetheless. And the passenger? Muriel, of course. It made him sick to his stomach.

Morton lowered his head and began the deep breathing techniques Harvey had taught him. He muttered something to himself, but it was too profane to repeat aloud.

All of a sudden the front door flew open. It was Joseph. Before the counselor knew it he was wedged in the entrance, blocking the Gestapo's way.

"Wait!" cried Joseph pushing out his palms. A fine terror was in his voice. He tried to backpedal but stumbled into Muriel, who was right behind him. Morton stepped closer.

"Please," pleaded Joseph. "Please don't shoot, Allison!"

Muriel was straining to her tiptoes to see over Joseph's shoulder. Both of them seemed terribly alarmed. An intense rushing sound was in the counselor's ears.

It took a number of moments before Morton realized what was happening. He was clutching the derringer. Inadvertently he'd raised his arm and pointed the gun at Joseph. Inadvertently?

The muzzle now pressed flush against the Gestapo's forehead, making two strange red indentations, over and under. Morton noticed the exotic, sulfurous odor of burnt gunpowder in the air, though the gun had yet to be fired. Curious how the brain worked.

The counselor's beard had grown wispy from neglect and marbled with pale blonde lanes along the cheek bones. Joseph's ebony five o'clock shadow reached high under his eyes, like the hoof prints of a goat who'd been stomping around the manure pit all day. The two men resembled a couple of desperado cowboys at the OK Corral.

Very deliberately Morton dragged back on the hammer. The derringer sounded its ominous clicks as the lock work advanced to the fully cocked position.

"Oh my God!" gasped the Gestapo. Slowly Muriel sunk to her knees. She was shaking.

"I saw you pawing her in the car," said Morton. "I was looking out the window. I saw it, Joseph."

'L.A. 2000:' Sex Asylum

The new Director appeared to want to answer, but his jaw was quivering too badly. His mouth opened and closed, but no words came.

"You're a rapist," continued Morton. "You killed Harvey. You broke Sally Featherman like a toothpick."

Joseph squeezed shut his eyes. So as to not jar the pistol, he remained still as a piece of dusty chrome in the salvage yard. "Don't do it, Allison. Please, I'm begging you. Please don't," pleaded the Gestapo.

"You molested Muriel. You're a criminal, Schopen. You've got to go."

Joseph's forehead skin wrenched as the counselor's finger tightened on the trigger. How much schnapps had he downed anyway?

"No, he didn't!" exclaimed Muriel. "He didn't grab me, Morton. We were getting out of the car is all."

Morton looked down at Muriel's supplicating form. It seemed such a humiliating position. A sadness poured over him. A river of tears for Muriel and for Sally, for Gordon, for all the hurt doves with whom he'd spent so much time splinting their fragile wings. For Annise too, in fact. Yes, for Annise too.

He lowered his arm. He was practiced at uncocking the gun by now. He did this.

A great sigh sprung from deep inside Joseph's muscular chest. Morton could smell the alcohol and tobacco on his breath. They bored into one another's eyes. The Gestapo's pupils were flood-gate dilated from Dexedrine, or from coke, maybe even from fear, assessed the counselor. He was straightening up quick though.

"You really would shoot me, wouldn't you?" said Joseph.

"Of course not. But I would turn you in to the police," returned Morton.

"What do you mean, the police? You're the one who put a gun to my head, Allison. I guess I'm not as smart as I used to be. I never thought of you as a killer. Maybe you're the one who did Harvey in. The police already have that idea, you know."

A jingle sounded as the Gestapo nervously delved for his car keys.

Muriel came to her feet. She edged carefully around Joseph and looked Morton up and down. She looked at the derringer. He could feel her panic.

"Don't make such a big deal of it," said Morton. "The gun isn't loaded for Godsake. What do you two take me for anyway?"

As proof he tripped the latch and broke open the barrel. Make an exhibit of it.

Darkness had fallen. The lights weren't on yet in the apartment. Outside the streetlamps had begun to glow. Morton angled the L of the opened pistol toward the road. The three of them stared feebly into his hands. For there, in the chromium glint of the stubby over-and-under barrels shone a pair of bright brass shells, the centerfire nipples of the percussion caps intact.

Morton's mouth dropped open. He had a sudden vision of Joseph's splattered apart skull, an afterbirth of blood and brains impregnating Muriel's dry sidewalk. In dismay he shook the *Smith & Wesson* like a salt shaker, and out dropped the two .38 caliber bullets. They clacked together in his palm, live as baby rattlesnakes.

Jesus H. Christ, thought the counselor. Annise had reloaded it. She *was* going to shoot herself!

Joseph glowered at Muriel. His eyes enlarged with— What? Lust, would you call it? A macho greed for her innocence perhaps? Conquer her and thereby gather a modicum of purity and strength for himself, like the cannibals of old eating the still pulsating heart of their bravest adversary to in some crazed way become the host?

Quickly he snapped the shells back into the bore and returned the gun to his jacket pocket. He made sure they saw. One's safety sometimes required being armed.

Joseph turned and walked toward his car. The counselor went inside and picked up the fifth of Rumple Minze. He returned to the doorway, and with a violent overhand delivery flung the bottle toward the Gestapo.

The Dexedrine must have kicked in, or the coke, because Joseph pivoted like a seasoned third baseman and snared the bottle in mid air. Miraculously he grabbed the neck, otherwise the glass would have hit directly between the eyes. The top hadn't been capped, and the alcohol spewed into his face, splintering like sliced diamonds in the streetlight.

Morton's heart sunk at what he'd done. Joseph's teeth were showing, but he didn't make a peep.

"Now *there's* a Snakebite," said the counselor.

Morton seized Muriel's wrist and pulled her inside. He was coming unglued, and he knew it. He whirled and kicked shut the door.

* * *

Chapter 66

Morton intended to return to Annise's, but under the circumstances he felt he could not leave Muriel alone. He was about to telephone, describe the situation and all, but he thought, no, better to let Annise take the reins for once. How else did you find the way a person honestly felt if you were always interfering with their possible kindnesses? He'd wait. She knew where to find him.

For the longest time Muriel stayed in her bedroom. Morton didn't bother her.

Around ten she emerged in a tattered red T-shirt and her holey blue jeans, the waist button undone in the new beachy style the girls were sporting.

She casually placed the Oregon brochures into one of the kitchen drawers. Then she fetched Little Morton from the closet and reclined lazily on the sofa.

Morton was sensitive to a kind of damsel in distress look about her, sleepy-eyed, yet frustrated. Though there wasn't a chill in the air she pulled the pink satin throw blanket, a housewarming gift from Wanda, over her legs.

Morton scooted a kitchen chair close to the sofa to be near her. He attempted a lead in. He was getting so much smarter. He'd found for instance that women, schizophrenics included, didn't go in a straight line toward a topic no matter what the gravity.

Muriel seemed particularly distracted tonight. Not distant exactly, but, well, uncomposed, say. They made small talk, but neither seemed very comfortable with it.

"Tell me why you were with Joseph, Muriel," blurted the counselor finally. Well, he'd tried.

"He got me off the bus stop in front of the Fraction House. I didn't even have a chance to run inside."

Morton shook his head in disgust.

"He started driving and I couldn't jump out. He was kidnapping me."

Muriel looked forlornly up. She made a suspicious gyration under the small patch of blanket.

"I told him not to come to my place because you were here and you'd take care of him," she said. "He didn't believe me. He was bringing me back for who knows what."

"I know what."

"What? Say it," she insisted. "I want to hear."

"Hear a bunch of dirty words?" he said.

Muriel squiggled nervously. "Uh huh," she said.

"Did he have a gun?" asked Morton.

"He can strangle people. He's got pills. I don't know. And now he's got one of those straight jackets they used to put on Gordon. I guess he found it in the old storage closet in C-Wing."

Morton jutted his jaw. "I wasn't here though," he pointed out. "I mean, you didn't know I was."

"Don't be so sure. Women know a lot of things they don't actually know," she said, her breath shortening.

Hmmm, where'd he heard that before?

"Kidnapping is a Capital Offense, you know. Or at least a felony. Why didn't you tell me this when you were at the door with Joseph?"

"Because you'd have shot him!" cried Muriel.

"Some people need killing."

"But you don't need life in prison for doing it. Or the electric chair either."

Morton thought it over. Muriel's eyelids fluttered. Vibes. Sex vibes, obviously running here. Reclining so weirdly on the sofa. Leg half cocked. She was making a move. He saw the hump of Little Morton under the satin coverlet. She pushed him onto the floor.

Well, sooner or later the counselor had to face the fact he wasn't pursuing her. Even a schizophrenic would be wise to this much. In more ways than one their history called for it. Was he ready?

Immediately Morton reverted to the hard details of Joseph's transgressions. That Gestapo was an enterprising son of a—

"Oh, Muriel!" he gasped halting, for he could see what was happening. "I'm sorry. I... I didn't realize—"

She held her breath for a long moment, then rapidly exhaled.

"It's all right. I'm just getting rid of tension," she said.

Morton sat there stupefied. She maintained the small circular movement of her hand. Her left leg was bobbing up and down.

"So how have you been?" she asked. "Tell me about you, Morton, nobody else." She looked over at him, her eyes smoked with a burnished iridescent tint, like little homes in a forest fire.

"I'm fine. Just fine really," sputtered the counselor. "But Muriel, is it all right for me to sit here like this? I mean, while you're... you're..." He was tongue tied.

"Masturbating?" she said.

Morton blushed red as a windblown stoplight. "Well, if you have to put it in those terms," he muttered.

"Oh, sure. I'm not nervous or anything, if that's what you're worried about."

"You do seem peaceful. I wish I could learn a few relaxation techniques." He wiped his brow.

"You're probably not feeling safe these days. If you're not protecting yourself every minute, Morton, you're not going to feel safe. Gordon taught me that much."

Swan-like, she rolled her head. Her hair V'd silkily around her cheeks.

Morton leaned on his knees. "Well, maybe I'm not. I've been trying to take things day by day. I really don't know what else to do."

Muriel scratched her head with her free hand. The other kept its rhythm. "What isn't taken day by day?" she asked.

"How about eternity? Eternity isn't taken day by day," he said.

"It's not?" She gave a quiver.

"Well, maybe it is. How the hell do you expect me to know, Muriel?" he returned waving his hand.

"You're the counselor," she said, breathless. "If you don't know how are you going to help me? *I'm* the one who needs a reason to go on."

"I need a reason too," he reminded her softly. "Things are happening out there. I can't ignore it all."

"You can't?"

"If I ignored everybody I thought was a nut there wouldn't be anybody left to talk to."

Her breaths were running short and quick. Out of courtesy he looked off to the side wall. This past week she'd done more painting. A blue and red rainbow arced downward from the ceiling and converged with the hardwood floor. Nice.

Then he heard the rarely published screech of female pleasure. He turned to see her hips driving upward, the pelvic area vibrating. The cover drifted away, and what was left was quite a sight.

~~~

Moments passed. By degrees her breathing began to even out. Morton reached over and touched her forehead.

"Ahhh, you feel good," she moaned.

"Tell me something, Muriel. I've always wanted to know why a woman does a thing like that." He felt himself flushing.

She shifted onto her side. "I think it does what Stacy used to do for you a couple of times a week. And Joseph says drinking does for him."

"Does what?"

"Lets him relax. No, *release*, that's the word. It makes time slow down. And at the very end it stops." She looked him in the eyes.

There was a dampness beneath Morton's arms. His chest had tightened.

"I guess I'm— Well, you know—" he sputtered.

"What?" asked Muriel looking concerned.

"Aroused," he said nervously.

"You're always so jumpy, Morton. I wish you'd try to let yourself go a little bit."

Muriel paused. With a ripple of her shoulders, she added, "A woman likes sex better after she's just had sex."

"Really? I didn't know that."

She rolled her eyes dreamily toward him. A cool, innocent blue they were, and lucid as sunshine.

"It's comfortable here," she said. She patted the sofa.

"Oh, no," objected Morton leaning far back in the chair. "You may be your own Guardian now, but there's this newfangled thing known as pregnancy going around. I'm sorry, Muriel. It's impossible."

"I wouldn't get pregnant on you, Morton. I'm trained in use of the Koroflex Press 70 cm diaphragm. It's not honest to trick a man," she said matter of factly.

"The diaphragm?" Morton felt a little uneasy inside. "Do you have one?"

"Oh, yes. Harvey said they can get lost real easy with us nuts. He gave me a bunch of them."

Morton looked up at the river with Annise's fish eyes in it. At the mountains with the snow covered peaks. At the cactus with its gnarly, humanoid arms and legs. Then he looked back to Muriel. She was a doll, no doubt about that. An immensely beautiful woman, when you really got down to it. Impeccable in the supple fragility of her mind, feather hearted but solid and independent as well, except of course for needing a man, a mate, like she'd said, who would look over her shoulder for her. And there were those fine sunshiny neck hairs...

"Don't worry, Morton, I'm safe," she declared taking him gently by the hand. "Completely safe."

* * *

Chapter 67

Morton did not join Muriel on the sofa. He was tense, like they all said. She wanted him to stay the night on account of the Gestapo's reign of terror. Naturally he agreed. Strange how he didn't feel afraid when he envisioned the ultimate confrontation. He feared for Muriel, yes, and he feared for Annise, but as for himself there was only the urge to do the next most important thing. And do it patiently by God, even if you were deep in enemy territory. Legal aspects seldom entered his head, which could be a problem. Would he have fired his weapon on the Director, given a sudden altercation?

The next day came and went. No call from Annise. No harassment from the Gestapo. Gordon telephoned to say hi. That was nice.

Morton and Muriel spent the daylight hours tuning up the surrealistic wall painting, the counselor passing brushes up to the artist as she teetered on the aluminum step ladder.

"Mind if I stay another night?" asked Morton.

"No!" cried Muriel looking down. "I mean, I don't mean no. I mean yes I don't mind at all. Not one little bit."

~~~

The following morning Muriel emerged from the bedroom wearing the counselor's button down shirt. It reached to high thigh. She was barefoot. Morton rolled groggily in the covers of the sofa bed.

"I'll cook us up some eggs," she called from the kitchen.

Morton stowed the covers, shut the louvered closet door, returned the bed to a sofa, and clip-clopped across the wooden floor. He pulled her to him and hugged her. Such a sweet thing she was, except for a bit of an odd smell coming. Hygiene problems, he wondered? But no, it was smoke!

He reached over and quickly pulled the pot off the eye. The four eggs, he could see, had turned a nasty brownish color.

"Are they done already?" asked Muriel.

Morton tilted the container. The eggs clanged against the sides.

"I don't see any water in here," he noted.

"Water?"

"Well, yes. When you cook eggs you can't just cook them, baby. You've got to *boil* them. You put water in here—"

Morton glanced wanly out the window. For a frightful second he wondered if this stumbling around reality's back roads with the likes of a certified loony was the right thing after all.

He dumped out the burned eggs, cleaned the pan, put new eggs in, added water, set the timer. Muriel watched carefully. He could feel her bubbling with enthusiasm.

"You're going to be my own private person now, aren't you, Morton? Not person," she corrected. "I mean like therapist and soul mate and everything we do all in the same man." She clutched him excitedly.

Morton raised his eyebrows. He took a moment to give her a calculated once over. Legs firm and young. Facial skin like a spring melon, smooth and gleaming through the sulfur-smelling egg air. Eyes pure and free, gazing up at him in her wonderful schizo way where everything no matter how old and worn was always brand new and about to send a fresh thrill deep into you. She took a tiny step backward.

"Don't you want to be my therapist?" she asked. Her voice was low and timid.

Morton said, "Only if I can get in the same tub."

She stared confusedly at him. The timer went off. He put the pan in the sink and began to run cool water into it.

"I'm joking, Muriel," he said.

The awareness hit and she broke into a wide grin.

"OK. I'll go fill the tub!" she said hurrying away.

Morton wasn't sure if you could call it right or wrong, this hanging out with Muriel. He wasn't sure about a lot of things these days. But at least he was taking steps, wasn't he? At least *something* was being set into motion.

~~~

In the afternoon of the second day at Muriel's, Morton said, "I need to run by my place. I've got to do a load of wash. Feed the cat."

"You don't have a cat."

"I feed the neighbor's cat sometimes. I give her leftovers sometimes."

"Don't go, Morton, please."

"I'm drifting in limbo, Muriel. I'm in the same grungy clothes, the same shitty frame of mind."

Morton slipped on his jacket. Muriel went to the drawer and quickly withdrew the travel brochures. She made an exhibition of spreading them out on the kitchen table. He watched as the leaflets, illustrated with slick glossy photographs of Oregon's shoreline and misty mountain ranges, unfolded across the Formica.

"It's so pretty up there," said the counselor checking them out. "But we all need a place to stay, Muriel. That's common sense."

"Not if you keep moving," she said. "Think about it. As long as a person keeps moving they don't need a place to stay."

What was this, streetwise Zen taking the place of regression therapy?

"I've got an apartment of my own, Muriel. Sooner or later I'm going to have to find work. I can't stay here forever."

Her eyes went big and searching. "Why not?" she asked holding out her hands. "Give me one good reason why not."

* * *

Chapter 68

At his apartment Morton found the message light flashing on his answering machine, a rare and exciting event. So she did care, after all. He nervously hit the play button.

"This is Wanda, Morton. Call me. It's regarding our mutual friend."

'Friend' was Wanda's name for patients turned loose in society. It had a socio-cultural ring to it. The next message began.

"Morton, this is Trina Lopez. I come by and find no one when I knock. You are all right? I must tell you, I have been fired. Joseph did something. He has found bad power since he becomes Dar/Neese Director. He black-eyed me with my boss, as I think you say. Be so careful, my friend. I have concern for you. I am sad, but I am angry too. We will fight together if you want. Please do not forget to take your Librium. You may have headache. You may get confusion or jumpy. Call to say you are OK, amigo. Gracias, and adios."

A third message buried under the last one perhaps? He fiddled with the machine, but nothing.

The counselor wandered through the rooms. No recliner. No coffee table. His TV set had gone to Muriel's weeks ago. Even his clothes were in other people's dresser drawers these days.

He began to fill his duffel bag. Unsure of his motive, he started gathering his backcountry camping gear. The Northface tent. His labyrinthine Gregory Mountain backpack. The flyweight Wilderness Experience sleeping bag, double stuffed with eiderdown.

As he went about lashing it under the bungee cords in the bed of his pickup he spotted a zipper broken here, a squall of feathers puffing through a ripped seam there. He sagged and leaned over the dented fender. Unhappiness. What was the definition? Yes, it was squandering your best years fixing busted stuff. Never getting a moment of simple enjoyment what with all the darning of toe holes in other people's minds. And then getting stuck with having to right godawful injustices, unbelievable homicides or incest, while simultaneously re-wiring the ancient corroded windshield wipers so you could see your way clear to the shoot-out.

He pulled away. Christ, what a nightmare. And rush hour traffic didn't even begin to thin until seven.

~~~

He drove to Vera's.

By this time the noise level at the Russian diner had lifted to a numbing roar on account of the many oldsters calling into each other's ears to hear. They were getting pre-pumped for happy hour down at Lost Weekend, the lounge they frequented.

"Leroy, how are you?" said Morton. "Benny, good to see you. The old lady still kicking?" And on down the line the counselor greeted them.

At last he found a seat at one of the booths. He needed a moment of privacy. Vera appeared for his order.

"Ah, Morton. Here is coffee. Here is water."

"Thanks, Vera."

"Why you have not been to see me?"

"I don't know. Problems, I guess. You know, with the new Director."

"But you are not there no more."

"I'm not supposed to be, but I seem to keep hanging around."

"You are tired. You have too many girlfriends. Vera knows this." She patted the counselor on the shoulder. "When you need therapy, come see me. Not girls. Not psychos. Me. I want to help. I am old, but I am a good helper."

Morton sighed and leaned back against the worn vinyl.

"Here is newspaper you forgot. I come with eggs. I not like it when you are troubled."

Buck Buchanan

The counselor opened the paper. He began to read about liver transplants. They were more popular than ever these days. The article next to it was about alcohol. Drinking, it said, was also more popular than ever, though it ruined the liver. Hmmm.

He squeezed his eyes. He was finding it difficult to read these days. Difficult to do much of anything coherently. Everywhere he turned it seemed something was already placed there to spin his head. And when he stopped spinning he landed in front of something else which whipped him hard the other way, gyrating the skull like a Roulette wheel. Muriel. Joseph. Harvey dead as a boot, even his bones powdered and gone to the wind. And Annise of course, the drop of dew he thought he could wade in who somehow evaporated the instant you tried to lift the shadow and touch her.

He folded the paper. On the back page was an article on erosion. Loss of topsoil was destroying the last vestiges of our great mid-western farms. When something started running over and over something else until you couldn't remember what either of you used to be like before it all started, and nothing could grow there but perverted cells and cold arguments... Well, he pondered, this too was erosion, wasn't it?

Someone was trying to get his attention from behind. When he looked around he was surprised to see Wanda Novice.

"I need to talk to you, Morton," she told him. "It's very important. Can we step outside for a minute?"

"Well, Vera's going to bring my eggs in a minute," he replied.

"I've been trying to catch up with you for days."

"You know where I've been, Wanda."

"Certainly I know where you've been. We're not fools, Morton. We're not going to call over there and embarrass you two."

"Embarrass us? For doing what? And what do you mean *we*?"

"It was a lucky break I saw your truck outside. You've got to hear me out."

The counselor's friends winked and slapped each other's backs as he moved Wanda to one of the quieter corner booths. It was then he noticed the curiously low-cut blouse she was sporting, and the tight black slacks with sexy loops for the feet.

"Annise knows you moved," said Wanda seriously as they took their seats.

"I haven't moved."

"She wants so much to see you, Morton. Only she's very very afraid right now." Wanda paused to assess his response. "Anyway, she definitely wants to talk. But she says you two don't have a good talking relationship."

"I'm afraid it's true," muttered Morton.

"So instead of contacting you she all the time goes for these long drives in the country. Except—" Wanda sighed.

"Yes?"

"Well, what she really does is drive over to Somerset and ride back and forth in front of your apartment."

"But I'm never there anymore," he pointed out.

"That's what I'm saying. She really has not been looking good. And you're aware of her, ummm, condition," replied Wanda heavily.

"I'll go over to see her right now. I'll straighten it all out."

"Now?"

"She's probably in need of support, Wanda. Emotional support, I mean."

"You don't have to keep touching me," suggested Wanda shrinking away.

"Sorry," he said removing his hand.

"I've been over there all afternoon," said Wanda. "She's crazy and upset. She's positive she has cancer. She hates being with all those men, Morton."

"Men? What men?"

"Well, all men, from what I can tell."

Silence.

"Don't act dumb," said Wanda. "She told me she told you about it. She's not at fault. Sex addiction is a disease, Morton."

Wanda's breasts moved inside her low-cut shirt. They were pretty nice ones. He hadn't noticed before.

"This last week I've caught her driving up and down in front of *my* house," explained the new supervisor. "And I'm hardly there either, ever since me and Stacy got—"

The counselor lowered his head.

"Incest is a terrible thing, Morton. It makes women like Annise and me, and Muriel too for that matter turn left a lot of times when maybe we should have turned right."

"Incest? Annise had incest?"

"Why do you think so many nuts go to Dar/Neese so they can work with nuts?"

"Why?"

"Because likes seek likes." She paused for a second. "Except for when opposites seek opposites, like you and Muriel."

"Interesting theory," said Morton.

"It's either the drunks or the religious fanatics," said Wanda. "They're the son of a bitches who do it to us. It's horrible, Morton. Truly horrible."

"Muriel's father was an alchy," said Morton. "He quit though."

Wanda said, "And Annise's father is a stone cold pent-up Catholic, *and* a drunk."

Morton scratched his head. It was true, you really did learn something new every day.

"Annise does want to see you, Morton. After all you're little Toni's—" Wanda halted.

Over his shoulder Morton could see the line of old fellows grinning and giving him the thumbs up. They'd mistaken Wanda's orientation. He drank his coffee.

"Anybody with any decent integrity would have to go over there and face her down," said Morton. "Or rather, I mean, work things out."

He clicked down his cup. He tucked in his shirt. He felt for his keys.

"But wait. I didn't mean right away. She doesn't expect you to come right away," objected Wanda holding up her hands.

"She doesn't?" Morton was put off. "Why not?"

"Well—" Wanda looked nervously around. "I guess she's probably— I mean, I think she's probably learned by now you never do what she wants. So, I mean, she's probably not expecting you right now. But like maybe tomorrow."

"Tomorrow?"

Wanda nodded. "Yeah. Like say in the afternoon? Around five or so?"

Wanda's cheeks began to turn red.

"Look, Morton, you could do something else. If you had the manliness you might swallow your pride for once and *not* go visit her."

"Not visit her?"

Wanda's cheeks went from red to a bright mottled magenta, a sure sign of desire in the face of embarrassment.

"She needs me so much right now. She needs someone to protect her," said Wanda squaring her shoulders.

Morton picked up a napkin and began twisting the corners. Vera appeared at the old table.

"Here comes the hag," said Wanda. "I've got to run. Let's both of us do the right thing for Annise. Consider it, Morton. You're in no shape to take care of a baby. On the other hand, I was like a wife to my father, taking care of my five brothers and sisters, feeding the babies at all hours..." Suddenly the Social Worker realized what she was saying and abruptly stopped.

"He's over here, Vera," called Wanda climbing out of the booth. "Think about it, Morton," she said quietly, and then she was gone.

Vera came. She didn't shake her head as he expected. Instead she was very tender and easy with him. She began to motheringly butter his toast.

"I always tell you. If you ever need favor come to me. I can help with crazies."

"Crazies? Wanda works up the hill, you know. In fact she's become the new supervisor."

"Perhaps," said Vera. "But I seen her eating soy curd cake and cabbage juice. She can't be all together, can she?"

"Maybe not, Vera, now that you mention it. Maybe not."

* * *

Chapter 69

Visit. Don't visit. Return home. Stay away from your home.

Morton's buddies urged him to pull a couple of hours with them down at Lost Weekend. Leroy tugged him along.

"I hear having sex every day with young girls will wear a person out, Morty," said the old fellow. "At my age I don't care if they do wear out." They laughed. "You know what they say, the more hair you lose the more head you get," joked Leroy slapping the counselor on the back.

Vera slit her eyes as they headed into the distance.

~~~

Morton followed Leroy in his truck to Lost Weekend. The place remained at full throb throughout the early evening. By eight the younger happy hour crowd disappeared, replaced by the red faced oldsters and the befuddled middle-agers. This was when the hard swallowing set in. Morton wanted to stay. They said they were his friends. But he sensed something squirrelly, something flimflamish in all the dart throwing and arm waving, a specialized nub of self-torture rattling the patients, the *patrons* rather. Their smiles were an eyelash too big for the jokes, as if hot air and sarcastic backbiting made for laugh a minute material.

The counselor left Lost Weekend. Friends? Admit it, they were barely acquaintances. He thought about visiting Gordon at the Fraction House. No, too politically charged over there, not to mention the injunction likely still being in force. What about Trina Lopez? He could drop by her place. And of course there was Roxanne down The Green Room. Hmmm, not a good choice.

Well, maybe he'd ride out to the beach, have a midnight swim. Take a stroll under the stars. He drove this way, made a turn, drove that way.

Before he knew it Morton found himself passing the street which happened to be only two streets away from the one Muriel lived on. What was it Wanda said earlier? It hardly seemed like the same day.

He stopped in front of Muriel's apartment. The lights were on inside. He could see her moving about through the large bay window. She was supposed to draw the curtains at night. He'd told her a hundred times.

Go on in, he wondered? Try to explain about Annise? He doubted she'd listen the way it had been going lately. Say, 'sorry, baby, but first thing in the morning I've got to take care of this little Toni thing. Annise isn't strong, you see. She'll need me there to, you know, to—' Already he could hear Muriel's head wagging answer.

As he was pulling away Morton glanced over his shoulder. He could make out his friend's face against the window, cupping her hands to it. He'd eased beyond the streetlamp. She couldn't possibly have seen him.

~~~

Morton drove to the beach. He wandered the S-shaped sidewalks the rollerbladers used in the daylight. A stone's throw behind him the nighttime cars raced furiously up and down the Pacific Coast Highway. He was living life in the fast lane all right, only with a junker thirty mile per hour pickup. The sea was out there crashing around, but he couldn't hear it. The sky was pure and clean, he knew, but he couldn't smell the freshness.

He drove back inland, stopping briefly for a six pack of the blonde's favorite beer, Guinness Stout. This punishing each other with no communication couldn't go on forever. Someone had to break the ice. Finally he parked in front of Annise's apartment.

He could see the green paper lantern glowing in the upstairs window. Just then it went out. Bedtime.

It was a black, moonless night. Morton fumbled with the keys and got turned around trying to kick the truck door closed. He started up the steps.

But wait, this wasn't Annise's building after all! Hers was the next one over. Lucky break, noticing that.

He started walking. Suddenly though he realized his mistake. Hers had been the *original* building. Christ, he was really losing it these days. For a moment he questioned whether he'd been drinking too much. He'd only had the one at Lost Weekend. No, he was *thinking* too much, that was it. He started back.

He was about to knock when he noticed the door a trifle ajar, though the dead bolt had been thrown. A little loose, he thought as he nursed it on open. Not like Annise at all.

No sense in startling the poor girl, he decided. He tiptoed down the hallway and peered into her room.

Annise's curved form was visible under the covers. He could make out the tiny jerks of first sleep taking hold. Those minute endearing twitches. Ah, we were all so much the same, he reflected as he moved to her bedside. So natural and free when we laid our bodies down and took in the night like we were meant to. Tenderly, so as not to frighten her, he touched through the sheets.

"Annise," he whispered. "It's Morton."

"Ahhh!" cried a voice.

Around whipped a head. Through the darkness Morton could see it was— Yes, it was a *man's* head.

"Wanda!" he exclaimed jumping back and reaching for the pull cord on the Taiwanese lantern.

But no. This one had a full complement of black hair.

"Joseph!" he corrected pointing down at him. "Joseph! Joseph! Joseph!"

"Morton!" cried Annise bolting upright. "You're not supposed to be here till tomorrow!"

The covers slipped free, exposing her voluptuous breasts.

As Harvey had taught him, the counselor took four deep, slow breaths. He didn't know what to do. At last he sat on the edge of the bed and opened one of the beers with the edge of Muriel's apartment key. If ever there was a time to drink, this was it. Erosion, he thought as he sipped off the foam. It was ruining our farms. All that fertile Pasadena mud slinking right off the side of the mattress.

"You're lucky you didn't get shot," announced the Gestapo jerking his leg away under the covers. "I'd have the privilege, you know. You're an intruder."

Joseph struggled up and began to dress. His clothes, noticed Morton, were stowed in Annise's top drawer, the one with her panties and bras and whatnot he never looked in.

For a long taunting moment the Gestapo stood there naked. His cramped muscularity idled under the funky green light like a field of granite, sunless white with a shadow of black hairs which built like fur toward his shoulders.

"Sneaking in here like some criminal," muttered Joseph disgustedly. He began to pull himself together, took a moment to step into his jockey shorts and run Annise's brush through his hair.

Morton looked around the room. The locking box was out. A couple of her magazines were hanging open. New, sadomasochism magazines, he reflected, not the harmless *Euro Follies* and *Swedish Sins!* he was familiar with.

Half exposed, Annise stayed put, her chest arched curiously forward. She was remaining silent too, an odd behavior for her. On closer look the counselor saw her wrists handcuffed to the headboard. In Morton's heart the venom flared. He ripped down the covers, and yes, her feet were bound with a shiny vinyl wrapping, like the kind used on Christmas gifts. There were obvious bruises on her upper thighs. He was reminded of the black and blue spots around Muriel's crotch when he first returned from the mountains.

"You son of a bitch," said Morton turning toward the Gestapo.

Joseph tucked in his shirt.

Slowly the counselor came to his feet. He put the beer aside. Joseph turned, squaring off at the shoulders.

"If you're going to call me a name, it's Dr. J. Schopen," said the Gestapo. "Or you could say, Director, if you'd prefer."

"You're no doctor. I doubt if you made it out of grade school. I contacted Johns Hopkins. They've got no record of you, Joseph."

One of the Gestapo's shoulders rose. He cocked out a leg.

Morton looked to Annise. "Was he forcing you?" he asked.

The counselor and the Director swept their eyes luridly over the blonde's bound, unclothed form. She remained silent. Possibly even stimulated, for all Morton knew. It wasn't every day two men stood between a chick's legs, ogling.

~~~

From what he understood of S & M, if she'd done it all voluntarily it wouldn't have been thoroughly sexy. Then again, if Joseph was taking her that way and it manifested hot and filthy it would likely have been *too* real, too dangerous.

Without losing his focus on Joseph, Morton began jerking the vinyl straps, stretching them enough to where Annise's feet could slip free.

"Take the handcuffs off her," said the counselor.

The Gestapo shook his head no. Then, apparently reconsidering, produced the key and went to the headboard. He crossed one arm between Annise's breasts and pressed his face harshly against her ear as he reached around for access. Morton heard the metal ratcheting. The handcuffs dropped to the floor behind the bed.

Annise wore a curious pouty frown. Did she want the handcuffs back? Perhaps sex wasn't as devilish for a Catholic once their own free will was involved.

"Satisfied?" said Joseph to Morton.

"The day you're in prison I'll be satisfied."

"Then you're going to be a frustrated puppy. There's been no crime, Allison. On the other hand, it's crossed my mind that somebody *could* have poisoned Harvey. Somebody like you, for instance. My door was always open. It had to be for the clients to feel they could reach me. I've been thinking about this, Allison. I know you snuck into Harvey's office during the fire alarm. You got the dangerous meds off my desk and poisoned him. Don't deny it. People saw you with a handful of pills when you pretended to hug him outside. Which was nothing more than swiping the evidence. The police might be interested in that, you think?"

"He wasn't poisoned," returned Morton. "He was killed because he *didn't* have his medication. You fabricated his pills, Joseph. And put Dilaudid in my Librium."

Joseph's mouth dropped at the depth of the counselor's knowledge.

Annise rubbernecked between the men. Who to believe when a new murder was about to occur, and perpetrated by either one?

"I know you were trying to string me out on Dilaudid, like you did Muriel," fired Morton. "Weaken me. Pull a bogus urinalysis to set me up as her abuser while you go ahead and kill Harvey, drug Muriel, rape Sally, rape Roxanne—"

"Roxanne! How do you know—"

"And rape Annise," tried Morton.

The Gestapo's eyes enlarged. So did Annise's, though she didn't move. Christ, how far had the counselor gone into the Director's life?

"I've got proof you put sugar in Harvey's pills. Trina's lab tested them for me."

"Shut up!" spit the Gestapo.

Annise didn't seem to know who to believe. She couldn't fathom Joseph spiking the Librium, or Morton going as far as phonying up Trina's tests. And anyway she had her own problems. Cancer? Too many lovers? Pregnancy? *And* she was in possession of the results of her own urinalysis—positive. Wow, what a word!

"And how come no new RN was hired to replace Trina?" persisted Morton.

"We've had agency nurses," said Joseph. "That's enough for the Arbitrators."

"So they won't be able to see what you're doing? So you can fuck people in the tub?" lashed Morton.

"You're talking out your asshole, Allison. You duped me into signing off on Muriel's Guardianship. But our lawyers will be in touch. I'll get her back. She's mine, count on it."

Morton had a sudden idea. "I talked her into signing a deposition against you, Joseph," he said. "Aggravated battery. Four or five counts of ethical misconduct. Rape. Kidnapping. Plus forced narcotic use when you took her to your place. You'll never get out of the stockade."

Annise gasped. Did she know something?

The counselor's heart flip-flopped at his fib. Then he remembered that lying to Joseph was akin to helping Mother Teresa save babies—good, not bad.

In the next second Joseph sprung like a cougar. He gripped Morton's throat with both hands and began squeezing into the arteries and air passages. The Gestapo's hands were sinewy and callused from weightlifting. He drove Morton downward onto the bed.

The counselor pummeled the Gestapo's forearms, to no avail. He could feel himself thrashing into Annise's nude body, who herself was being powered back by the struggle of the two males.

Morton was going dizzy. In a surge of desperation he swung a fist into Joseph's ribs. The blow did nothing. In the flailing and thrashing the derringer he was returning to Annise flung free of his jacket pocket. The Gestapo's eyes bulged as the little chrome L bounced across the mattress.

Joseph lost interest in his chokehold and snatched up the pistol.

"I can blow you away right now, Allison. You're an intruder," he said gripping the gun.

"No, Joseph!" cried Annise. "I'm a witness. I know he didn't break in."

The Gestapo placed the barrel tip on Annise's stomach, a mere inch above her pubic hair. For the first time she seemed ashamed of her nakedness. The three of them were jammed close against the headboard, each for their own reasons gasping for air. Morton edged away, nearly tipping over the end table.

"It doesn't matter," said Joseph to Annise. "The fact is he broke in here and I'm protecting us. This is better than I'd hoped. Murder made legal for once, eh Allison?"

Joseph turned the gun on Morton. He leaned forward and placed the barrel flush against the counselor's forehead, as Morton had done to him on Muriel's porch. He cocked it.

"No!" screamed Annise.

Joseph sucked his breath. With a mini lunge that shook the bed like a deadly orgasm, he pulled the trigger.

Click!

He cocked it again, hoping for the second chamber.

Click.

Unloaded! It had to be to return it to Annise, she being suicidal at times.

Morton was enraged. He grabbed the plaster Madonna off the end table and roundhoused it at the Gestapo. It struck pistol, hand, and the side of Joseph's head, flew free of the counselor's fingers and exploded into millions of pieces against the far wall. Those Madonnas, they were made cheap, he reflected.

The gun was knocked free. It pitched onto the floor near a broken piece of the baby Jesus.

Joseph's head was bleeding from somewhere above the temple. Morton considered running to the kitchen for a knife, when he realized Annise had crab walked across bed. She'd found the pistol. She was reaching into the locking box for a bullet and beginning to load it.

'L.A. 2000:' Sex Asylum

Morton dove across the mattress, but the Gestapo was back to himself, his muscles double engorged it seemed. He blocked the counselor with a violent shoulder to the diaphragm.

Annise bobbled the second bullet. Joseph launched toward her. Morton was right behind. The three of them battled for the pistol, when all at once it discharged. A blast through the gasping silence of the struggle. A shattering explosion ringing out twice as loud due to the short barrel and the closeness of the room.

They peeled back from this thundering center of gravity like leaves off a three leaf clover. Morton came up with the gun. Immediately he cocked it against the Gestapo's chest.

"I don't know if she got the second bullet in," panted Morton. "But if you don't get out of here right now I'm pulling this trigger."

Joseph stared at the pistol. Blood was streaming down his right cheek from the deep gash somewhere in his hair. The combat must have cleared his head, for like an animal with hypothermia he was shaking from the inside out. Or perhaps, considered the counselor, he was simply withdrawing from his daily supply of designer drugs.

Joseph inched to his feet. He glared at Annise. His fingers were drenched with blood as he pressed his wound. He walked to the front door. Morton followed.

"I'm going to kill you," said Joseph outside.

The counselor nodded.

"You better marry that cunt and get a fat insurance policy right away," continued the Gestapo. "Widows need money, Allison. And little Toni, or whoever the fuck it is, will need a new father. Think about it next time you see me."

Morton lowered the gun. His arm ached from aiming it so long.

"I'll remember," said the counselor. "I promise."

* * *

Chapter 70

When Morton returned to the bedroom he found Annise still huddled among the jagged, blood tipped shards of plaster. In the fray she'd been knocked off the bed and pinned in the corner. She was staring up at the silver dollar size gash in the ceiling where the hollow-point cartridge had blasted through the drywall. A mixture of both combatant's blood was painted in smeary swipes from her chin to the top of her bright blonde pubic hair.

For the strangest of moments Morton forgot the recent brawl and worried she might be miscarrying. He rushed to her. She seemed in shock.

"It's all right. There's no one up there to hurt. We're already on the top floor," he soothed.

As if they had a silent understanding, Annise rose and slipped on her red gown, the one with the lace at the wrists and neck. They sat on the bed and talked quietly, which in its way was quite delicate and touching.

"Joseph's gone now?" she asked finally.

This was an indication of her state. "He's been gone for thirty minutes," said Morton.

The counselor's jacket was ripped along both sleeves. There were deep lacerations on his forearms. A series of slices on his neck pulsed out small, half-congealed clots from Joseph's digging fingernails. The Madonna was gone. That helped. But Morton was wise to the ongoing notations on her calendar. He kept eyeballing the conception date. He could almost recall the round. Something seemed amiss in the logistics, or the timing. Something off center, or undone maybe, the way you'd feel at sea with a load of wind but no waves in the water.

"I didn't do anything with him," said Annise low.

Morton leaned against the headboard.

"Please quit lying, Annise. You've been lying all along. Why do you expect me to believe you now?"

"Lying?" She came back to herself. "Haven't I gotten this through to you, Morton? If a girl is forced it means she didn't actually do the thing of her own resolve, or intent, or whatever they say in court. Didn't I explain this to you before? It's like she didn't honestly do it whether she did it or not."

"That's an intriguing twist."

"Isn't it though?"

"What if she *isn't* forced?"

"Humans are supposed to do what's best for the other person, Morton. Not for themself. You have to suffer and turn the other cheek, and a lot of times just plain lay down in the back seat and take it. After a while you learn to look at yourself as a giver by receiving what's put on you in life. Job did that in the Bible. I'm only following suit."

"Screwing is the best thing for the other person?" he wondered.

Annise nodded big. "Don't you think so? All the guys say it is."

Morton jutted his jaw. At least his stomach had quit fluttering during these revelations. He was very tired. Maybe that was softening him to her intricacies.

"If you confess it really fast," she added, "you can blow the whole mess right off the hard drive and it's like it never happened. You get a clean slate. The old phone numbers evaporate right out of your back pocket. It's similar to being annulled."

The counselor scratched his head.

"Even if you got pregnant from it?" he asked. "Without an abortion how do you clear the machine? I mean, uh, the womb? That's what we're talking about, isn't it?"

"Well, of course there's the Immaculate Conception argument. You know, where somebody must have done it but you claim nobody did it to you. Even I'm not flaky enough to use that one."

She paused. She was getting so conciliatory these days.

"I guess you're right, Morton. I guess pregnancy is so goddamn real it cramps even the Lord's style."

"No offense, Annise, but this is all sounding a bit hypocritical," he noted.

"Maybe. But you've got to remember hypocrisy is the very foundation of Christianity. Even Jesus had doubts. And he wasn't even a real Christian."

"He wasn't?"

"He was a Jew, Morton," said Annise with a shrivel of her nose. "They didn't have Catholics in those days. But if they would've, I'm sure he'd have been a Catholic."

～～

The place was a shambles. The spilled bottle of Guinness Stout lay sideways in the wet part of the bedspread. Morton lifted it and swallowed the last of the foam. Annise turned dead serious. Things flipped back and forth so many times there wasn't any use trying to predict it. He kept silent.

"I need the church, Morton. I get afraid about things and it helps me. Don't you ever need help?"

The air had thickened. Her disheveled beauty was there and coming out of her.

"Yes. Lately I've felt like I've needed a lot of help," he admitted.

"At night? Is that when you need it?"

He thought about it. Yes, it was mainly at night. When he was alone with himself. When he knew he was strong and healthy and couldn't think of a new country which wasn't like all the other countries he'd thought of.

"You know, Morton, you mystify me sometimes," said Annise. "In a lot of ways you're the most spiritual person I know. Everybody's aware of how you made the Fraction House shape up and vaccinate the clients during the hepatitis-B rigmarole. And you didn't even get mad when Joseph took credit for it. Plus how you fought to get Gordon his own room and solved so much of his paranoia. Yet you won't give in like everybody else and go to mass. I don't get it. You need a higher power, for Christsake. Every one of us needs a higher power."

"I keep the faith though," he returned with a smile.

Annise frowned.

"There are lots of higher powers, Annise."

"Like what?" she asked tilting her head in the puppyish way she used when she truly didn't comprehend something.

"The electric company," he said. "The Upper Chalmouth river. The Arbitrators. Porsche engines. Hell, just about everything's higher than me. Even you're higher than I am, Annise."

"Me? How can you say that?"

"Because I don't understand you. Everything I don't understand has to be higher than me."

She thought for a moment.

"Well, as long as it keeps you humble," she said at last.

"I try to stay humble," said Morton.

"It's much harder for Catholics," continued Annise. "We can get God seeing our way if we pray to exactly the right saints. Which can screw your ego up if you're not careful. I mean, thinking you've got an *in* to God." She wriggled close beside him. "I often wonder how a person like you can figure out right from wrong as if it's simple, everyday arithmetic."

"When I worked with Stacy it was a lot easier," he said thinking it over.

"Oh? Why?"

"Because I watched her like a hawk. Once I pinned down what she was doing, I'd do the opposite. I think most of my growth came during that period."

"Interesting," said Annise.

"Lately though it seems like I've been more and more on my own. It's a scary feeling. I don't know, I guess when you get your hands so deep into somebody's life..." He trailed off.

"Muriel's, you mean?" asked Annise.

Morton looked into her eyes. She pulled a leg up under her, then blinked a couple of times.

"Yeah," he said abstractly. "Muriel's life."

Annise leaned forward. She made her voice sensitive and confidential sounding. "Let me tell you something, Morton," she said. "You're not really afraid. So stop pretending you're afraid. You know what you're feeling?"

He shook his head.

"Guilt," she said tapping the back of his hand. "I'm being honest now."

"I know you are."

She touched under her breast where her heart was. "I know about this, Morton. It always starts right in here. Later it gets down in your stomach and makes you almost sick." She grimaced at the thought.

"Yes," he said. "I've felt it."

"And when it gets up here—" She rubbed her forehead. "Behind the eyes, I mean. Well, then you're ninety percent ruined."

"Is that where it is in you? Behind the eyes?" he asked.

She looked around for her cigarettes. "Yes," she sighed.

"Where does it go after the eyes?"

Annise reached out and touched in his crotch. "It goes there. It goes right there. I may not know a lot, but I know about this," she said softly.

Morton's nerves had sprung raw. Any other time he'd have craved her fingers there. But not now. No, not now, after... after the Gestapo? Slowly she removed her hand.

"Tell me, Morton. What are *you* guilty about these days?" she asked staring deep into him.

* * *

Chapter 71

The counselor started cleaning the room, putting the stuff back in the locking box. He came to the Librium pills, the ones stuffed with Dilaudid rather. And what was this? A blindfold? He reached under the bed for the handcuffs. He picked up the pistol. He was about to put it in his pocket, but wait, break the barrel first.

Morton breathed heavily as he saw the empty chamber. No, she hadn't managed to slip a second bullet in. Joseph had been chased out on sheer bluff!

"Leave the gun here," said Annise.

Morton turned. "Why? So you and Joseph can have another sex device?"

"Not me and Joseph."

"Oh my God! Not... Not you and Wanda!"

Annise shrunk. "If you have to know, it's for when I'm in private. Women still have *some* rights, don't they?"

"Is that a right?"

"It's the pursuit of happiness, Morton. The founding fathers weaseled it directly into the Constitution. You can't take it away from us."

"No, I have to keep the gun. I can't trust you with it, Annise."

"Me? It's you and Joseph who have the problem."

"I found it loaded when you were sleeping the other day. I was afraid you were going to shoot yourself. You've certainly hinted at it enough."

"Bullshit. You make up things."

"It was in your hand after I walked Wanda to her car. Why?"

Annise reddened. "Morton, please don't make me go through this again. I told you why I need it. I got excited when you two went out to talk."

"Excited?"

She turned away. "All right then. *Aroused* is what I got. Does that satisfy you? So I went for it on my own. Understand now?"

"Oh," said Morton gathering her meaning. Appalling how many gaps between the sexes could fuzz up a man's mind.

"I'm still taking it," he said. "I can't risk Joseph getting hold of this thing. You saw what he did."

"What'd he do? It wasn't loaded. Nothing at all happened."

"Joseph didn't know it wasn't loaded."

"Things meant to be, Morton, are meant to be. You act like Joseph is the worst thing ever happened to this country. I don't think you realize he's on your side in a lot of this."

"In what?"

"Well, he wants me to have an abortion, for instance. He says I could take this special abortion pill and I wouldn't have to go to a butcher. He's got access to certain drugs, I guess. You pop two or three and pretty soon it's all over with. No doctor. No dirty men around."

"No man around?"

"Nope. Just me and Wanda."

Morton felt ill in his stomach. "Why does Joseph care?" he asked.

"He doesn't want me to have a baby."

"Why not?"

"I don't know. Maybe he wants me all to himself. Or maybe he respects my right not to have one of those slash and burn abortions. It's hard to say about him. He keeps pressing, but he knows I've got too many morals to go through with it."

Morton had the room halfway in order. Annise said, "God, look at you. You're filthy!"

It was true. He was caked with drying blood. He'd been in the same clothes for days now. His mind was far south of understanding this as telltale symptoms of an impending mental breakdown.

"Come here, Morty. Let me help you," said Annise.

She got to her knees on the bed and helped him off with his jacket. She undid the front of his shirt. With two dainty fingers and a well placed thumb she started to unhitch his belt and work his pants down. Jesus, what momentum these modern day sword fights could take on. There came a small clinking sound as metal met metal.

"What's this?" asked Annise.

She'd found Muriel's silver hairpin, the one he's slipped in his pocket earlier as a souvenir of her warmth and kindness. Annise's eyes grew large.

"Oh, that."

Annise looked naïvely up. Her lips curled slowly into a smile. He could see the sense of thrill race into her. So swayable. So girlie and cute.

"It's a gift, isn't it? You broke down and bought me something, like I've always wanted. It's silver too. Probably an antique, the way it's all tarnished and old looking."

"Uhhh, Annise—"

She beveled her palm to the light to see it better.

"You're the kindest thing. There's so much about you I ought to be grateful for."

"Well, no, you really shouldn't—"

"Oh, yes I should. Wake me up for Christsake, will you! Thank you, Morty. It's beautiful. It's really and truly beautiful."

Morton was exhausted. Annise flopped him onto the bed where he worked into a sort of modified S of the fetal curl. His pants were gone. Annise crawled around and lay in front of him. She was being sexy again, he could tell. What the hell, mulled the counselor. After all this time and talk what was there to lose? But as soon as he thought this into the foreground roared the Gestapo's grotesque image.

"I understand women like sex more right after they've had sex," he suggested low.

"Wow. Quite an insight. You're not as primitive as you seem sometimes."

"Is that why you're interested now?" he asked.

For reasons he couldn't define, Morton had a stray thought regarding Wanda Novice.

"It's been Wanda too, hasn't it?" said Morton over her shoulder.

Annise moved sheepishly fro, then to.

"You only asked about seeing other guys. And anyway, I thought that kind of thing got guys going," she defended.

"In the movies it does," said Morton. "Not in my wife's bedroom."

"Your wife's!"

"I mean my girlfriend's. My girlfriend's bedroom."

"But you said wife. I heard you."

Annise set the hairpin aside.

"You're so fabulous, Morton. You're the only man I've ever known with half a chance to understand a woman."

"I am?" Despite himself he was flattered.

"Uh huh. Which is why I'm going to say this next thing to you." She worked backward, narrowing the space between them.

"About this intercourse business. You should know women get kind of like ashamed about doing it when they're pregnant. It's as if the child is sacrificed for lust. Do you know what I mean? Or sacrileged. Or compromised. I'm not sure exactly what I'm saying, but I mean with the man still hammering and sawing and making a mess when the apartment's already been built."

"I think I can understand, Annise. You're saying—"

"Oh, that reminds me," she interrupted. "Take a look at this."

She reached into the drawer of the night stand and handed him a pink paper.

"Isn't this exciting! I got it from the O.B. the other day. They did an ultrasound. I'm seven weeks. Do you believe it?"

She pointed behind her as he tried to read. It did all appear valid. "See there at the bottom? It's signed and dated and all. Like you're always saying things should be if you really want to nail somebo— I mean, you know, prove something."

Morton slid the paper back onto the night table.

"I want you to know, Morton, we're going to be here for you. Both of us will be right here whenever you're ready for us."

"Here?" he said. "In this place?"

"Always," she told him. "You're the center of our life now."

"But why do you want me so bad, Annise? What's so special about me?"

She looked around the room. "I guess it's because you won't completely take me. Nobody likes to be rejected. Think how you'd feel if I wouldn't want you."

"But we've had so much trouble."

She looked away.

Morton said, "Everybody knows you can't turn a big emotion around in your fingers. You've got to at least see both sides of it first, don't you?"

She shrugged. "Can't an emotion have more than two sides?"

"Like how many?"

"How many sides does the soul have?"

"Two," he said. "The good side and the bad side."

"I think it has three. Your side. My side. And," she patted her belly, "our little Toni's side."

Perhaps she was right. You couldn't crush it all out with the side of your knuckle and get on down the road. No, there was far more to it. He was going to have to pay better attention. Feel it all closer to the gut if he wanted to get a handle on this thing.

"Please," said Annise pushing back toward him. "Please lie here with us."

She was playing the seductress. Next would come the big sex scene. Should they be racing to bed in hopes of the best round ever?

Christ, this Annise *was* a hot tamale. Could there be a titillation factor for him because others wanted her? Her admissions had cleared part of the bad air. Cleaned her heart, probably. The way she worked it the greatest purgation was somehow mixed in with the dirtiest part of the soul. For Annise

Chastain, classic L.A. blonde right down to the painted toenails, there was only one way to solve the great mystery—orgasm.

When they began Morton did not resist. Only after a moment he discovered this was not to be the conventional way. She'd really meant it about not compromising little Toni. Apparently there was a loophole where satisfaction could be had without sullying the embryo. What a notion! But did she really want it this way? Likely she did, since anything to do with the Devil fired her up. In lieu of the Pearly Gates, this was Satan's most preferred passageway. Hmmm, speculated the counselor.

Well, a case could be made for her deserving such a fate. But no, that wouldn't be right. On the other hand, there was something to be said for Morton himself deserving it, in a sort of secularized erotic way, particularly considering all the hell she'd put him through. Yes, they *both* deserved it in their quirky ways.

The pillow was damp. Morton could smell Joseph's stinky *Paca Roma* cologne rising from it. She snuggled close with her buttocks. "Will you make this special love to me?" she whispered.

He hesitated.

"It's you we really need, Morton. You're the one who has to accept us for what we are."

"I don't know, Annise."

"Are you saying you don't love little Toni?" she asked. She stretched her neck to see him. Her eyes were full of sincerity.

"Well, no. You know I'd never say a thing like that," he replied.

"I didn't think so," returned Annise. "And you know what, Morton?"

"What, Annise?"

"She loves you too."

The blonde snapped the string on the paper lantern, then eased up the already high hem of her gown.

* * *

Chapter 72

In the wee hours Morton prepared to return to Muriel's. He was in the process of writing out a note when Annise stirred.

"What's up?" she asked.

"I haven't been able to sleep," said the counselor. "I'm worried about Muriel. Joseph might show up over at her place if he thinks I'm not there."

Morton expected opposition, but Annise said, "OK. Be sure to tell her hi for me." She rolled over.

～～～

At Muriel's apartment Morton quietly let himself in. He cracked the bedroom door. She was safely asleep, thank God.

He spotted something new on her dresser. The small floor level night lights he'd put around illuminated it. At first he thought it was the Madonna, a statue like Annise's. But no, this was a mini potbellied Buddha, like the one they'd seen in Venice. Was she a Buddhist now?

He shut the door, rolled out the sofa bed, and in seconds was in another world.

～～～

When the counselor next opened his eyes crisp bars of sunlight were slanting across Muriel's whitecapped river. It was afternoon already. Had she been hovering over him as he slept? He sensed sounds of her scurrying away as he came to.

He lay there staring at the walls. Pondering the various predicaments he was in.

Finally he rose and wandered into the small backyard. He found Muriel using the aluminum can to water the tomato and pepper plants. There was so much foliage. A couple of potted palm trees. Ferns hanging from the guttering. She was turning into a real green thumb. When had all this happened? And why hadn't he seen it the other day?

Morton plopped into the lawn chair.

"Sleep good?" asked Muriel.

He shook his head.

"I don't think I like plants with flowers," she said continuing her work. "I mean, I like them, but I think I like food plants better."

Muriel eased a few steps along the tiny walkway, reached into the foliage and snapped off a fully ripened tomato. She shined it on her T-shirt. "Don't you?" she asked taking a bite. "I mean, like the eating plants better?"

Morton looked closely at her. Eyes bright and lucid. Skin clear as a chunk of ice blue sky. Schizophrenia had never seemed so profoundly normal to him. In return Muriel conducted a survey of her own, squinting her eyes over his slouched facade, much the way he used to assess her in the old days.

"What's happened, Morton? You've got blood all over you!" she cried dropping the can.

She hurried to him and peeled back his collar, exposing the encrusted fingernail gashes. She unbuttoned his shirt and gazed fearfully at the palm painted smearings of blood.

She left, and a couple of minutes later returned with a gallon jug of white wine. Afternoon sunlight and tart white wine, that was California for you. What a thoughtful girl she was.

"No glasses?" wondered Morton.

Muriel wore a grave expression. Quickly she removed her Grateful Dead T-shirt, doused it with the wine and began to bathe him. She had a bra on underneath, so it wasn't a blatantly inappropriate move. She operated quickly, checking the severity of his wounds as she worked.

"Wine to clean with?" wondered Morton.

Muriel paused. "You used vodka on me at your apartment. I thought alcohol was supposed to be for this," she said.

Morton closed his eyes and let her attend to him. Had the tables somehow turned when he wasn't watching? These counselor and client roles were somehow blurring on him. Muriel the nurse guru? Well, maybe he could use a guru about now.

"It was Joseph, wasn't it?" she said.

Morton nodded.

"Tell me. Is he hurt? Did the police get involved?"

Morton muddled through the scenario, trying to assemble his words in a way which wouldn't disturb her unduly. It didn't seem to come off.

"You look sad, Morton. You've been upset for so long now," she said.

A full minute passed. "Muriel, I have to be honest with you about something," he said. "I don't want to hurt you. I realize this will probably ruin everything we've established, but I really feel you should know. It's about Annise."

"Yes?"

"Well, the fact of the matter is—" He sighed. "The fact is Annise is pregnant."

Muriel stared blankly at him.

"She's telling me she's something like seven weeks now. She says I'm the father."

"Yes?" said Muriel.

"Well, aren't you surprised? My God, I've sweated out two or three eternities over this thing."

"But, Morton, don't you remember? You told me about this last week. You had a plan. You said you were going to sneak a needle out of the Fraction House and get blood from her."

"I did?"

"You said if you got blood Trina could send it to her lab and have it tested. Then you could prove for certain it wasn't your little Toni."

"Hmmm," he said, though he could feel himself trembling.

"You were very sweet to me that night. You really don't remember?" added Muriel laying her head softly against his chest.

"Oh, yes. Of course I remember. I'd come from the Lost Weekend with all those old guys, hadn't I?"

"No. You'd been at the beach someplace. Or maybe it was Vera's. Anyway, the blood idea wouldn't work."

"Why not?"

"Because you'd need the baby's blood. I don't think you could get little Toni's blood, could you?"

Morton raced quickly through the possibilities. She recapped the wine jug.

"I just can't remember fathering anyone's baby," he said absently. "I've been a little out of it, I know. Taking all that Dilaudid, and then coming off the Dilaudid..."

"What's Dilaudid?" asked Muriel.

"It's a nasty narcotic Joseph spiked my Librium with. He wanted me strung out so I'd have a guilty urinalysis. You know, so he could make me look bad to the Arbitrators. He wanted them to think I gave you drugs and I did the rape. This all went down at your Termination Meeting, remember?"

"What's spiked mean?" asked Muriel.

The counselor squeezed shut his eyes. He gave her his best explanation.

"I've got this powerful intuition. Or instinct or something telling me I'm not little Toni's dad."

"All men have that instinct. It's the cut and run to south Florida philosophy."

"How do you know all this, Muriel?" he asked her. "I mean, about the blood not working?"

"Easy. I called the Fraction House and talked to Wanda," she said. "It's OK, though. She didn't think it had anything to do with you and Annise."

"She didn't?"

"No. She thought I was talking about you and me."

"Wanda thought *you* were pregnant?" Morton's heart fell.

402

"I guess so. I'm not really sure. You stay at both our places. I have kind of a hard time knowing what other people think."

The counselor slumped. "Me too," he said.

This was calling for a straight rum. And with a tequila chaser on the side. Or how about the new thousand-and-one-proof liquor they'd invented—yes, Afterburner! That's what was called for here. Maybe it'd spin his head counterclockwise and end up on a number facing forward for once.

But alcohol had never worked well for him. Mix it with Dilaudid, or a Dilaudid withdrawal, as Trina had warned him, and in an L.A. minute all your systems were down like lead off the end of a gangplank. He was staggering along like a floppy old hobo these days, yet in the next instant frozen in his tracks, ossified as a busted up skyscraper out of the long-forgotten 19th Century, all weak and shivery inside at the slightest threat of the next California quake.

"I know you're worried about Annise finding out this stuff," consoled Muriel. "You don't have to though. Wanda cares for Annise. She promised not to tell her. And anyway, I'm not pregnant to begin with."

"I don't know. Gossip is thicker than mud. And those two have gotten very close lately," said Morton.

A terrible anguish washed through him. Like the way a tree must feel when someone started chopping at it. The whole thing had gotten to be too much. More than his bruises from Joseph, more even than betrayal by Annise, he was torn to the quick at remembering he'd given away Muriel's silver hairpin. He must have had perspiration under his eye, a patch of wetness, for Muriel reached out and brushed it away with her fingertips.

"I suppose I told you about Annise's tumor too," he muttered.

"No. But everybody at the Fraction House knows about it. She hasn't been keeping it a secret."

"I see."

Minutes passed. Who he'd told what to had become a pure fog.

The sun was lower. The air had begun to cool. Nevada, he wondered? At least there weren't many people there. And it didn't rain much. But no, the desert was where they'd tested the atomic bomb. Deadly radiation lingering in the dust and the cactus needles. Big problems for a blooming family, mulled the counselor.

"You don't smell so good, Morton," Muriel noted softly. "When's the last time you showered?"

He shrugged. "I've had a long history, Muriel. I'm a worrier, I guess. It seems like I worry about a different problem every few minutes."

"Not me. I worry about the same problem over and over."

"Which one?" he asked quickly, lost inside himself as to the workings of the female mind.

"I'm going to run you a tub," she said starting inside. "And I want you to use lots of soap, Morton. You haven't been keeping up with yourself. This would be a good place for us to start."

* * *

Chapter 73

The counselor lingered amongst his plants while Muriel ran the tub. Well, his ex-plants.

When he entered the apartment she was at the table opening a new series of travel brochures.

"Montana? I hear it's nice there. Are you thinking of moving?" he asked glancing over her shoulder as he headed toward the bathroom.

"There are other places in this world than L.A., you know," she said.

Muriel must have squirted dish soap into the bath water, for a small mountain of bubbles was climbing over the rim of the tub. Morton undressed and eased in. He was a soaker, not a scrubber, and after a spell Muriel appeared with a cup of coffee for him.

"This tastes great," complimented the counselor. He experienced a dose of pride in her skills. At last his efforts were paying off.

"We ran out of paper coffee filters, so I used a piece of cloth," said Muriel.

"Good thinking."

"Thanks," she smiled. "I dug up an old pair of panties and made my own strainer."

"Panties?"

"Uh huh. Cause of how they're cupped and all to hold the coffee grounds. Did I do good?"

Morton's nose wrinkled. Slowly he set the cup in the soap dish. This was Muriel's way. Win you with her honied glove of affection before you realized the flowers weren't in the vase yet, but still out there in the field, growing wild. She perched on the edge of the tub. She was still in her bra and jeans.

"God, look how dirty I am. Mind if I bathe too?" she said. She began to undress.

"Well, uh, I'm just thinking—"

But already she was in. She faced opposite him, lacing her legs outside of his and reclining far back in the bubbles. Morton stared at her.

"I'm going to soak a bit," she informed him, her voice high but controlled.

He could feel the slippery laminate of her skin sliding over his. Under the water he noticed his feet extending quite a ways in her direction, almost grazing the faucet, so to speak.

The tub. From a psychological viewpoint this wasn't so unusual, perhaps. People followed things up in ways they knew. Muriel, being acquainted with tub sex at the Fraction House, and thereby accustomed to her breasts knifing in and out of the suds as she swirled the water... And with your Freudian rebonding theories causing Morton, the counselor, to take on the role of surrogate father figure... Which, let's see, he feared, would make sex between them akin to sex with dad. Or worse, with Joseph. No, this wouldn't do at all!

The water was unbubbled in spots, and not dirty enough to conceal his accidental arousal.

"Uh, Muriel, may I have your attention for a second?" Her engine at low idle, she lifted her chin. "The way it's going here something could happen," he said.

"Like what?"

"What do you mean, like what? Like lust. Like sex. That's like what."

The white bar of Ivory was floating near his hip. She reached for it, bumping him slightly.

"You're supposed to have lust when you like somebody," she said.

"But if I've rebonded with you it's the same as having sex with your father. You already did that and it didn't work."

She said, "I don't think there's any such thing as rebonding. It's something that Freud guy thought up when he was taking all the cocaine Joseph says he took. Anyway, it's dumb."

The counselor thought it over. She had a point there.

"This is reality grounding, Morton. It's what Harvey always wanted for me. A good cup of coffee. A nice hot bath." He felt her toes wiggle. "And right here in the same room a great big—"

"Muriel!"

"Feeling of peace," she said low.

Morton sighed deep. Well, she was young. There were a lot of sticky adult-minded things she didn't know about yet. Funny though how he'd become more student than teacher these days.

He looked across the foam at her. Yes, she was a real person all right. With a variety of personalities as down to earth as they came. Not crazy. Not schizophrenic at all. Hell, she even knew how to be upset at the right time, which was a lot more than he could say for himself.

"By the way, I saw the Buddha in your room."

"Goofy, huh?" said Muriel.

"Yeah, pretty goofy."

"Wanda gave it to me. It's the one from Venice, remember? She lives up there, you know."

"Wanda's been seeing you? Christ, this place is becoming a freeway."

"I think she bought it for Annise. But she didn't want to interfere with the Madonna. Especially with Annise praying so much about the pregnancy and all."

"So you pray to the Buddha?"

"I would if I prayed, I guess. I haven't learned how though. Wanda says it's good to pray, as long as you're not talking to some stupid Christian God."

"Since when are you and Wanda so close?"

"Wanda needs somebody to confide in, Morton. I'm trying to help. A person can't stop themselves from being in love."

"In love? With who? Wait. Shit, don't tell me."

"I think I'm a lot like you, Morton. I worry about people too. Not just Wanda. I was thinking about this pregnancy thing. Imagine how hard it's gonna be for Gary, you know, Annise's new Assistant Priest, hearing her Confession."

"I don't think it'll bother him. A lot of those guys secretly want to be parents," said Morton. "That's why you have to call them 'Father' all the time."

They were talking along like this when a moment of clarity hit the counselor right between the eyes. He was attracted. He'd come clean in his mind and could feel the genuine heat of excitement for her. She was gorgeous. Not in the Fraction House way. Not in a quirky, cute-faced way. She was gorgeous in the way of the world at large. Anyone, by God, would have seen her as a fine fox of a girl, particularly in the tub, a cocktail only a fool wouldn't devour if he had the chance. He felt rise the cough-like tickle in his throat he sometimes got at challenging moments.

Morton reached for her. Their lips met in a kiss as sensual to the brain as the slick sheen of nakedness was to their bodies. Steam rose off the tiny popping bubbles. Their chests and groins began to work in a harmony of finger molded ovals, their tight, dark underwater hairs like a scribbling of dirty words coarse in each other's skin as they drove together, a couple of kids from the playground seasoned at last to full blooded man and maiden.

They would not need toys for this game. The future wasn't an infinite month away, nor an hour, no, not even a second away from the fullest acceptance of their vulnerability, when the telephone rang. They both surged rigidly back. Much water sloshed onto the floor.

"We've got to get it!" exclaimed Muriel.

Then she changed her mind. "Forget it!" she cried diving back into his arms. "Let it ring."

"We have to answer," said Morton. "What if Joseph's done something? What if somebody needs help? He's a murderer, Muriel. Anything could be happening."

They looked longingly at one another. The phone continued to toll. By degrees Muriel went lax in her muscles, as if a gloom were entering her.

"It's Annise," she said drawing away. "I know it is."

Morton frumped his lips. "You women and your intuitions. It could be anybody."

The counselor waddled into the kitchen. Muriel bustled in behind him.

"Please don't answer, Morton. She'll have a reason for you to go over there. Can't you see how she's always jerking you around?"

"Since when did you turn into a psychic?" he asked lifting the receiver.

"Hello?" said Morton.

"Good God, what are you two doing!" cried Annise.

The counselor's mouth fell open. He whipped his head toward Muriel. She stood on the kitchen tiles, naked and dripping. He could hardly take his eyes off her.

"Morton? That's you, isn't it?" said Annise.

"Yes, it's me."

"Listen, I realize it's late, but I got a call from Aphie. She's flying in from San Francisco tonight. She's finally coming to visit me."

"Great," said Morton.

"The thing is, her flight gets here at two this morning. I mean, it's not really safe for a single girl to go driving around L.A. in the middle of the night."

"Probably not," he agreed.

"Getting you two together would really tell me a lot."

"I'm looking forward to meeting her," said Morton.

"By the way, my Miata can only hold two of us, you know."

"Yeah, I know," said Morton.

"Wonderful! So we can go in the truck? It'd be too late for drinks, but maybe we could all go to Vera's or something."

"Vera closes at one."

"Oh, and Morton, I know how you have trouble with new people," she said. "But would you please not wear that ugly looking cast this time? Aphie's a beautiful human being. It's not going to kill you to shake her hand."

"OK," said Morton.

"By the way, I found out what you've been doing with Muriel," added Annise.

"You did?"

"I know why you've been hanging around all summer. A lot of it's been because of her, am I right?"

"I guess so," he muttered.

"You could have told me, Morton. Anyway, I want you to know I think you've done a very honorable thing. I mean, moving in so you could supervise her and watch out for her and all. You can be so decent sometimes. Why do you always try to keep that from people?"

"I guess I shouldn't," he said feebly.

Annise's voice took on a humble, God fearing quality. "Christ, you really are good. Taking care of a nut and not even getting paid for it! And giving of yourself and all. I mean, when you could be here with me. What's more, you didn't want me to find out what a good deed you were doing. Jesus, Morton, what's next out of you?"

"I don't know, Annise. Might be anything."

"I have claims on you too though," she went on. "I mean, I'm going to need to see you more and more."

"When?" he asked nervously.

"You mean you're willing to see me a lot more?"

"Well, I, uh—"

"I know you'll want to keep abreast of how baby's coming along."

"Sure I will. I mean—"

"Anyway, about Aphie. Will you come now? We don't want to be late for this."

"I'll get there as soon as I can, Annise."

"Thanks, Morton. You're a dear. You really are."

They hung up.

* * *

'L.A. 2000:' Sex Asylum

Chapter 74

For a long moment Morton and Muriel scrutinized each other's unclothed forms. Naked as peeled fruit they were, yet he experienced not the first shred of shame. Then again, this place wasn't laden with those Garden of Eden snake and bite the apple vibes like Annise's apartment harbored. No, this was merely pseudo west side L.A., where the whacked out working people lived and made their working man's love.

Muriel put her robe on, pulled out one of the kitchen chairs and began to once again eyeball the travel brochures. Morton went to the livingroom closet and started to dress.

"Why don't we get out of here for a couple of days?" called Muriel after a minute. "Why don't we take time for ourselves? Maybe go up to the mountains."

He looked around. "Leave here?" he said.

"Only for a few days. We've got your tent, and the camping gear. I think it would be good for us."

"When?" he asked.

"Anytime we want. We'll pick up and go whenever we're ready."

"I don't know," objected the counselor.

To his surprise he could sense the old fears coming out. It was the infamous Roselawn rigidity, and he'd never been a patient in Roselawn. Change. Damn if it didn't terrify everyone.

"People say it's so beautiful and clean up there," she went on.

Muriel lifted her arm and pointed eastward through the walls. Morton went to the window. Way in the distance he could almost see the gray silhouette of the mountains rising up out of the nighttime haze.

"It's pure too," she told him. "Nothing but forests. Huge gigantic forests. No cities. No crap. No people swarming all around you. See. This pamphlet here explains it all."

He glanced reluctantly at her.

"Please. I need your help, Morton. I want us to do something real. Can't we for once break free and do something that isn't phonied up with documents and perfume and shitheads everywhere we look?"

A lot of time went by. Morton touched along his ears.

"Won't you help me?" she asked finally.

"Of course," he said low. "Of course I'll help you, Muriel."

"Great!" she exclaimed coming to her feet. "Can we go tonight?"

Morton put his hands on his hips.

"OK," agreed Muriel. "After Aphie leaves. I can wait. I think I can, anyway."

"I'll find out where Joseph is. That way I'll know you're safe while I'm gone to the airport," said Morton.

He dialed Joseph's home.

"I'm not going to let anything happen to you, Muriel. I promised you protection a long time ago," he said over his shoulder.

Joseph's phone rang and rang. Finally the answering machine came on. He had to think fast. He needed to make Joseph pick up if he was listening.

"It's Morton, Joseph," said the counselor. "I've got Annise and Muriel with me. They're all dolled up in miniskirts and tube tops. They want to be dropped at your place for a couple of hours while I help out over at Vera's. Can you handle it for us?"

This was a lie. And lying wasn't good. But sometimes the good got in the way of the best, of the truly right, and you had to juggle the stakes.

No answer from the Gestapo's place.

Morton dialed the Fraction House. The night shift was arriving. Stacy answered the phone.

"Joseph hasn't been in all day," she said. "I'm worried. Usually he calls. Wanda's not around either. I guess I'll have to cover for him."

Morton hung up. "Let's see. Where else could he be?" he said to Muriel.

An instant of extra sensory communication strung taut between them. He could almost visualize her lips forming out the words, "The Green Room." A sudden sense of betrayal ran through him, an intuition which cut deeper than real knowledge.

He got the number from information. A woman answered.

"Green Room. Roxanne speaking," she said.

Morton jutted his jaw. "Is, uh, Mad Dog around?" he said. "I've got an important message for him."

"Who's calling?"

"A close friend," said Morton. "I've got something he ordered. Is he there? His package just came in from Peru."

A long pause in the lines. "You're not Rooney," said the woman.

Rooney! The same Rooney from Carney Apothecary?

"I don't know if you remember me, Roxanne. This is Morton Allison. We met a while ago—"

"The counselor!" she exclaimed. "Of course I remember you. It's not every day somebody cops a feel right over the bar."

"Yeah... Well, it's about Joseph. I need your help."

"You need *my* help? Listen, right about now we're the ones need *your* help."

"Why? Is he there? Has he hurt anyone?"

"He's here," said Roxanne low. "It's a godsend you called. I'm afraid something bad's going to happen. If I call the police we'll be closed down for weeks."

"What's he doing? Do you want me to drive down there?"

"He's been drinking all day. And he's pumped up with Peruvian snow at the same time. He's in his bully stage where he grabs and laughs and slaps at people. It's going to get worse. I know him. He's about to go insane."

"I'll come there right away," said Morton.

"No," barked Roxanne. "He's lost interest in us. He's got a new one to chase. Some nut he does his therapy on. He's been raging about her all night."

"What's her name? Is it Muriel by any chance?"

"Yeah, that's the one."

Morton flashed on Annise's pistol. What he might be capable of doing with it.

Roxanne said, "It's not her I'm worried about. It's the *ex*-girlfriend they always stalk. I guess she's pregnant or something, because he keeps saying he's going to beat the baby out of her."

"The ex? Do you know what she looks like?"

"Sure. Blonde. Twenty-three. A box of L.A. candy. She's been in plenty. Came in with the nut one time."

"With the nut? What do you mean?"

Morton looked to Muriel. She lowered her eyes. Betrayal? What rights did he have anyway? And Annise with all those J.S.'s on her calendar. Therapy schmerapy, that's what it was with your shifty suicide blondes, and maybe with your double-stepping schizophrenics too.

"All I know is when he gets done with one he knocks the shit out of them," said Roxanne. "You saw my scars. And I wasn't even pregnant. I thought maybe the blonde and you— I mean, from what you said—" She trailed off. "Look, I gotta go."

"Roxanne!"

"Somebody ought to protect the dumb bitch," said the barmaid. "I don't care who they are they don't deserve their eyes kicked out." She hung up.

~~~

Muriel returned to the brochures. She did not look up when Morton said he was leaving. He went to the closet. His Dodgers jacket was ripped and bloody. It was cool out and looking like rain. He had no choice but to select his loud purple blazer.

"Don't worry. Joseph won't come here tonight. I know him too well, Muriel. He's got other things in mind."

"I'm not worried," she said quietly.

He went to her. "I've got a plan. Would you like to hear it?"

She wouldn't look at him, just kept turning the colored pages of the pamphlets.

"I've got to try to clear these things up," Morton began.

He could have broken a chunk off her she was so icy. Sweet Muriel Gonska, the oriental sex philosopher turned to cold American steel. Romance, one noticed, tended to have this effect on people. Well, she had the right. And yes, she was becoming more predictable all the time. No longer was she stonewalling. He walked around in front of her.

"I've really got to do this," he said. "It's Annise Joseph's going to hurt first. I can't let her roam around L.A. like a mosquito with the Gestapo's boot waiting to come down on her." He paused. "You do understand this, don't you, Muriel?"

As if in answer, she picked up the paring knife and slit open another envelope. The sound it made caused him to shiver all the way to the bone.

* * *

Chapter 75

Morton collected Annise and they began the long drive to the airport, the LAX, as it was called by the locals.

"I'm so excited," she bubbled. "After all this time Aphie gets to take a long hard look at you. I'm glad you decided not to wear the cast. But Jesus, Morton, that wild purple jacket. And it's velour too!"

Mortified at his dress code, she stared intently out the window of the truck at the passing concrete median.

~~~

At the airport Annise contrived a bow as she made the introduction.

"Aphrodite Chastain, meet Morton Allison. Morton is a graduate of Johns Hopkins University."

"Annise, I'm not really—"

"Now you two hug," insisted the blonde.

Aphie and Morton embraced. Little sister held on an extra second, he noticed. Warmhearted girl.

At last she pulled back. "Hey, what a *fine* sport coat," said Aphie. "I've always thought good taste lies a couple miles left of center." She caressed the lapels. Yes, she really meant it.

~~~

When they pulled in front of Annise's apartment Morton had a fright. "The lights are on. Somebody's in there," he said driving slowly by.

"Oh, it's probably Wanda. I loaned her a key," said Annise. "See, she's waving at us."

"Wanda? At 3:00 a.m.?" Morton jutted his jaw.

As usual, Annise was radiant. Inside, she donned her pink satin housecoat and her gold, filigreed slippers. Her permanent was beginning to unkink, and her hair fell in long loose curlets. And so clean looking!

"My but you look sultry today, Wanda!" said Morton from the kitchen. "Don't you think so, Aphie? With the pretty bow in her hair?"

An awkward moment of quiet. Morton bent down to pet Sassafras. Lately they'd become quite tight.

"Thank you, Morton," said Wanda.

They chatted a while. Although it was 3:30 a.m., Annise got out the Ouija board.

"I think I'll pass," opted Aphie.

"Me too," said Morton.

Wanda and Annise folded their legs yoga style on the carpet and started asking the board supernatural questions. Morton and Aphie stayed on the sofa. She leaned toward the counselor. "My sister can scare me sometimes," she whispered. "When she gets upset she tries to act twice as confident about everything."

"You're quite perceptive," said Morton tapping Aphie's knee. "I was wondering, are you familiar with her, uh—" He searched for a way to put it.

"No hanky panky back there, you two!" cried Annise playfully slapping at Morton's hand.

They all giggled. The floor level search into the great beyond continued.

In many ways Aphie was extremely attractive, but fortunately not in the mind breaking body and face way of Annise. Yes, she did carry extra padding in a few spots, but they happened to be sites Morton respected on a woman. As the morning wore on the counselor detected a real rapport building with Aphie.

"Uh oh!" exclaimed Annise. "It looks like you won't be having any children, Wanda."

Wow, that one *was* funny. Even Wanda smiled.

The telephone rang. Annise and Morton glared suspiciously at one another.

"I'll get it," volunteered the counselor.

Annise said, "That's Muriel, I'm sure. Let the answering machine pick it up."

"It's the middle of the night, Annise. What if something's wrong?" he said.

"You know she'll want you to go back over there. At some point babies have to learn to sleep in their own beds," countered Annise.

The ringing stopped. All except for Morton breathed a sigh of relief. Then it started again. Sassafras gave a single sharp bark. The blonde dashed to the jack to pull it from the wall, but the counselor caught her wrist and held her back. Annise's greeting clicked in on the tape.

The message began. It was Joseph.

"You better take those pills, blondey," he said. "Or Dr. Schopen himself will do the butcher job. If you don't you're gonna to lose a lot more than the baby. I'll blow your ability to work in this state. Your reputation. You know I'm holding the videotape. You'll be dragged through the mud, gorgeous. Your family will see it. You're *going* to do what I say. Don't forget, Monday is D-day. Bring your beach pail and we'll fill it up with little Morty's blood and guts behind the bar. Love ya like a father. Bye now."

The vicious snap of the hang up caused all four listeners a white-knuckled start. A frigid silence ensued.

"Little Morty? What's he mean?" asked Aphie at last.

"Yeah, what *does* he mean?" said Morton. "What was all that about the butcher job?"

Wanda looked around for her fanny pack. "It's late, Annise," she said. "Time for us to get to bed—I mean, for me to head on home."

Wanda kissed Aphie on the cheek. She hugged Morton and kissed the air beside his ear.

"I'll walk you out," offered Annise.

When they were gone Aphie said, "I want to thank you for talking to me tonight. To tell you the truth, we get worried about Annise sometimes. My sister hasn't always picked the best men in the world. But I can see she's trying to change."

"Thank you," said Morton. "Only there's something I think you need to know, Aphie. A very important, ummm, event of anatomy, I guess you'd call it, has been occurring for awhile now. It's hard to talk about. I guess I'm probably part of it myself."

In his earnestness the counselor leaned over and unconsciously placed his hands on Aphie's full thighs.

"Is it about sex?" asked Aphie. "I know with her other boyfriends—"

"No, no. What happened is, a while back— A couple of months ago I guess it was—" Morton went on to describe the tumor.

Was it gossip, he wondered, if you spilled such secrets to an in-law—or rather, a member of your girlfriend's family? Aphie was incredibly understanding. He considered sharing the pregnancy issue with her as well. He could use a little sympathy, advice even. But as they conferred the counselor found himself more and more apprehensive. About what? Little Toni? The upcoming surgery? Some fictitious shoot-out with Joseph Schopen?

No. It was the idea of leaving for the mountains with Muriel that was disturbing him. Was there such a thing as a non-dirty liaison? Would he be running toward something new, or away from something old?

At bottom Morton simply didn't have the heart for big farewells, voluntary or otherwise. He seemed to be clinging to everyone around him. Joseph included. Co-dependence. It truly was a prison, as Harvey always said. Set the hook hard, but don't dare reel the quarry all the way in. Muriel? Well, she was different, he reflected, always so alert to finding pertinent ends and fresh beginnings. She got worried when she *wasn't* leaving places.

The front door opened. Annise trotted back into the living room. Morton looked down. His fingers were inadvertently squeezing into her sister's jeans.

"Morton, may I see you in the bedroom for a moment?" said Annise turning quickly away.

The counselor sighed, got slowly up and walked into the bedroom. Annise yanked the door closed behind them. He knew of course what it would be. First the scolding for molesting Aphie. She'd insist he find an excuse to limp on out for the night. Save face with little sister, who'd be sure to report this nastiness back to the rest of the Pasadena clan.

"Listen, Morton, I don't know what your plans are, but you absolutely have to do this one gigantic favor for me," said Annise nervously.

She went to the window and pulled closed the curtains.

"First, though, I want to thank you for being so nice to Aphie tonight. She worries about her weight, you know. You didn't? Well, she does. She's always thinking men don't like her. What a darling gesture the way you kept touching her and all." She gave him a hug.

"It was nothing," he waved.

"Anyway, what I'm going to ask is *the* most important thing right now. So please don't make a big stink about it," she pleaded.

"What do you want me to do?" he asked cautiously.

Annise hesitated. "I want you to promise you'll stay here with me tonight. I want you to sleep right there all the way till noon." She pointed at the mattress.

Morton shrugged. "All right," he said stepping toward the bed.

"Wait. I don't mean sleep like closing your eyes and actually going to sleep. What I really want you to do is—"

She went and listened at the door, then tiptoed back.

"What I really want you to do is get me all loud and squeally like I can sometimes get. OK? Will you *please* say OK and not make a stink about it?" she whispered.

"You want to get loud and squeally?"

"I have to. Aphie will know if I'm faking."

"But she's your sister, Annise."

"I'm aware of that, thank you. But you have to remember she's a terrible liberal too. She wouldn't respect me for the first minute if she thought we didn't get it on."

"She wouldn't?"

"Hell, no. And if there's one thing I really truly need from my family, Morton, it's respect."

~~~

Annise went out to the livingroom to do the final clean up. Morton could hear her speaking quietly with Aphie, then moving into the bathroom where the sink water started to run.

When she returned he tried to initiate things.

"Not yet, Morton," she said. "It's too soon. Aphie likes a lot of slow foreplay."

"Sorry. I didn't know."

Annise lit a candle and they waited for the time to pass. They talked in the low, sexy sounding tones they thought Aphie might respect. She asked about Muriel.

Morton explained how when they'd gone downtown last week for her annual I.Q. test she came out thirty points higher than the year before. If this continued she'd be a genius in another six months.

"You don't want her to come too far," advised the blonde squeezing his arm. "Because when people get extra intelligent about life they can become very lonely inside. You better be careful, or else she'll turn out half depressed all the time like I'm starting to feel."

Morton tried to see into her eyes. They were lax, almost happy in the candle light.

"You're beautiful, Annise," he said stroking her forehead.

"Don't say that," she replied.

They were quiet for a moment.

"You don't talk much during sex, do you?" she asked lazily.

"No, I guess I don't."

"You were talking the night I found you with Muriel," she reminded him.

"Only because I thought it was you," he replied gently.

Annise was wearing little pink socks. She reached down and started to peel them off. "I feel like talking sometimes," she said balling them together. "Would it be all right if I talked?"

"What do you want to say?"

She lit a cigarette. "Prayers," she said exhaling. "Well, not prayers exactly. Chants I guess is what they are. You know, like the kind monks use. Only dirty ones with a lot of kinky cuss words in them. I don't know why. It's just how I feel."

They were lying on their sides, facing each other. As they talked he traced down her backbone. Every now and then his fingers would graze the rim of the lump.

Morton said, "I doubt if you want to talk about this, Annise, but Joseph's call out there—"

"You already know about it. He wants me to take the abortion pill. RU-69 it's called, or something like that. He says he can smuggle it in from France."

"But you're not going to, are you?"

"No."

"And the butcher job? He's saying he's going to cut little Toni out of you if don't take the pills?"

"He thinks she's yours, Morton. He can't stand that."

Out of the blue the counselor fired, "Or else he thinks she's his, and he can't stand *that*."

The covers were off and he could see the fine contour of her lines in the flickering light. Morton felt guilty. He stroked her back. Desperately he searched for a telegraphed response regarding the Gestapo. But no, she simply lay there, supple and warm as a piece of morning sky, awaiting his embrace.

After a minute she went to the bottom drawer for the locking box. As usual she dumped the contents onto the carpet. The batteries. The bullets. The Librium.

"Give me that vial," said Morton. "There's Dilaudid in those pills. I don't want it around here."

"Dilaudid? You said that the other day, didn't you? They're very powerful, I hear."

He heard a kind of skeptical excitement in her voice. Morton stooped to get the pills, but Annise quickly slapped shut the box.

"They're a good high, aren't they?" said the blonde putting her arms around him. "People say they take your mind off yourself. Off life, I mean."

"They take your mind off death, Annise. Off dying. Which is why they work so good."

"Perfect," she said. "Lay a couple on me."

But this was all make talk, for she was already locking the box and putting it away, only the critical rubber and leather pieces left on the floor.

Annise said, "One thing though. I want you to run say good night to Aphie for us first."

"Do what?"

"Go say good night. Give her a bedtime kiss if you want. We need her to relax, don't we?"

Annise grinned softly at him. Long blonde wisps snaked forward over her shoulders.

"A bedtime kiss? In my undies?"

"Why not? This isn't dirty, Morton. It's sexy. There *is* a difference."

He cracked the door and stuck his head out. Aphie was in her gown and reclining on the sofa.

"Good night, Aphie," he whispered with an elfish wave.

She smiled through the dim light. "Good night, Morton," whispered little sister in return, giving a hip finger wave of her own.

Buck Buchanan

The counselor was experiencing a moral discomfort. Over on the calendar little Toni's conception date sparkled with colorful stars and moons and happy faces. Annise had mounted June and July side by side for convenient tracking.

From the edge of the bed Morton scrutinized the dates. Yes, he could recall them having done it that day, yet something about the scenario struck him wrong. It was only an intuition. But men didn't have legitimate intuitions, did they?

He began to congest a bit. Possibly from emotion. A cough he'd come to recognize as his little Toni hack flowered at the back of his throat. Gradually it built into a full-fledged, tubercular sounding fit. This was distressing, for it signaled an upcoming period of impaired concentration, which he knew from experience could mean impotence. Hmmm, the calendar?

When she needed to Annise could interpret a mood in a split second. She went to the calendar and methodically turned each page around to face the wall.

"I'm sorry, Morton," she said. "I'd forgotten how much this thing bothered you. Strange, nobody else minded it."

Without his permission Morton's jaw jutted.

Annise came to the bed and pulled the switch on the green lantern.

"What I said before. I mean, I really do want to show my sister where I stand on this."

"I'll do my best," he said.

"It's probably about time," said Annise. "If we pull this off just right I'll make enough noise to scare the Devil all the way back to heaven."

She angled her head so far into the pillows it was almost upside down.

"Love me for Aphie, Morton," she cooed. "Please. It's what all three of us need tonight."

* * *

'L.A. 2000:' Sex Asylum

Chapter 76

The next day the three of them went down to the religious cafe, Matthew's Place, for brunch.

The girl who came to wait on them wore a dangerously low-cut blouse. Annise sometimes flashed these types the hairy mug, but with this person she was downright cordial.

As the waitress leaned to serve their miniature bread loaf, Morton had to take evasive action, for the girl's huge Jesus-on-the-Cross medallion swung pendulously over his coffee cup. She smiled and jiggled. And it suddenly became plain as day to the counselor how her cross was actually validating the boob show.

"I liked that girl's necklace, didn't you?" said Annise.

"Absolutely yes I did!" returned Morton a little too enthusiastically.

Annise glanced into her own cleavage. "I've been thinking of buying myself one of those," she said. She adjusted the sparkling chains already around her neck. "Mine aren't the heavy-duty, take-charge kind like that girl's wearing. They're nice, but the thicker the piece the better. A big Jesus would really look impressive with my smaller necklaces. They'd compliment each other. Don't you think?"

"I guess so," said the counselor.

"You guess? This stuff is almost solid gold, Morton. It's quite valuable."

"I've never really understood all the hoopla about gold," he admitted. "I think of people going down in the earth with dynamite and blowing it out. You can't build a house with it. It's even outdated as tooth fillings."

Annise pursed her lips. "I doubt this has occurred to you, but in actuality gold is the word 'god' without the L. I can see by your expression you haven't considered that. Well, it is. And anybody who's anybody wouldn't dare underestimate the value of money."

Morton drank his coffee. Aphie pushed hers aside.

"Dad said a very important thing to us girls once," continued Annise. "He said, 'You'll never have your cake and own it too, unless you can get clear title to it.' And that's where gold and silver and drachmas and all that come in. The whole damn country is on the gold standard, Morton. I'm afraid you're a little out of step on this one."

The waitress brought their soup. The sisters chit-chatted while the counselor read the newspaper. Before long he came to a disturbing article. It was about the increasing willingness of nuns to be surrogate mothers. He showed it to the girls.

"I can't put this together," he said scratching his head.

Annise mounted her elbows on the table. "Christ, Morton, you're so naïve sometimes. Don't you realize how perfect nuns would be? They could get inseminated, you see, without intercourse. With a long needle or something say, so there wouldn't be any sin," she said.

"Please," said Morton. "I'm trying to eat."

Annise began to smile. Her perfect rows of teeth were showing for the first time in a long while.

"If you think of it, it would almost be like an Immaculate Conception," she said thrilled.

The blonde put her fingers to her lips in thought. Morton looked over to Aphie, who was wearing the same troubled expression he was.

"It says here more than a third of Catholic priests are sexually active despite vows of celibacy. 'Sexual misconduct as related to the clergy is a very hot issue,'" he read pointing to the headline.

"What do you expect?" returned Annise. "You've got to remember, Morton, those young nuns are completely nude under their habits."

"They are?"

"Absolutely," insisted Annise. "A woman can only hide it under a bushel for so long."

"I guess. Only it says here the priests are usually gay."

He waited, but she didn't reply. Aphie sipped her coffee.
"Homosexual," clarified Morton.
"Well," grunted Annise waving for the waitress. "It's never too late for a queer—I mean, a clergyman to change."
"Ladies can be gay too, you know," he noted cautiously.
"Ladies with ladies aren't much of a problem for God. It's the sword fights with men leave a girl stained and defiled," explained Annise. "Nobody can be snow white, Morton. But a couple of girls are going to leave each other a lot less ravaged when their dry cleaning bill comes due in purgatory."
Morton jutted his jaw.
"I've got to hit the restroom," said the blonde.
She left, on the way pausing momentarily to confer with the bosomy waitress. Hmmm.
Aphie whispered, "When my sister gets extra religious we know she's going extra crazy. I hope you can help her through this. It's obvious something big is going on with her."
Apparently Annise didn't have to use the restroom after all, for he saw her talking on the pay phone under the plastic replica of Moses and the Ten Commandments.
Whoever she was communicating with, she was smiling. It wouldn't be Joseph. It definitely wouldn't be Muriel. Aphie was here. Which left—yes—*Wanda*! No, Wanda Novice wasn't a novice at all. More like an Immaculate Deception for your waif-like blondes, decided the counselor. A serpent in bulldog clothing disguised as the female gender. That's what they said the Devil could do, wasn't it? Change shapes and body forms and whatnot in order to seduce the meek?
Jealousy. It was the ugliest of emotions. Even a nice person like Wanda could seem a threat if you were seeing through the torn pupils of the green-eyed monster.
Look to yourself, boy. *Inside* is where the answers are.

~~~

Aphie had to make her afternoon flight back to San Francisco.

At LAX, the sisters sashayed sexily toward the boarding gates. Morton stepped over to the telephones. He must have waited through twenty rings before she picked it up.

"Muriel?" he said.

"Yes?"

"It's Morton."

"Hello, Morton."

"Are you all right?" he asked. "Your voice sounds strange."

For many seconds there was no reply.

"I've been painting this morning. I'm probably tired now," she said at last.

"Painting? I thought the walls were finished."

"I'm redoing them."

"You're what?"

"I was reading too. I sent away for more pamphlets, so I was reading them," she added lackadaisically.

"I wanted to give you a ring. Make sure you're OK and all."

"I'm OK."

"Good. That's good."

"I got a call from Joseph. I'm frightened, Morton. He says he's got videotapes of me doing bad things."

"What bad things?"

"Well, I did bad things one time. But only one time. Anyway, he's got videotapes and he's going to keep me from going free. No matter what happens I'll never get away as long as he's got those tapes."

"Tapes of what?"

Silence.

"I'm ashamed, Morton."

"Of what?"

"Joseph gave me vitamins. He said they were vitamins."

"Did you take drugs? Is that what you're saying?"

"Not on purpose. I know I got high though. I got nauseous and puked."

"Dilaudid!" cried the counselor. "I knew it. Joseph's been tampering with the pills, Muriel. He's probably been doing it for years."

"I'm so scared, Morton."

"I'll be there as soon as I can."

No answer.

"I really will, Muriel. I'll protect you. I promised I would and I will."

Another long silence. "I'm going to finish painting anyway," she said.

Annise was returning from the boarding gates.

"Look, Muriel, something's come up. I can't talk right now. I'll try to get back to you later."

No answer.

"I'm sorry," he said. "I've really got to go." He hung up.

It wasn't wise to make important decisions around people who had an opinion of you. Particularly if she was a sizzling Hollywood blonde. Addled your vision. While the counselor understood this, he also knew the time had come to act.

"Who were you talking to?" asked Annise.

"You know I've been in touch with my mother this last week."

She shook her head.

"You didn't? Well, I'm sure I mentioned it. She's down in Palm Springs. I've decided to visit her for a day or two. Try to clear my head a little. Don't worry. I won't be away long."

Annise looked idly up. She had her emery board out and was filing the nail of her middle finger. "OK," she said.

Morton experienced a twist of the gut. Black lies. Pseudo-lies. White lies. They all had one thing in common: they made you feel bad when you said them. Morton swallowed his pride.

"Wait. That's not true, Annise. The truth is— The truth is I've decided to go up to Big Bear with Muriel. We're going to camp and fish. I have to get away. We both do."

So there it lay, the bitter truth, for what it was worth. The blonde looked placidly up from her fingernails.

"OK," she said blithely. She blinked a couple of times, then continued her filing.

* * *

Chapter 77

Throughout the morning Annise had been so up she seemed almost euphoric. Now, however, with Aphie gone, a gradual change of mood crept in. They were both quiet as Morton pulled onto the freeway and headed back to her place.

"Didn't you think it funny, Aphie flying down for only one day?" asked Annise as they rode.

"Kind of," admitted Morton. "But you Chastains can be funny sometimes. I think I'm getting used to it."

"It's important you know I had her come for one reason, and one reason alone."

"Yes?" Morton tensed.

"There's something special about sisters and their gentlemen callers. They can know freaky stuff inside each other without having to say a word."

"Gentlemen? Are you referring to me?"

"It's only a phrase, Morton. I'm saying when siblings hate each other's boyfriends you've usually got a lifelong match there. They'll hang on to the worst guys out of sheer spite. They'll marry them and bring them around the family and generally try to irritate each other as best they can."

"I didn't realize how complicated it was," he said.

"Family values are very complex, Morton. People who try to skim read eighteen years of growing up in the suburbs miss out on so much of the weird infighting it drives me crazy sometimes. Two sisters in the same house are like two vacuum cleaners with no bags inside, the dirt flies out the back side fast as it's sucked up."

"I wish Harvey was still around," said Morton. "He'd know what to make of that."

Annise put her back against the door and crossed her arms.

"I'm not sure if I was seeing it right. But I have this suspicious feeling Aphie might have liked you," she said. Her eyes were corset tight in their sockets.

"Yes, I think she did," agreed Morton.

"I feel you ought to know my sister and I have totally opposite tastes in men," said Annise solemnly. "To be frank, it doesn't seem possible we could ever both like you. She actually admired that stupid purple coat. Do you see what I'm getting at?"

Morton pursed his lips. The blonde thrust her hair straight back and held it hard against her scalp. Very austere.

"I suppose you know what I did last night— Well, it was for Aphie. Not for myself. Not for myself at all. It was for my goddamn sister!"

She shivered at the recollection. He could sense her tearing at her chains. She glared fiercely over at him.

"How do you think that made me feel, Morton? Doing something for her I could never stomach doing for myself?"

"You couldn't stomach it?" Morton took a deep breath. "But wasn't I helping you, Annise? I thought I was helping you with your problems."

"How the hell could you help me when ninety percent of the time you *are* the problem?" she returned.

"That's cruel, Annise. I might be my own problem. A lot of people are mixed up inside. But I've been fair with you all along."

"Fair? Do you think it's fair to look right through somebody to their dirty linen? Especially when they're breaking their back to camouflage themselves? Do you think it's fair to make a person feel like some see-through oyster shell all eaten away by maggots?"

"I make you feel like a shell?"

"You know when people get those big conchs and blow in them and it makes a loud horn sound?"

"Yeah?"

"Well, I'm that sound after it's hit the rafters of a gigantic church and comes echoing back. You've got no idea what it means or why it did it. But at least it's out there bouncing around. And believe me, Morton, sooner or later somebody's going to catch it."

"Sounds like a disease," noted the counselor.

He felt bad though saying that. The speedometer was up to eighty. The engine shook like a terrified animal. He eased off the gas and looked behind. Yes, his camping gear was still there, lashed firmly to the truck bed. For unknown reasons he felt a sense of relief.

"Look at us," continued Annise. "I've always respected the most implausible mysteries known to man. But you! You act like you can't see a thing if it's not right there in your face. Well, what about wind storms? What about supernatural fusion and fission? I bet you don't even believe in aliens from other planets, do you? Admit it, Morton. You don't!"

"No, I guess I don't."

"Which proves my point. Because neither does Aphie. And it doesn't seem possible the both of you could be in such idiotic agreement and be related to me. God. Men!"

Quite a talk it was. The counselor had considerable difficulty wording his feelings. He'd heard a hundred times over how love and hate were necessary co-anchors in the age-old bride and groom wars. Many claimed if you didn't have hate you likely wouldn't have love either. What, exactly, *did* he love about Annise?

He found himself cringing in recollection of last night's round in front of the calendar. It hardly seemed real, since he was forever dreaming up the backdrop scenario to sustain the flow. Perhaps a wayward notion of Aphie dressed in fishnet stockings, hitchhiking on a dirt road out in front of the Pearly Gates; or of Muriel, say, in a platinum wig, dancing naked with rock and roll singer tattoos of red vipers curling upward along the inside of her thighs.

He calculated the tangents as they traveled the freeway, until at last he arrived at Annise's breasts. Yes, this was what he loved—those immortal Annise Chastain breasts. And likely so did the other five million red blooded males of L.A. county.

He snuck a glance at the coy turn of her lips. At her long, dark eyelashes and her way of crossing her legs which made them seem uncrossed and somehow open to your advances.

Jesus Christ, fretted Morton! He really was letting the one dangling eye below see for the two above. Well, Annise had a perfected system of putting a person's brain on the blink, then asking a trick question about whether the Devil wore gold buttons on his fly or merely a low rent brass zipper.

You got deflected from your own reality and caught up in hers. Ambushed, so to speak, as much by what you couldn't comprehend as by what you could. Was he really able to see through her, like she feared? Or was she a distant ship walking the smoky horizon, stranding him forever at a minute to midnight in the wake of her hot tropical air?

Was he truly little Toni's father? He looked over at Annise through the smoke of her freshly lit cigarette. Copulation. Would he have even become aroused without the magazines and the vibrators and the sharp evil of the pistol as accessories?

Annise had the radio up loud. Morton clicked it off.

"I want to know about the videotapes Joseph mentioned on the phone, Annise."

"What about them?"

"I want to know what they are. And I want to know where they are. I want to see them."

"God, you're pushy. Since when did you get so pushy?"

"Since Harvey got murdered."

Annise rolled in her shoulders. "Those tapes are confidential, Morton. They've got private Dar/Neese information on them."

"Like you and Muriel over at Joseph's apartment? Like you and Muriel at The Green Room?"

Annise sucked violently on her cigarette.

"You don't know what you're talking about. Those tapes have never been out of Harvey's safe. And they never will come out. Not as long as Joseph's alive anyway."

"Don't be so sure," said Morton.

"Why do you say that? It's because you have the missing set of keys, isn't it?" she said accusingly.

"What missing set of keys? What are you talking about, Annise?"

"I'm talking about crimes. I'm talking about thievery and about like stressing Harvey out so bad his death is all of a sudden mysterious."

Morton refused to be deterred. "Were you with Muriel?" he pressed.

"What do you mean, *with* her?"

"Take it any way you want. I'm going to find out sooner or later."

"I wasn't with anybody. Not Muriel. Not Joseph when you always thought I was. Not even Wanda. Now lay off me, will you?"

Like two lions who had to fight for their sexual rights, they stared each other down.

Annise said, "Go on to the mountains with your schizophrenic. I'm sure she can take a rape with the best of us."

A strange instant passed. Annise was sheet white. "I feel ill," she said. "I've been having a lot of morning sickness. I think... I think I'm going to throw up."

Morton veered to the shoulder of the highway. He reached past her and flung open the door. Annise lunged toward the pavement. Sure enough, she began to vomit. He held her.

When she finished there remained debris in the ends of her hair. The counselor found a handkerchief and swept it away. He cupped her face. Tears were streaming down her cheeks. He almost said, 'I'm sorry, Annise. I didn't mean what I said before. I'm so sorry.'

But he did not say this. Instead he held his tongue, and found himself thinking of Muriel, whether she was safe. Thinking of the mountains and about fishing in a clear pond with a wide-brimmed hat to fend the sun off.

He helped Annise back inside, then drove her on home.

* * *

Chapter 78

At Muriel's the counselor parked by the front curb. Right away something struck him as odd. The calico curtains, one of the first items they'd purchased when she moved in, weren't hanging in the front windows.

When he opened the door Morton saw cardboard boxes stacked along the baseboards. Coat hangers lay haphazardly across the bare floor.

He stepped inside. A roller and paint pan were in the sink. He realized what she'd done.

The rainbow. The forest. The great river with the frantically leaping fish—all those dazzling pictures she'd spent so many hours creating had been blotted into nothingness.

Painting? Yes, she'd been painting all right. The room was now a bland off-white latex. He was stunned.

In the kitchen the counselor saw the travel brochures fanned across the table. On certain ones he noticed how she'd highlighted the distances from L.A.

Morton checked the bedroom. No Muriel. He put his hands in his pockets and wandered out to the backyard.

There she was, sitting in the lawn chair, still as ice.

"I, uh, saw the walls," he muttered.

But nothing from her. Not even a nod of the head.

"Those brochures. Has anything caught your eye?" he asked.

They looked deeply at one another. Muriel's hands were folded over a white legal-size envelope. He could make out fancy, calligraphy style typing around her fingers. She tapped absently at it.

"Listen, baby, I realize you're probably upset with me. First, I want you to know about Annise."

"I'm sorry, Morton," she interrupted holding up her hand. "I told you before, I'm not going to listen to any of that."

"But, Muriel, this business with Annise is coming to a head. I really have to tell you this. Now look—"

"Morton, please!" She came to her feet. "You're the one who taught me to get firm about these things. You of all people should understand."

Morton dropped his head. "I do. I do understand," he said humbling himself.

A horn sounded out front.

"Oh, there's my cab," said Muriel.

"Your cab? Since when do you go around in cabs?"

"I never know if you're coming or going, Morton. I went ahead and made plans."

"Plans for what?"

"I'm going over to the Fraction House. I have to talk to Wanda. She's the supervisor now."

"To Wanda? What about?"

"Dar/Neese is about to get me back anyway. I want to make sure Wanda lets me have my old room. It's the only one with a window, you know."

Muriel passed through the white gate. She started walking toward the cab. Morton rushed to catch her.

"Wait!" he cried. "There's something I have to say to you."

She stopped.

"I want to promise you something."

"You do?"

"Yes, I do." Morton took her hands. "Happiness, Muriel. A really wonderful happiness," he said. His heart was pounding in the smoggy heat.

"Happiness?"

"Don't you want it?"

"Well, I—"

"Please don't do anything drastic," implored the counselor. "Give me a chance to get these things—"

Another blast of the horn cut off his sentence.

"I'm sorry, Morton. I really have to go."

437

She shouldered her purse. He watched helplessly as she climbed into the back seat of the cab. The door closed.

He strained to see her through the tinted windows. It drove off.

~~~

Morton returned to the backyard. He fondled the leaves of the pepper plants. They were moist and supple. He put his fingers into the soil and rubbed them together. His head dropped far back on his shoulders. Tears were welling in his eyes.

"What have I done?" he moaned aloud. "What have I done, what have I done?"

Depression. It was like a nicad battery. You had to deplete the unit totally for it to recharge properly. If only drained part way it continued to function in an excited way, accidentally almost, though it was actually in the process of dying out.

Did a person have some mystical body memory of how many bad things had happened to him? If there hadn't been enough good—then depression. Or worse, if the nicad hadn't been run dead, fully killed enough, just half killed, you acted like an ass and called it moving forward. No, to get better you had to kill it super low, a real breakdown, a bottom.

Morton squeezed the droplets from his eyes. A car was pulling up out front. It was the cab. Muriel stepped out. He watched as she paid and walked toward him.

Such was the great thing about your recovering schizophrenics—they were comfortable reversing themselves. Why couldn't normal people do this? Simply undo it if it rubbed the wrong way and come on back home? That Muriel Gonska. He respected her style.

~~~

She entered the backyard and stood beside Morton at the cement block wall. Together they looked silently toward the faraway humps of the mountains, which shimmered like lazy camels in the distance.

"Thanks for coming back," said Morton.

Muriel smiled. "You're welcome," she said.

He noticed her hair. How close to full red it was turning from the sunshine. He ran his eyes over the heart-shaped curve of her hips.

"I know I've been behaving a little backwards lately. I'm not sure what to say," he offered finally.

"You don't have to say anything."

She turned toward him. "I was thinking, Morton. Do you remember when I got scalded so bad at the Fraction House?"

"Sure. I was the one drove you to the hospital."

"Well, I was running the water. And it took the longest time before I knew hot was going on me and not cold. I was berserk, I know. But it always feels cold first if it's hot. I mean, it fools everybody right at first, doesn't it?"

Morton scratched his head.

"Do you know what this makes me think?" she asked.

"What?"

"It makes me think you're supposed to feel the wrong way first. When you really start understanding it you stop and turn the water off."

Neither of them spoke for a moment.

"I think that's why a person can get burned so bad before they even know it," she added quietly.

"You're talking about Annise, aren't you?" said Morton.

"Maybe I know her better than you think I do," said Muriel. She turned to him. "Morton, a terrible thing is happening. Look at this letter. It came in the mail."

She handed the envelope to him.

'Marshmont, Peterson & Liam, P.A.—Attorneys At Law,' was inscribed on the letterhead. This was the top drawer legal team Joseph had swindled away from Dar/Neese. They had a city-wide reputation for making mincemeat of their foes.

Muriel said, "There's a form here I'm supposed to sign. I've got to turn my Guardianship back over to Dar/Neese. They're going to lock me up forever, Morton."

The counselor read over the letter.

Attn: Muriel Elaine Gonska:

Dr. Joseph Schopen possesses videotaped evidence of narcotic abuse involving one Morton Allison and Muriel Gonska. Further evidence of sexual misconduct, including the crime of forcible rape by Mr. Allison upon Ms. Gonska is in Dr. Schopen's possession.

With an eye to Ms. Gonska's safety, we at Marshmont, Peterson & Liam believe it to be in her best interest to return Ms. Gonska's Guardianship to Dar/Neese forthwith. Be aware that any charges proffered through the State Arbitrators could cause Ms. Gonska to be immediately remanded to the rehabilitation ward of Roselawn State Mental Institution.

Dr. Schopen requests Ms. Gonska's signature be placed in the three designated boxes of form 490A on or before 4:00 p.m. July 29th. This will insure her voluntary return to Dar/Neese, where she can be looked after properly.

Your immediate response is required, Ms. Gonska.

Cordially,

*The Honorable Marshmont,
Peterson & Liam*

Morton wrinkled his nose. "What's this mean? Do you think Joseph knows we were in the tub together? Could he be using that as blackmail?"

"Not the tub, Morton. Come inside. Something else was delivered today. It's a videotape. UPS brought it. It's probably illegal to send this stuff through the mail. Joseph would know that."

"Pornography?" asked the counselor half jokingly.

Muriel lowered her head. "I'm afraid so," she said.

* * *

Chapter 79

Morton drove out to Blockbuster Video and rented a VCR. He got his television set from the closet and rigged it all up. They began to watch.

Yes, this was pornography. Genital close-ups filled the screen for many of the early minutes. Soon it became clear three people were involved. One was a blonde with a bombshell body. The counselor breathed deep. It was Annise Chastain. She was as well traveled as Rodney had suggested. Here though she seemed different, not the frozen fire she usually exhibited, but groggy and uncontrolled in her movements.

"Turn it off," said Muriel. "I'm afraid to see the rest."

Morton let it run. The tape was choppy, filled with erratic stops and starts.

There came a close-up of a pair of gleaming handcuffs. A woman was locked to the headboard. Her feet were tied spread-eagle to the posterboards with electrical cord. The sound was gritty. She thrashed against the restraints.

"No! No! Please, no!" she screamed.

The woman was Muriel. Her pleas were slurry. Her eyes bloodshot and lolling three-quarters closed. She'd obviously been drugged—even nerds like the Arbitrators could have seen that much.

"I'm so sorry, Morton. I didn't mean to do wrong," said Muriel gripping his elbow.

"What did you do wrong?"

"I did sex. It's so bad. I didn't mean to do it."

"Now listen to me. A person doesn't do wrong if they're forced. Joseph did it. He's the one stole something you can't get back."

"I can get it back. A good man could give it back to me, couldn't you?"

"Did you know you were being taped?" asked Morton.

'L.A. 2000:' Sex Asylum

"I guess I did. But Joseph always taped everything. It didn't seem unusual. And I was so blasted."

"Do you think Annise knew?"

"Joseph gave her vitamins too. I don't think he took any though. He likes to stay up on Dexies."

"Couldn't you tell you were being drugged?"

"I've been drugged for the last thirteen years. They make us take whatever they give us, Morton. Priscilla was a pill pusher big time. And Joseph's been feeding me all kinds of chemical dope since I came to the Fraction House."

"Not narcotics," objected Morton.

"How do you know? All those pills make me feel funny. But I feel funny when I don't take them. I'm sorry, Morton. I know I'm not much help."

They didn't speak for a minute. The grotesque movie continued.

Muriel said, "That's why Joseph wanted you out of the way when he pushed you down those stairs. You'd have known for sure if I was getting out of whack. But with you busted up and away from the Fraction House he could stuff my Tofranil with heavy narcotics. I think that's what he did. I really do."

There appeared hard to swallow girl-on-girl scenes. Annise was half out of it. Not even in enough control of herself to act out her repulsive part. Morton could see the telltale signs of narcotic use. The dose the Gestapo had administered was far too concentrated for a neophyte like the blonde. Yes, Joseph had drugged her. It was plain as the nose on your face. He'd drugged them both. Annise was flopping and licking like a drunken sailor.

"I didn't do those things!" objected Muriel dashing toward the TV. Morton seized her around the waist.

Odd, he reflected, how Annise likely wouldn't consider this a rape, since it was the way she preferred to get off. Handcuffed. Strapped to the bedposts. There was something important to learn here.

"I feel ashamed," said Muriel.

"It's OK. Women don't get themselves as dirty with each other as when they're with men," consoled Morton.

The next shot was of a man. To their amazement it appeared to be Morton himself. He was naked. Or at least his torso was naked. Muriel's face and exposed breasts appeared on the screen over his shoulders. The counselor's eyes bugged in dismay as he watched himself begin to penetrate Muriel.

The film sputtered and crackled, then began to track. She was helpless. Thrashing and screaming and helpless. Again and again a fist rose and slammed into her face. Morton's fist? Impossible.

On the videotape Muriel was weeping and crying out for all she worth. It was rape the likes of which Morton had only read of in the papers. Hideous, back-alley womb-ripping. Shots of the counselor's face flashed in super magnification, then of Muriel's contorted, bloody grimaces as she suffered the vicious impalement.

~~~

Morton collected himself. He held Muriel in a bear hug as he analyzed the film.

The counselor's own face was on the screen, but it wasn't hard to figure out that Joseph's body was doing the dirty work. The tinted mat of black hair layered across the shoulder blades, the double torqued contraction of muscles—it was all unmistakably the Gestapo.

Was Annise doing the taping now? She couldn't be, all narced and gooey-eyed.

Together Morton and Muriel watched in horror as the assault continued. For the first time in his life the counselor felt he had the ability to kill. A frightening calm entered him, a robotic passion to lift the knife and run it through the heart of the rapist. He knew he could do it. He could hardly speak. At last he opened his mouth.

"This is unbelievable," said Morton.

"How did they get you in there?" asked Muriel. "Is it magic or something?"

"I guess Joseph must have filmed me at some point. He probably spliced the footage into this crap at his apartment."

"Look, Morton, you're not wearing a shirt. And do you see there on the table? It's your bottle of Sopov."

The tape sputtered and clicked, chewed up from Joseph's home brewed editing job. The bottle of vodka, barely visible, bent in the shadows at the edge of the screen.

"That's my apartment!" cried Morton. "Those shots of you and me together are from when I found you all busted up when I got in from the mountains."

He had a sudden awareness. He turned Muriel toward him.

"I've been wondering how Joseph got to my place so fast. I wasn't home fifteen minutes when he showed up."

Muriel's eyes opened wide.

"He'd just dumped you there, hadn't he? He watched for me to come home. Or had someone else watch. Maybe those snoopy neighbors. It was all a setup to make me look like the rapist. And he's still setting me up."

"But he's got this evidence," said Muriel. "He'll give it to the Arbitrators, Morton. You'll go to jail and I'll go back to Roselawn."

"It's phony though. This tape is hack work. I'm sure I could prove he pasted the thing together."

Morton pushed the eject button.

"In a law court maybe you could," countered Muriel. "But if the Arbitrators see this they'll do what Joseph wants. They'll never let a porno tape get out and screw up their precious program, even if it is phony."

Morton thought it over. She had a point. Above all the Arbitrators protected the state's image. Damn, it looked like Joseph had him over the final barrel.

"It's all getting very clear, Muriel. Joseph wanted me back to pin the rape on me. And probably Harvey's murder too."

"He always hated you, Morton. He wanted Stacy when you had her. I think he only went after Annise because you were after her. He even wanted Sally to fall apart, but you helped her get better. You messed up every wrong thing he tried to do."

Morton shook his head in frustration.

"And of course there's me. He knows I've always loved you."

"You've always loved me? How did he know? I didn't even know."

"He was my therapist. I wouldn't lie to anybody about you."

What a revelation! Morton felt his sinuses thicken with emotion.

"He held it over me though. That's why I couldn't tell you things," continued Muriel. "Joseph said he'd kill you if I ever let on what he was doing in the tub. I know it was wrong, but I didn't want you killed either."

"I'd have killed *him*. You underestimate me, Muriel."

The counselor paced the floor.

"They hired me back so Joseph could make your regression look like it came from me abusing you. But you were breaking down because of what he was doing."

"It wasn't a regular thing. Not at first, it wasn't. I don't want you to think it went on regular for years. It did some. But after you left your job it was all the time. I started going a lot crazier. Except when I got around you. When I got around you I was happy. I was myself."

Morton smiled. He leaned and gave her a tender kiss on the lips. Seeing her naked on the video hadn't done much for him. Now, however, with the real sun and sky flavor of her mouth he felt a sudden urge to take her into his arms.

"Let me get this straight," he said collecting himself. "When you came to my apartment and spent the night—remember? You were supposedly going manic."

"But Joseph told me to spend the night."

"I know. And he told me I had Temporary Custody. It was all a trick though. I'd signed the blue Custody Repeal form. I had no Custody at all. With you spending the night he was nailing down the coffin."

"He's horrible," she said.

"He had to make it look like I was following up on the first time I raped you. It was easy for him. He looked at his sins and transferred them to me. And it worked. You were going crazy because of Joseph. He hired me back to take the blame. That was the point of firing me in front of Priscilla and the Arbitrators."

"We got even," said Muriel. "You stole me right from under his nose with the G-F and those raffle tickets and all."

"I'm afraid it didn't help much," sighed the counselor. "Joseph's got his hot shot lawyers on it now. Plus this sick video."

He jerked the cassette out of the VCR.

"Let's throw it away," said Muriel.

She snatched it from him, wedged her fingers into the plastic and started jerking out the brown reel of tape.

"That won't help. I'm sure it's a copy. You can bet Joseph's keeping the original."

"Where?" said Muriel.

"In his safe. I didn't have a chance to tell you, but he called when I was at Annise's. He mentioned the tape. Annise let something slip about it being in Harvey's safe. You know, the old clunker under his desk. She said it'll never come out of there as long as Joseph's alive."

Muriel slumped. "There's nothing we can do."

Morton thought hard. "Right this minute you're still your own Guardian. We could fly you to—I don't know, Venezuela or someplace. I doubt if his lawyers could do much to us there."

"To us? Oh, Morton, you're going with me after all!"

"I mean, to you. Extradite you back here is what I'm saying. Damnit, Muriel, this is all so confusing."

She lowered her head. "I don't know how to talk Venezuelan anyway," she said.

A lonely silence rose like a flood across their lips. The coiled bunches of videotape were balled in Muriel's hands. She walked to the kitchen and dropped it into the trash.

Morton went to her and took her hand.

"Come on. We're getting out of here," he said.

He led her into the bedroom.

"Pack your clothes. And do it quick. I can't take another minute in this miserable cesspool."

"Where we going?" asked Muriel stumbling behind him.

"To the mountains, baby. We're going to the San Bernardino mountains. It's another world up there, and I'm gonna show it to you."

"You are?"

"Absolutely yes I am. Starting now we're forgetting everything and everybody we ever knew. Including the Gestapo. And including this ignorant tape."

"Including Annise?" asked Muriel carefully.

Morton jutted his jaw. Then he unjutted it.

"Including Annise!" he cried throwing up his arms. "Now let's go!"

* * *

Chapter 80

Morton wanted everything right. A new wick for the lantern. Sew the rips in the tent and paste seam sealer over the stitches. Air out the sleeping bag—they'd only need one, unzip it and use it as a blanket.

But there wasn't time. An urgency had mustered in the wind. A squall line he'd been shooting high caliber bullets at, to no avail. You had your valleys and your still-life deserts, like in Muriel's wall paintings, but you had your thunder too, and your wildfires of passion and hope.

To thine own self be true, this was the prescription, yet more and more the counselor was treading a fine blue line of mascara between selfishness and honesty.

In certain instances, though, a man might have to be true to someone else, mightn't he? To his woman, for example, assuming he could determine which one she was. Sometimes you had to use the back of your hand to sweep onlookers out of the way for the big rescue, didn't you?

Perhaps mother nature's wrath ought to be left to take her course. Or maybe he should try to help her out by running the lightning rod straight down Joseph Schopen's fly to where the evil resided. Then, when the storm brewed up, grab the Gestapo by his rosy red, uh, ears, and force him to stand there until justice bolted through.

~~~

Most days in Los Angeles were clear, but this afternoon the sun was double bright, as if reflected off a giant mirror hovering over the city. Scary almost.

He hadn't gotten around to unpacking his camping gear. It was still lashed tightly in the back of his truck from the last trip a couple of days ago to his apartment. Muriel worked inside stuffing paper grocery bags with clothes and food.

"Ready?" he asked.

"Ready," she said.

At the last minute Morton returned to the closet in the livingroom for his alligator-skin briefcase. One never knew when the need for an important document might arise. Especially the way things were shaping up with Joseph and his hot shot legal team. Better to be safe than sorry when it came to affidavits and flashy rubber stamps.

Annise? No, he couldn't just drive off scot-free of guilt. Not with the Gestapo's threats hanging over her. He went to the phone.

"I told you to go on and do your business. Didn't you hear me?" said Annise.

"I can't leave you alone. Not after what Joseph said on the phone about cutting the baby out."

"I'll be fine, Morton. I won't be here anyway. I'm going to my parents' place in Pasadena for the next few days. It's been planned for a long time. I'll be safe there."

"You're sure about that?"

"The Bible says never to throw pearls before swine. That's a principle I believe in. Now just go the hell to the mountains and quit causing me grief."

"If you're the pearls, then who's the swine?"

Silence.

"Joseph, right?" said Morton. "That is what you meant, isn't it?"

She didn't answer.

"Annise? You there?"

No, she wasn't there. She'd already hung up. At least, he thought, she was going to her parents. There was some comfort in that.

~~~

Morton and Muriel surged up the ramp onto the eight lane Santa Monica Freeway. They skirted smoggy downtown L.A.

before cutting eastward through the suburbs on the San Bernardino Freeway.

Soon they passed the sprawling complex called Failsafe Polymers, which had been cited for massive chemical pollution last year.

Muriel tensed, for ahead loomed a giant billboard advertisement for Dynasplice Genetics. This was Wojeck Gonska's firm where they froze embryos, or reconfigured sperm counts—something too avant-garde for the counselor's shopworn mind to comprehend. Neither mentioned it.

"Isn't this where Annise is from?" asked Muriel. She was referring to the opulence of the suburbs.

"Someplace north of here, I think," said Morton.

"She seems to get prettier every day. Don't you think?" Muriel glanced at him.

"Yes, I guess she does. But you're incredibly pretty yourself," added Morton quickly.

She was too. Not merely physically, but inside she carried an intriguing gravity which at any instant could switch fluffy pink and little-girlish. It was as if her heart could endure only so much pushing along of the blood of the child, and was finally beating out the steaming mirage of woman.

"Annise is so beautiful," said Muriel. "It doesn't seem like she could have such a bad tumor."

"Tumors are similar to mental illness. They don't care about a person's looks," replied the counselor.

Muriel squinched her nose. "Are you saying she's got a tumor *and* she's mental?"

Morton scratched his chin.

"I think Annise has a good core," said Muriel. "Except for when she lies."

"She lied the night they took you away in the ambulance," noted the counselor.

Muriel was quiet.

"She knew I didn't rape you," continued Morton. "She knew Joseph brought you to my apartment. She danced up like nothing on that videotape happened. Joseph planned the everything, didn't he? He'd coached her."

Muriel bit her lip. "I guess he did," she muttered.

"You deceived me too," persisted Morton. "I asked you over and over and you didn't make a peep."

"I think I had more dope than they did. I didn't know much of anything."

"You knew you weren't telling me the whole story."

"I couldn't, Morton. You'd have cut Joseph's jewels off that very instant. And if you'd known he took us to the lounge—" She thrust her hand over her mouth.

"The Green Room?" he said.

"Uh huh."

"So that's what Roxanne meant about Annise coming in with a hot redhead. You were the hot redhead, weren't you?"

He watched as Muriel considered stonewalling.

"I'm afraid so," she said at last.

~~~

It was a crowded, rush hour drive out of the city.

The pickup droned loud in the desert air. Modernistic vehicles shot like diamond-honed chips of silicone between the orange lane reflectors.

In the rearview mirror Los Angeles receded into the distance like a futuristic madman, his hair the mercury sided skyscrapers ignited with sun flame in the crimson smog, and wearing a Pinocchio nose as long and red as Hollywood Boulevard.

The pedal was hard down as the counselor powered across the body of the state. Ah, what a sweetheart, this California, the automobiles like thousands of masculine hands running from the hips of L.A., through the narrow waist of desert, and up to the bare, majestic breasts of her mountains. Yes, the mountains, by God, the place where no one could invade you!

He looked to Muriel. He wanted to tell her what he was thinking, but she'd fallen asleep.

Outside the city of San Bernardino Morton took a left on Route 30 and began the slow climb around Harrison Mountain. Soon they approached the small town of Running Springs.

Morton motored past the souvenir shops and the cocktail lounges. To his surprise the parking lots were overflowing with racy looking cars, reminding him of the kind Annise drove.

"Are we there?" asked Muriel coming around.

"Not yet. I thought we'd get something to eat."

In the diner Muriel operated on her sandwich. She separated the pieces of bread and stacked them on the side of her plate. She forked the alfalfa sprouts away from the chunk of avocado. As she'd always done as a schizo, she proceeded to eat all of each item before going to the next.

Morton had a flutter. He checked over his shoulder for gawkers. Suddenly he realized this was the first time they'd actually traveled together as a couple. He risked a second look behind. No, nobody was watching. And anyway, she had the right to eat the way she wanted, didn't she?

He touched his head and wondered for a moment if he'd remembered to comb his hair today. He had a notion it might be himself who was the troublesome one.

"You don't feel funny being out with me like this, do you, Muriel?" he asked nudging his plate away.

She set down her fork. "Oh, Morton," she sighed. "How do you come up with these things?"

After a moment Muriel said, "I guess we all have our foibles." She glared sideways at him. "But you don't seem to have any."

This was odd. It seemed to Morton he had nothing *but* foibles. It was a matter of interpretation, he guessed.

"Plus," she added, "your foibles are what endear you to people. It's a talent you have."

Morton smiled. A few contradictions here, he noted, but nothing to take seriously. The counselor patted her shoulder. She was a good kid.

~~~

They traveled deeper into the wilderness on the road known as the Rim of the World Drive. Morton saw green milemarkers indicating they were now inside the San Bernardino National Forest.

"Isn't it beautiful here?" said the counselor.

Muriel lolled her head back. "God, yes. And it smells so *green*," she said.

At the wooden signpost for Heart Bar Campground Morton squeezed Muriel's leg and navigated toward the registration office. A number of expensive RV's were backed up at the gate. Each made a U and returned to the main road.

Beyond, inside the campground, plumes of black smoke from the barbecue grills shrouded the trees. Litter blew across muck-mud mosquito ponds. Particle board firelogs blazed beside the pump out station. Annise might have called this the Apocalypse, but it looked to Morton like a bunch of sloppy campers and bad river management.

He idled up to the window.

The ranger said, "Sorry, buddy. All booked up. It's been a zoo around here."

"Anywhere else to camp?"

The man named several other places, but they too, he said, would likely be full.

"The mountains, huh?" murmured the counselor with a twinge of disgust in his voice. "Feels an awful lot like Tinsel-Town to me." He gave a shaky laugh as he pulled away.

The sun had fallen behind the trees. Long shadows spiked down across the road as they pressed ahead.

"Do you think we'll find a place?" asked Muriel looking worried.

Morton gnawed at his fingernail.

They continued, the air becoming icier by the moment. Finally he spotted a small opening in the trees. It appeared to be an old fireroad leading up the mountainside.

The counselor slowed and nosed off the pavement. Risky maybe, but worth a try, he felt, given the late hour.

Ruts of dried mud lined both shoulders as they bounced crudely up the steep grade. Dangerous scraping sounds rose from the chassis. The wheel jerked in his hands as the pickup dragged through the underbrush. Muriel gasped. Morton sucked his breath.

"I don't think we can make this," she stuttered nervously.

Night was upon them now. The fireroad became still rougher. Nevertheless the counselor forged into the darkness, twisting in a switch-back pattern up the slope. Yard by yard the truck proceeded.

As Morton was about to turn back, when the trail seemed most impassable, they emerged onto a wide, rolling plateau of grass dotted with small groves of pine trees. The full, late summer moon cast a dynamic white florescence over the sprawling plain.

Muriel pointed excitedly down the hillside.

"Look, Morton, it's a lake!" she cried.

Shocked at their good fortune, they stared awestruck across the high savanna. For the longest time the two of them sat there in wonder at the splendor, each gripping the other's hand.

* * *

Chapter 81

They dug a pit to put kindling in, then set about gathering wood for a campfire. Morton struck a match.

"Blow underneath," he said.

Muriel huffed on the small flickers. They had firelight, and warmth against the frigid night air.

Pitching the tent was more complicated. Morton kept hearing a harshness in his voice as he dictated instructions. Hold this. Hammer on that.

"I'm sorry if I was short with you," he said later.

"Short?"

She looked at him in confusion.

"You know, giving those orders and all."

"But you have to tell a person how to do something if they haven't learned it yet. I don't mind," she replied.

"You don't?" He was amazed.

"Not at all."

That Muriel. Naïve to a fault, wasn't she? Marry her up and you'd never have a squabble.

They settled cross-legged before the fire, the eiderdown sleeping bag draped in a giant wrinkle over their shoulders. Golden flash points from the embers materialized in the moonlit lake below, then snuffed black again. Every once in a while they heard a fish jump.

"I'm so happy, Morton," said Muriel softly. "I think this is the happiest I've ever been. In a way, it's like the Fraction House doesn't even exist."

They were slightly higher than the peaks of the other mountains. Beyond their gray silhouette Morton could see what appeared to be tiny fireflies blinking on and off way in the distance. He looked harder. He could hardly believe it. They weren't fireflies, they were the lights of Los Angeles! What, a hundred miles away? All sparkling and vibrating in tiny neon pinpricks. Picture perfect, at least from this distance.

'L.A. 2000:' Sex Asylum

The counselor was antsy. Stray, citified thoughts kept besieging him. Against his better judgment he started talking.

"You know, Muriel, this thing with Annise hasn't been feeling right. I think I told you about her calendar. I haven't been keeping close track or anything, but her boyfriends have these letters over the days they, uh, well, visited, I guess you'd say. Rodney's a yellow R for instance." He paused. "Do you see what I'm driving at?"

She shook her head.

"I don't even know what I'm saying," sighed Morton. "I guess a man can get kind of lonely for himself is all. Like thinking about his old friends or something. Then you see a shirt you haven't worn for a couple of months and you start thinking of it as somebody else's shirt. Like a person who's dead or something. It's like— It's like it's not even your own damn shirt anymore." He scratched his cheek.

"Whose shirt is it?" she asked blinking.

Muriel lifted a stick and stirred the coals. They could hear the spooky sounds of the night animals beginning to forage through the leaves. Just then a tremendous roar ripped across the plain. Morton leapt into her arms.

"It's only the wind," consoled Muriel rocking him.

Her breath was hot against his ear. He pulled back to look at her. Those eyes again. Always her eyes shining like gems through the altitude.

Inside the tent they snuggled close against the chill. Stones were in all the wrong places beneath them.

Morton gazed through the mosquito netting into the sky. The treetops were swirling and the early stars came down like impossible dreams through the high pine branches. An unexpected whiff of Annise's ritzy *Heroin* cologne floated in on the westerly breeze. Like a startled puppy he raised his nose.

"That's her scent. Smell it? I know it is!" exclaimed the counselor peering nervously out the front flap. "Annise Chastain is around here someplace. I'm sure of it."

Muriel leaned on her elbow. "No, Morton. It's only the juniper bush we've been burning. But Annise *is* close by. She's stuck inside your hard head."

Muriel stroked at his febrile brow. She placed her fingers on his trapezoids and began to massage.

"I only wish I could point the way for us," she said. She paused and ran her hands across her breasts. "Curves. There's no direction to a curve, is there, Morton? A woman just is. She doesn't point the way in life like that big thing a man has does."

"I thought a curve was *all* the directions," said the counselor. "I thought a woman pointed every way at once. Isn't that what's so exciting about them? Never knowing what angle they're coming from?"

"Lay back, Morton. I'm going to take care of you whether you like it or not."

Sweet little Muriel the guru. Putting down the law plain as day. He kissed her on the forehead. He was feeling much better. As the minutes passed his shoulders began to unbind for the first time in months.

The counselor reclined and cuddled up to her. The eerie night wind whipped through the edges of the tent. Morton placed his thumbs on her temples. He kissed her eyelids. Beneath her clothes he could feel her heart beating a mile a minute. The natural sea spray odor of her skin mixed with the sweet perfume of the juniper branches crackling outside in the campfire.

Muriel had the presence of mind to rotate the sleeping bag beneath them.

This time it would not be a case of one beckoning and one pulling away. Of one being dense and hopping out of the tub and the other half loony and accepting it. No. This time, at last, they were on equal ground.

"Give me a second," she said.

It seemed a miracle of female evolution the way they could somehow wiggle free of a pair of poured on jeans without breaking the gaze. Plus take care of the diaphragm and the jelly, and whatever other stuff they had to do. The male was clumsier, but when he wanted a thing, as Morton did now, the same headstrong urges were there to strip away the incidentals. He smiled. They were buddies, after all. And yes, he *was* going to like it.

"I love you, Morton," whispered Muriel.

God, but she was loose with those words. A shudder ran through him. A twist of beauty and confusion. It was cold as hell, yet he was sweating buckets.

"Love. Funny how it makes you see everything so clear," she said.

Morton remembered the time in Annise's bedroom when she'd exclaimed, "Love! My God, it's so *blinding*!"

Right there was the difference between the two. One clear as a bell. The other blind as a bat.

"You... You love me?" he echoed low.

"I've told you a million times."

"But how?"

"How?"

He couldn't think more, and he said, "Yeah. How?"

"Well, like say if you were swimming and I was the water you were in. Everywhere all around you," she answered playfully shrugging her shoulders. "That's how I love you."

Morton caressed her. The firelight licked softly at their exposed bodies. To his amazement he was at last able to feel the breast, the silky cresting of warm flesh into the rare hot find of her nipple. He sucked her like a baby, hard until his lips tired, then gently. His touches were so sincere he was hardly aware of how his hands had opened her, or at how seamlessly she moved to accept his slow shoulder roll and the untenable weight of his body driving upon hers.

It was improbable as hell, this event. Like every snowflake being different. Like each gene coming up perfectly unique, and only you having it. And only you, friend, with the right to share it.

Lust? Yes, it was lust all right. The hot and cold winds streaking like whitecaps over the counselor's undulating buttocks. What was it she'd said about the sea? "It might be ancient, Morton, but it's not old. It's fresh as a daisy every time somebody jumps into it."

And boy, was it! At each squeeze of the accordion came another explicit grind of Muriel's hips. She *was* talented. Hmmm. Maybe this wasn't an act requiring experience after all, just empathy. Absolutely yes, that was it! A little decent empathy and, well, like maybe commitment too?

The counselor was awash with emotion, yet he also showed talent. It had gone beyond the mere need to feel wanted.

Who knew what to call this phantom rush slipping back and forth between their legs? Screwing? Yes. But it was another thing too, which like those great swirling pictures of the atom circled up faster than the speed of thought to encompass their hearts. Well, perhaps this was the real making of love. Manufacturing the stuff out of naked bodies and half blown minds.

Morton gripped her shoulders. Muriel drove her knuckles into the small of the counselor's back the way she'd done the time on Annise's sofa.

Finally, as it was meant, Santa Claus got ready to come down the chimney. And when he did there was a big meeting at the fireplace, and in their tent under the stars all heaven broke loose in a trigger-happy spewing of sparks and burning logs.

Morton lifted to see her. He watched through the moonlight as her lips slowly returned to their soft pout, a curl accentuating the corners.

"I love you, Muriel," whispered the counselor. "I know that now. I've loved you ever since you first came from Roselawn."

Muriel pulled him to her. "Oh, Morton," she squeaked, her voice laced with emotion. "You're the best thing ever lived."

"No," said Morton. "You are."

* * *

Chapter 82

Afterwards he lay beside her, panting. His throat was dry, and as sometimes happened at these moments he started to cough his little Toni hack. His mind spiraled with worries of Annise and her multitude of emergencies. He recalled the time, one of many, she'd become annoyed with him over a minuscule gaff of wording.

"Have a heart, will you, Annise," he'd pleaded.

"I do have a heart. Actually, I've got two," she replied petting her midsection. "You're outnumbered, Allison. Maybe you better wake up and start towing the line."

"Two?" he said, worried.

"Uh huh. Yours and mine make one. And little Toni's is right behind."

He wasn't positive, but Morton thought he detected a hint of Joseph Schopen in her tone.

The counselor's mind reached back to those early, inept sessions of lovemaking with the blonde. By now he'd committed the calendar and its exotic notations to memory, so often had he eagle-eyed it. The 6th of June was the culprit date. Had they really scored such a successful round that evening?

Morton cleared his throat.

"Honestly, Muriel, I cannot remember becoming little Toni's father. Something is way out of kilter, but I can't seem to put my finger on it," he said.

He thought hard. The whole business had occurred a matter of weeks ago. Why was it so foggy? Psychologically, one had to consider early senility, a sudden bipolar attack, generalized nuttiness. What with his eccentric ways the counselor suspected he could fall prey to some burned out mental bankruptcy.

"I had a thought, Muriel. Remember when Annise gave me the Librium up in Venice? Well, it wasn't Librium. It was Dilaudid. I'd already been taking it. So I kept on taking it. And sometimes, especially at night, I'd get so groggy—"

"From the Dilaudid?" asked Muriel.

"Trina explained I was going to have a withdrawal problem. She gave me a prescription for *real* Librium. I used it like she said. I think I'm back to normal now. But there were times with Annise—"

Morton grasped the sides of his head and tried to wade through the haze.

Let's see. Annise had gone to lunch with Joseph, hadn't she? To The Green Room, as a matter of fact. Which had been circled on the calendar. Yes, now he remembered. They'd painstakingly worked around to the romance. It was to be a great body shattering union of white hot Catholic and drug addled, wet-behind-the-ears counselor.

"It's coming to me, Muriel. I swear it is!" exclaimed Morton. "I think something really *didn't* happen that night."

"It really didn't?" she said.

Her eyes were open and shining blue-white through the darkness. She could feel Morton's thrill. A revelation was nearing and she knew it.

The counselor sifted through the details. By degrees he was at last sneaking up on the truth. For when they'd lugged the ammo up to the firing range, so to speak, metal ordnance box and all, and prepared to commence firing, he'd come down with— Yes, with a fit of coughing! As it happened, he'd coughed his way right through the climax. Not through it, *instead* of the climax. At the moment it had been rather disappointing that nothing happened. Besides— Well, face it, besides impotence. And, well, a kind of spastic hacking, which Annise must have construed as the trucking in of little Toni's fertilizer.

Unsuccessful romance was always a bummer. Now, however, there welled an immense joy in Morton's thumping heart. He was not little Toni's father after all! And for once he knew he had the math right.

He shot bolt upright, like an Indian chieftain in fast-forward recognition of nirvana.

"It wasn't me!" he exclaimed. "It wasn't me, Muriel. I just figured it out!"

"Figured what out?"

"I'm not little Toni's daddy. I'm sure of it!"

In his excitement to explain it all to Muriel he nearly took a bite out of his tongue.

Then a new awareness poured in. If the sixth was her ovulation day; which she'd said it was; and if the counselor wasn't the culprit; which he obviously wasn't; and with Joseph's initials inked in over the same day; and supposing Annise and the Gestapo exercised more than their mouths during the lunch date; for which you didn't have to be Perry Mason to make such a supposition; you were left with one major fact in your hat: It was *Joseph's* little Toni.

Morton tried to relate it to Muriel in a way she could understand. Something though felt fuzzy in the translation. She wasn't quite getting it.

"Sex with Annise isn't exactly sex," he clarified. "Not always, anyway. Rather, not exactly intercourse, if you know what I mean."

"I don't know what you mean," said Muriel.

"I'm saying if she's pregnant from the day she claims it couldn't possibly have been me. I'm absolutely positive I didn't, you know—" This was embarrassing. He trailed off.

"Ejaculate?" asked Muriel.

Morton nodded sheepishly. "Jesus, you're blunt," he said.

"What did you do if you didn't—?"

"Coughed," he answered quickly. "I told you."

Muriel was like twelve men jammed in the jury box. She needed every shred of evidence before agreeing to his innocence.

Finally she nodded and said, "Maybe this will work out for the best."

"I doubt it," said Morton. "Joseph wouldn't be much of a father figure."

"Wanda's the one who's always wanted Annise. She's loved her more than any of us."

Morton pursed his lips. "I thought it was Joseph wanted her," he said.

"He probably did at first. And he never lets anybody go. But I think Wanda knows she'd be the better father, don't you?"

That Muriel. No prejudice. No judging. Spit it out like Jonah from the bowels of the whale.

"Wanda's doing a lot better, Morton. Ever since she broke up with Stacy she's gotten stronger and stronger."

"Broke up with Stacy! I've heard rumors. You mean Wanda and Stacy have been... been..." The counselor jutted his jaw.

"Together," said Muriel placidly.

Although he wasn't standing, a weakness came into Morton's knees. Everywhere he turned females were beating him out. He took a moment to compose himself. Did he have to let go of *all* his ego?

"Everybody says Stacy's after Joseph now," revealed Muriel. "You know how much she likes money. I guess Joseph promised her my father's fifty thousand when it comes in this year."

"Kinda figures," admitted Morton.

"Wanda says Stacy is even perverser, I mean, perverteder—or whatever the word is—than she thought. Stacy keeps telling Wanda she needs excitement, like in spy novels. Crime. Intrigue. She wants to find it in Joseph."

"She will," said Morton.

"Once you know these people it all starts to make sense," said Muriel.

The counselor was eating a lot of humble pie these days. The chase for Annise, after all, had been between Joseph and Wanda. Not between Morton and anybody.

Muriel said, "I guess Wanda found out Stacy was messing around with Joseph. So she started messing around with Annise to get even. It got shabby real quick."

"It sure did," grieved the counselor.

'L.A. 2000:' Sex Asylum

"Are we gossiping?" wondered Muriel looking concerned. "You always told me gossip is bad. We don't want to do anything wrong, Morton."

"We're conferring. It's all right to confer."

"Well, OK," said Muriel relieved.

"And Wanda? What's her story?" he asked.

"I think we both know what Wanda wants."

The counselor wagged his head in despair.

"Don't feel bad, Morton. Wanda is perfect for Annise. Think about it. Two girls can have all the sex they want without facing any of those immortal sins. They never have to—"

"If you don't mind, Muriel, I'd rather not go into this," interrupted Morton.

Moments of silence passed. He found their plastic liter of Coke and took a swig.

"I've been wanting to ask you something, Muriel. You never say anything about it." He moved to sit cross-legged in front of her. Her eyes were big and free, and he said, "Weren't you ever jealous? I mean, there's no secret about what's been going on, is there? Because sometimes I guess I feel like I might be—I don't know, maybe like I might be cheating or something."

"Cheating?" she said quizzically.

"You know what cheating is. Women call it disloyal if you go to other people. I mean, you know, go to women who aren't them."

"To Annise, you mean?"

"Well, yeah."

"Does Annise feel you're cheating?" she wondered.

"I don't think so. I'm only now starting up. You know, this is the first time we've..."

"But Annise cheats, doesn't she?"

"She used to. She says she doesn't anymore."

Muriel wrinkled her nose. "But if you're still going over there you're not cheating her, are you?"

"Well, uh—"

"If you weren't going to Annise she'd be cheated even more. I mean, she wouldn't see you at all. So when you think about it she's cheated a lot less this way. That's how I figure it." Muriel looked innocently over at him.

"You do?" Morton was shocked.

"Oh, yes. I'd feel extremely honored to have you cheating on her all the time. Otherwise where would I be? And anyway, she's only a piece."

Morton nearly spit out his soda. How could the mentally ill peer so deeply into these issues?

"I only mean if you don't have a whole person somewhere you'd probably go around looking for enough pieces to make one up." She gave a nonchalant wave. "If each one on their own wasn't enough, I'm saying."

Yes, he decided, this was reasonable. Quite reasonable, actually. Only now, suddenly, Muriel had somehow become that very person, the one who wasn't missing any pieces. He leaned forward and kissed her on the forehead. He was feeling much better.

Morton was comforted. It was always heartwarming to have a comrade join you in a squirrelly thought. Added credence.

"You're trying to find yourself in a woman, Morton," counseled Muriel. "Unless— Well, unless you've already found yourself in one."

A moment of quiet passed while the counselor assessed the data.

"You're fabulous, Muriel. Absolutely and utterly fabulous," he told her.

He cupped her face and kissed her deep and pure. A river of heat flooded out of him for her. It had all gone right for once. Incredible how distinctly you could see a thing when you looked through the proper person's eyes.

He uncrossed his legs. Muriel uncrossed hers. The fire was out now. Blackness everywhere. All they had left for warmth was the inside of each other. That would do fine.

As they kissed she held his face to hers by the scruff of his beard. It felt good the way it hurt a little.

In return he clawed her rump. Sensually though. Not violently. For in the sex wars it was looking like the heart had to go through its own reverse osmosis, nail down the purification process before you were allowed to unsheathe your saber—certainly a new concept for Morton.

A mighty cleansing was coming over him. A kind of baptism by emotion.

They started another round. No, this was not your dictatorial blonde. This was a pliable, even-tempered girl. Not a lover of mankind who couldn't see the forest for the trees, but a lover of one man, of him. So put that in your pipe and smoke it, Annise Chastain!

* * *

Chapter 83

The next morning Muriel was invigorated. Her face glowed bright red from sitting too close to the fire the night before. Morton dabbed her with the ointment he kept in the glove box. She gave him a funny look.

"Isn't that your hemorrhoid medicine?" she asked.

He checked the label. "Um, yes, I think it is."

He worried she'd be mad, and carefully capped the tube.

"You're so cute, Morton, the way you do things," she said reaching out to hug him. "And sweet too."

Cute and sweet? Would this ever have come out of Annise's mouth? Or anybody else's either, for that matter? No. It was—only a fool wouldn't see it—a whisper of love.

~~~

For breakfast they ate the Pop Tarts Muriel brought along. The sun sprung up behind them. They joined hands and headed down the hillside to the lake. California's early sunlight blasted the surface of the water with exotic purples and reds, majestic and surreal. And best of all was their solitude, their moments alone together to take it in.

Muriel hurried to the pebble-stone shoreline. Morton watched as she took a bobby pin out of her hair, bent it into the shape of a hook and began dragging it slowly back and forth under the thin layer of water. She was pretending to fish. So spirited, that kid.

They kicked off their shoes. The counselor came up behind her and squatted in the sand.

"Morton?"

She touched softly at his face.

"Yes?"

"I'd like to catch a fish one day. I don't know how though. Would you help me learn to do it?"

They looked out over the acre-wide lake. He felt like crying, he was so happy.

"Of course, Muriel. Of course I'll help you," he said.

He kissed her. Solid and self-reliant. And lusty, as well. Morton could feel her oven warming. He flashed on a reckless lovemaking session there on the edge of the lake. Buck naked and steam-cleaned with their own perspiration. A fine wallow it would be too in the sparkling, morning glory arms of nature, where everything in their world was both private and wide open to all creation.

Inadvertently they'd waded in up to their ankles.

"It's wonderful here with you," said Morton. "I feel so free I can't even remember the date."

Muriel thought it over. She couldn't remember either.

Back at the truck Morton got the mini calendar from her purse which had come with one of the travel brochures.

"Jesus Christ, Muriel, it's July 28th!" he cried, alarmed. "Do you know what that means?"

"What?"

"It means Annise's surgery for the tumor is tomorrow morning. I completely forgot about it."

"Tomorrow?"

"Yeah. Across from Cedars at nine in the morning. It's been scheduled for a while."

With a philosophic demeanor Muriel turned the counselor to face her. Morton felt a flutter invade his chest. She'd never tolerate his return to the old mistress. He couldn't blame her.

Muriel said, "Annise is probably flipping out by now. I don't think she's strong enough to face this alone. We've got to go back for her."

"We do?" Yet again the counselor was put on his heels. When would he figure this girl out?

"I'm sure Wanda will try to help. But she's not you, Morton. She doesn't have your strength."

Muriel possessed a magical existence all her own, separate from the living and breathing world. A kind of penetrating, organic understanding Morton often missed out on. This was how she was—catch you completely off guard, yet at the same time make you feel like she was part of your upcoming destiny.

"And anyway," she added, "Joseph might hurt her. He could do anything, Morton. He could even kill her."

"I know he's tried to make her take the abortion pill," he returned. "She refused. And on his message the other night he said he'd cut the baby out of her if he had to." Morton shook his head. "What have I been thinking about driving around the countryside like this? You're right, Muriel. He could do anything. We've got to get back there right away."

~~~

They started taking the tent down, stowing the gear. Morton crammed it into the truck bed.

With a new focus the counselor crab-walked the truck down the lumpy fireroad. Not once did they look backward to their campsite or the lake. A bad premonition riddled the air. It was a mood only a bloodthirsty werewolf like the Gestapo could imbue.

"I'm very worried, Morton," said Muriel as they pulled out onto the highway.

"Me too," returned the counselor tightly. "Me too."

* * *

Chapter 84

At a desolate turn in the road they came to a telephone booth. Nothing else. Woods everywhere, and this newfangled, oval-shaped chunk of Plexiglas intercepting impossible voice configurations as they streaked out toward L.A. Morton pulled over.

"I need to call her," he said.

Annise's phone rang and rang. The answering machine had been turned off. What did this mean? Maybe that she couldn't handle another vile threat from the Gestapo, like the one he'd heard with Aphie and Wanda.

Morton hung up and dialed his apartment. He punched in the remote code to hear the messages on his own answering machine. He wondered, vaguely, how many days had passed since he'd been home.

He listened to the playback.

First was Trina Lopez.

"I do not hear from you, Morton. I worry very much for you and Muriel. And for the blonde lady too, I worry. I told you Joseph did something and got me fired from Shearer-Kaplan. He is friends with ugly people all over this city, Morton. Yesterday he called and said I would never work again in Los Angeles. I live here, Morton. I have to have work. Let us help each other. Tell me you are safe, amigo. Remember, I am your ally. Goodbye for now. Oh, I forget. I am in a new apartment. 432 Lorraine St., in the back. Joseph will not find me there."

Immediately Morton called Trina. Luckily, she was home.

He updated her on how he'd freed Muriel at her Termination Meeting, and on the Annise, Joseph and little Toni connection. He told her about the videotape, how the Gestapo had doctored the scenes to make it look like Morton was the rapist. He told her about the letter from Joseph's hot shot lawyers, how Muriel could be forced to return to the Fraction House.

"I don't know how you're going to take this, Trina. I want you to understand something, I'm with Muriel now," he said.

"Yes?"

"No. I mean, I'm *with* her. You know, we're, um, together."

A long moment of silence. Trina said, "I am terrible happy for you, Morton. You two have deserved this since the day Muriel came. Everyone knew so."

"Everyone knew so?"

"People cannot hide big feelings. Love is the same no matter what angle we look from."

That Trina. She was no nonsense to the core.

"Thanks," said the counselor. "I'll contact you when we get back to L.A."

He re-dialed his home phone for the rest of his messages.

Gordon came on, but being unfamiliar with the tones and beeps and whatnot nothing much was intelligible.

The next three recordings were all from Wanda Novice. Her voice became progressively shrill with terror. Joseph had been harassing Annise. He was demanding an abortion. He'd gone completely off his rocker.

"He says he's going to beat the baby out of her, Morton. Please come and help us. I'm chanting in hopes you'll call your machine. I'm at Annise's now. She's not here. I don't know where she went. I'm scared. Really scared. And Sassafras..." There was pause.

"Listen," she continued, "I know I never got on top of this Joseph thing. I hurt you, Morton. I was a coward. Please accept my apology. There's no one to help us now except for you. All last night was pure horror. I'm frantic, Morton. Call me as soon as you get this message."

Morton telephoned Wanda's home. No answer. He called Joseph's old number at the Fraction House, the one for the Clinical Supervisor.

"Hello?" said a gruff female voice.

"Wanda?"

Silence.

"No, Morton. This is Stacy."

"Stacy? Where's Wanda? She's the new supervisor, isn't she? Or has she been fired already?"

"Supervisor? You must have dialed Harvey's number by accident. You've reached the Director's office."

He could feel Stacy's smug, authoritarian vibes right through the lines.

"Joseph isn't in right now. He asked me to handle things for him till he gets back. Actually, I think he did leave a note here for you. Let me check."

Morton waited while Stacy rummaged through some papers.

"Here it is. You wanna hear it?"

"Certainly I want to hear it."

"It's just two words. You sure you're ready?"

"What two words, Stacy?"

"Get fucked," she hissed.

Morton took a deep breath.

"It's from both of us," added Stacy. "And you can give the same message to Wanda. Here, I'm putting you through to her."

The intercom phone rang in the background. When Wanda answered Stacy Lung slammed down her receiver so hard it shook Morton's teeth all the way up in San Bernardino.

"Wanda?"

"Morton?"

"Thank God you called. Joseph hasn't been in for two days. I went to Annise's this morning and the place is a wreck. I mean, her furniture is all smashed up. You don't think she would do something like that, do you? I mean, we've got to admit she's not always a hundred percent with it."

"You know as well as I do it was Joseph," said the counselor.

"I'm so afraid for her. He's going to kill her, Morton. At the very least he'll kill the baby. He hates it for some reason. Maybe because he hates you. Maybe he thinks if he kills the baby it's the same as killing you. I don't know. I'm only a Social Worker."

"At least you're trying, Wanda."

Very quietly she said, "All this is because it's your little Toni, isn't it?"

"It's because it's *his* little Toni," corrected the counselor.

Wanda sucked her breath in shock. Morton expected her to question this, but she said nothing. It was as if she'd known it in a subliminal way all along.

"We've got to take action, Wanda," he said. "Those desperado types murder their families all the time. They've got an instinct for not wanting their scrambled up genes in the world, so they draw their magnum and blow them away."

"How'd you get so smart?" asked Wanda.

"Muriel's been helping me," said Morton looking through the windshield at his friend. "She's a secret genius."

Wanda said, "I've tried everywhere, Morton. I've even gone to your place thinking she might be driving back and forth in front of your apartment like she used to do. Joseph's changed her schedule around. She was supposed to be in today at noon. She didn't show. Nobody's seen her. Nobody's seen Joseph either."

"I know where he is. The Green Room."

"What's The Green Room?" said Wanda.

"Annise never mentioned The Green Room to you?"

"No. Should she have?"

"How about the tapes?"

"What tapes?"

Ah, those dirty mysteries again. And lurking behind more bushes than lined the Pasadena Freeway. The counselor wisely held his tongue.

"One last thing," said Wanda heavily. "Over at Annise's this morning I found something."

A tension mounted. Morton lingered while he heard the rustle of her shifting the receiver to her other ear.

"Sassafras is dead," said Wanda finally. "It looks like she was poisoned."

"What?"

"There were a bunch of capsules around her bowl. She was lying on the kitchen floor. I didn't know what to do, Morton. I just left her there."

Dilaudid! suspected the counselor. A lethal dose of Dilaudid.

"Capsules? What did they look like?" he asked.

"I don't know. I was so upset." She paused. "You don't think Annise would—"

"I've got to go, Wanda," he said, feeling crushed. "I'm in San Bernardino. I'll be in touch as soon as I can."

Morton returned to the truck. By the time he'd situated himself in the cab his sorrow had turned to humiliation with a touch of rage thrown in.

"He killed Sassafras," he said staring hard out the windshield.

"Her little beagle? Joseph... Joseph killed her?"

"Sassafras was a good friend of mine. I don't mean to be harsh, but in a lot of ways she was a better friend to me than Annise ever was," said Morton.

Muriel scooted over and hugged him. He began to quietly weep.

"Joseph has murdered for the second time in two months," said Morton. "He's a psychopath. He's like a roving executioner. He's got to be stopped."

After a minute Muriel slid back to her side.

"I feel like I've got a temper tantrum stuck inside me," he said. "You ever feel that way?"

"Start the engine, Morton," instructed Muriel. "Let's get back to L.A. and take care of business."

"I'm no policeman."

"You've got to be. The police are hog tied," she said.

Morton squinted. "Uh, you mean their hands are tied, don't you?"

"Whatever. There's no evidence for them. You and me have to be the police."

"You and me?"

"Who else?"

The counselor gave this deep consideration.

"I'm afraid you're right, Muriel."

An unfamiliar surge of ego entered him. A kind of high from the belief that you and your best friend could accomplish virtually anything. Morton slowly lifted his head. He blinked out his tears, and without hesitation fired up the old V-8.

"All right," he said. "Only be warned—there's no backing out now. We understand this, don't we?"

Muriel smiled at the old Fraction House lingo.

"Yes," she said. "We understand this."

* * *

Chapter 85

Out of the mountains and back on the freeway.
Did it really matter, in the big picture, where a person went anymore? Leave L.A. Return to L.A. The world was merely one small town these days. And why was the trip home always so much faster than the inch by inch crawl that got you away in the first place? Such riddles!
It wasn't long before the flaming head of the L.A. madman appeared on the western horizon. The skyscrapers. The burning smog. Morton felt as if a bull's-eye had been painted on the truck hood and a sharp wooden stake was hurtling toward them at megasonic speed. Was it a unique California syndrome that the ultra-modern kept fumbling the ball to the prehistoric, though neither team knew which way to the goal line? And how did weirdo vampire style superstitions get so laced up with plain old day in day out living, with your BLT on rye down at Vera's, where the blonde, on any given day, might mutter a heated prayer to Count Dracula as quick as to the Holy Father?
Being Sunday, it wasn't rush hour on the highway. In a way though, there was hardly an L.A. minute that didn't come with its own pre-installed accelerator chip. No longer were counselor and client traveling fossilized asphalt, no longer in covered wagons with a couple of swayback mules dragging the load, though he couldn't tell it from the way his pickup bucked and sputtered when he gave it the spurs.
Those sentimental horse and buggy days were gone. Travel over the ground was simply outdated. Face it, running scared across the tundra had been an illusion to begin with. A nightmare, where your feet spun in place and Mad Dog Joseph Schopen kept catching up anyway. As for powering to your destination, that notion had been tossed out decades ago by your acid-eyed visionaries up in Berkeley who'd swapped it for, yes, *mind travel*, for the screaming swiftness of the information superhighway.

There followed improvements in lifestyle, for nowadays two incurable hyperactives like Morton and Muriel skimming the far edges of the lanes weren't so far out of the mainstream. They made for an unusual sight—a couple of brain bent tourists escaped from the loony bin, heading back to the big city for a final game at the barroom of who'll drop the hand grenade.

In the end, pondered the counselor, maybe a person had a kind of intrinsic, black magic right to choose a schizophrenic for a soul mate, and the rest of society be damned.

It was a difficult question. There were the Arbitrators—your suit and tie throw-backs to pre-punk rock whose idea of a hot tamale was Priscilla Daddio with her braid let loose. You had your Harvey Muellers, gone to the dogs himself on account of too much sensitivity. And of course there was the inevitable Joseph Schopen driving the data train. Joseph Schopen about to make the counselor and his genteel client part of his drug-pumped road kill.

On the Gestapo's highway, if you weren't demolished after the first violent hit and run the next turbo powered bloodmobile laid you out flatter than a pancake for good measure. In which case not even God's silver hammer and chisel could hold a fine enough edge to peel your stubborn soul off The Green Room floor.

The Green Room, considered Morton. When people developed habits, whether they were rape or religion, they didn't die out easily. The chemically dependent person would likely be where you expected him to be. He had no choice, really. His behavior too, you could expect to take on certain predictable characteristics. Which gave Morton an edge, didn't it?

Back to L.A.? Christ, with thinking like this maybe he needed the asylum after all. Maybe they were all lost in their broken truths. Disenfranchised, like poor refried Harvey Mueller, like big wheel Sigmund Freud himself. Like all those who chased their sanity in a secret, wrong-headed garden—in another human being, for instance.

'L.A. 2000:' Sex Asylum

He was thinking of a person so isolated they couldn't bear to share themself even with themself. Joseph? Yes, this would be Joseph. But despite himself Morton kept thinking of Annise Chastain, the most perfected of L.A. blondes, yet one of the most hurt. Ah, your boll weevil of co-dependence chewing the soul out of the biggest box of rain in her attic.

But to look at it straight on, pursued the counselor as he drove, there was only one way you could find your heart in someone else—which was to die and have the bugger transplanted into them.

Veer right and bolt north to Oregon? Take a sharp left and slip south across the border into Mexico? Be realistic, Allison. Mexico was too damn hot. Too dusty and reeking of tequila and the underarms of people you didn't know. Was life really a slow-motion getaway toward death? Wait, boy. This was your old thinking. Open your eyes for once and see the sun through somebody else's window.

He glanced over at Muriel. She wasn't expressing herself. Just riding along, gazing at the scenery. All at once he realized the enormity of the change taking place inside him. He could feel what she felt, he was certain. A bit bold perhaps, this thought, and yet he was more positive of it than of anything that had ever happened to him.

But what, exactly, was she feeling? Prove your insight, if you had one. Then and there he met himself, for he was both leaving and arriving at the same instant. Yes, he recognized what she was experiencing. It was love, the most massive of all concepts, *and* the most contemporary.

Joseph had always sneered when this topic came up. "A riot in reverse, that's what love is," he'd say. "Why you think you gotta pull it back out the minute you stick it in?" The Gestapo and his porno philosophies. He was a man gone criminally insane.

"Golly, Muriel," said Morton aloud. "We're coming up on Hollywood Boulevard already."

Night had fallen, and sure enough there were the bosomy ladies of the street, dressed to the hilt. Perhaps Joseph was right. In terms of love, there wasn't a shop on the Strip didn't carry the stuff. Only—well, they all happened to be out of their decent stock right now. It'd be coming in soon though, along with those new vinyl whips and the designer bottles of *Paca Roma* cologne the customers were in such need of.

Morton soared back down to the here and now. At last he hit on it. It wasn't what he'd become, it was what he'd gotten rid of. Suddenly he realized he wasn't lonely anymore! Not lonely? God, what a long, strange trip it had been.

At the stoplight by Filthy McNasty's he spontaneously said, "Wanna get married, Muriel?"

She jerked her head toward him. Light from the streetlamps refracted into the side window, dappling her face with a sharp new reference to the artificial.

"You're your own Guardian right now. Maybe we better take advantage of it before something new happens," added Morton.

"Get married?"

"Yeah. Tomorrow say. Or maybe the next day at the Courthouse. What do you think?"

She bit her lip. "OK," she said.

He reached over to take her hand, but she was already reaching for his, and their fingers waved miscellaneously around at mid seat. Then they entwined like braided hair on a magnificent blonde, silky and warm. Muriel squiggled over and sat so close the other drivers cut their eyes in censure.

Muriel said, "I just thought of something. If I was married, I wouldn't have to go back to Dar/Neese. Or Roselawn either. Would I?"

Morton lifted his eyebrows. "I guess not," he said. "Joseph's lawyers would probably fight for an annulment though."

"What's annulment?"

"It gets canceled. Like it never happened. You get married, but they reverse it and you're not married anymore."

"I'm sure learning a lot about life in this world," said Muriel.

"Screwy as hell, isn't it?"

"So even if I was married Joseph would still have the videotape and everything would be the same."

"It's worth a try," said Morton. "I want you to be my wife, Muriel."

"And we shall be together as two," she said quoting her self-invented spiritual program.

"Uh, as one, I think it says."

"But we can never be one, can we?"

Morton itched his beard. "Right," he said.

Already she was playing the acquiescent spouse, for not once had she mentioned their destination. Odd, he thought, how moments like this never needed explaining. It was something you knew—that you both knew.

Muriel held very still. Her ears had gone red. He could feel a trembling in her knees.

"Do you remember what I promised you in the courtyard?" he asked.

"What?"

"You know you remember," he chided in his old counseling tone.

"It was happiness," she said meekly.

"I've taken a hundred steps to get you free. And to get myself free. Now we can finally have it. I'll take you—I'll take you to Panama. Or Costa Rica or someplace when this is all over."

Morton breathed deep.

"I got scared before," he admitted. "And fear, Muriel—when it gets you in here—" He touched his crotch the way Annise had shown him. "Well, then you're really done for."

"That's true," she said amazed.

"I love you, Muriel. At first I didn't recognize it for what it was."

"I love you too, Morton. I've loved you since 1930—Ummm, since 1960, was it?" She looked confusedly at him. She'd never been good with numbers. "Well, for a long time," she said.

"Maybe we should run away together," he said seriously.

Muriel squeezed his hand shakily. He could feel her tightening bit by bit, like in the old days.

A minute passed. Two minutes, as he waited for her to curl into the rigid fetal position he'd spent two years trying to unravel her from, when out of nowhere came this horrific, animal-like groan. An incredible gasp it was from someplace deep within her heart. Morton reached to hold her as everything—eyes, hands, all of it—fell lax and drooped in exhaustion. It was like someone who'd faced the holocaust coming out of a hypnotism with a new, liberating knowledge of their past.

Becoming very measured, she rotated her head toward him. Lucid? Loving? Crazy? Liberated from the surrogate chains of the dazzling blonde, Morton wondered? From little Toni? From Joseph Schopen, brutal Mephistopheles of the Fraction House?

Impossible, of course, to know these things. With anyone really. With yourself even, he thought, as he blinked and looked ahead to the cars which had now switched on their headlights. He heard her mumble something.

"What?" he asked.

She leaned and placed her head softly on his chest. "I said, I want to run away with you."

It seemed an hallucination almost as she huddled into the blanket of his body. He had his arm around her. He could tell she was back to herself. It wasn't like in the old days when it sometimes took weeks for her to recover. Here, now, she'd done it in a matter of moments. Which was, he realized, like a normal person. She lifted up and began to adjust herself there beside him. Rubbing her eyes. Stroking down her hair.

She looked up at him. For a quick second her brow furrowed.

"We could go to Oregon," she said. "They sent me nice brochures. It gets cold there though. Do you think—" She hesitated. "Do you think you would mind that?"

* * *

Chapter 86

The truck chugged farther down the Strip. Soon they approached the small urine-puddled parking lot in front of The Green Room. As Morton expected, Joseph's flashy Jaguar sat cockeyed in one of the spaces. Close beside it was an over-chromed Harley-Davidson Sportster. This was Rooney's motorcycle. A perk from high-end sales of the famous Peruvian marching powder. He'd be hanging out inside with his main buyer.

Morton parked and killed the engine. A second later however, he fired her back up.

"What are you doing?" said Muriel.

"I've got to get hold of Vera, or Trina, so you can be safe while I take care of this. I'll drop you off."

"Drop me off? No way. We're going in there together."

"Not we, Muriel. Me."

"But you'll be shot, Morton. Or strangled. He's a strangler, you know. Something terrible will happen. It's how you men are."

"Us men? You heard Wanda say that, didn't you?"

Muriel frumped her lips. She reached over and switched off the ignition.

"I don't care who said it. I'm not leaving your side. I'm your right hand chick now, Morton. I'm standing by my man no matter what."

A warmth welled in him as big as the state of Florida. She really would be his wife one day, the one beside him in all his future fiascoes—er, endeavors, rather. For better or for worse, that was the vow.

He squinted over at her. She was going in with him. The whole of the Salvation Army couldn't have kept her out.

The counselor reached behind the seat for his bright purple blazer, which might be necessary in a crisis for purposes of distraction.

Together they exited the truck and headed for the propped open doors of the Green Room.

~~~

Morton and Muriel crossed the short stretch of pavement to the entrance. There was no cover charge. The place wasn't that high class.

Inside, they paused to get their bearings. Tobacco smoke and old perfume drifted in the air.

In the low light the counselor began to shoulder his way toward the bar. He'd never known The Green Room to draw a crowd, but this evening there was standing room only.

"It's Sunday night," said Muriel over the pounding drone of the music. "They're having a last fling before Monday, I guess."

On the stage, gyrating like ribbons of flesh before the life-size mock up of the vanity, were the girls. One was naked. Another was rhythmically peeling out of her skimpy cowgirl outfit. Morton's mouth hung open.

"What are you feeling?" asked Muriel wedging in beside him as they found a spot at the bar.

"Amazed," he said.

"Aroused, you mean?" asked Muriel.

The counselor gripped his chin and attempted to crack his neck. It didn't work.

"It's OK, Morton. Dirty girls should arouse you. I'm going to learn how to be like them."

"You are?"

"Sure. How can I please you if I don't have my priorities straight?"

"So you like being dirty? Even after that horrible video?"

"Dirty is different from ugly, like with Joseph. I want to be as dirty as I can. As long as I'm honest with you about it."

Morton was elated. What a future to look forward to! He thought of the novelty stores along the Strip... of buying her a sexy gift... And when they were at last safe down in Guatemala...

"When Joseph first brought me here he told me this was mainstreaming," Muriel said. "I didn't know any better. It was the first time I'd been out. It's not mainstreaming though, is it, Morton?"

The counselor shook his head. "No, Muriel, it's not mainstreaming."

~~~

At first Morton didn't spot the Gestapo. With Rooney's bike outside they'd likely be huddled in the back room, divvying up the cut.

Roxanne was behind the bar, pouring drinks fast and furious. Morton pawed at the cigarette smoke and tried to see through the murky lighting. He noticed a motorcycle helmet on the bar top. Rooney was on the right of it. Joseph, he saw, was on the left. And, God forbid, Annise Chastain was pressed between like a feather pillow, parts bulging out the opposite way when one of them slopped against her.

The three were dead center before the stage, ogling the dancers. It didn't take a genius to see the two men were high as kites, whistling and cat-calling the way they were. Maybe Annise was loaded too, it was hard to tell. He knew she could play vixen or angel at the drop of a hat.

With Muriel beside him, the texture of even the most familliar places changed. For once there was nothing wishy washy in Morton's perspective. Nothing romanticised or exotic. The pictures on the walls, the people milling around—they were all merely what they were. Reality without your myopic baggage was a hell of a thing.

The set of songs on the jukebox came to an end. The girls bustled offstage and trotted over to Rooney and Joseph, not bothering to don the blue satin gowns on the rack.

How was it, wondered the counselor, that macho addicts generated such charm with these so called exotic dancers? The deadened eyes of the drug trade, there was the answer. Anybody on Hollywood Boulevard would tell you so.

As Morton glared across the bar one of the Gestapo's knifing phrases came to mind. "You're dead meat, Allison. And after today your girls are *my* meat."

Unfortunately, this prediction had come true. The videotape had been the final straw.

Roxanne appeared. "Can I get you two a drink?" she asked Morton over the music.

He started to answer, but she recognized him despite his beard, and jerked her head nervously toward Joseph.

"I know. I saw him up there," acknowledged the counselor.

Roxanne nodded to Muriel. "Hi, honey," she said.

"Hi," said Muriel.

"I'm sorry I couldn't help you that day. I—"

"It's all right," said Muriel.

"You two have to get out of here right away," said Roxanne. "They're on Dexedrine and coke both. And who knows how many Snakebites they've downed."

Dexedrine *and* coke? Why these people didn't drop bug-eyed dead of heart attacks had always mystified the counselor.

"We've come for Annise," said Morton. "We're taking her out with us. She's got surgery tomorrow. She'll be needing her rest."

"Surgery? The abortion, you mean?" said Roxanne.

"No. She's not going through with any abortion."

Roxanne said, "Somebody's going through with it. Joseph's been talking all night about the D and C she's having tomorrow morning. I never heard her say any different."

Morton looked to Muriel. "That's why he kidnapped her," he said. "To make sure she has the abortion."

Muriel's jaw stood rock solid with resolve. "We can't let him get away with this," she said. "He killed Harvey, Morton. He killed Sassafras. He even tried to kill you on the steps. And now he's going to kill little Toni before she's even born."

"That appears to be the case," agreed Morton.

"Do you have a gun?" she asked.

"Of course not. You know I don't carry a gun."

"Joseph might have a gun," said Muriel. "Well, he might, Morton. We need equilibrium. You're always saying so. A person has to have a gun to equal a gun." Then she said, "Annise has one. Let's go get hers."

Morton quickly considered it. He thought of Sassafras, dead. And there was the time factor.

Muriel turned to Roxanne. "Have you got a gun?" she naïvely asked the barmaid.

Joseph's gruff voice boomed out. "Roxanne! Get your ass down here. Now!"

The Gestapo bored in on Morton and Muriel across the distance. The background noise condensed eerily as a slow hush began to infect the patrons between them. Joseph's eyes lit up in a perverse, bursting at the gills way. Vibes. When they were this hairy anybody could read them.

Morton narrowed his gaze in return. Roxanne eased away.

"Before we get too deep into this, Muriel," said the counselor, "I want to know why you kept it from me about you and Annise in bed. I see why you didn't say anything about Joseph, but if I'd known about Annise it might have saved a lot of needless hell."

"I wanted to protect you," she said.

"Protect me? From what?"

"From if you fell in love with Annise. I didn't want that ugly sex game to bust up your feelings for her."

"You were trying to protect my feelings for Annise?"

Muriel nodded. "I didn't know whether you were falling for her. You might have been. Plus, it's bad to say rumors about people."

"Rumors! It's not a rumor if it really happened."

'L.A. 2000:' Sex Asylum

What revelations! And what dedication this woman had, to let his love go where it would most naturally, while all along she'd been seeking it for herself.

No, love was not a riot in reverse, Joseph Schopen.

Rooney and the Gestapo looked like a couple of linebackers embedded in a huddle of unbelievably pink skin.

Another set of songs began. A new bevy of dancers shimmied up to the stage. Making a flash about-face, Joseph turned and stomped into the back room.

~~~

After a minute Annise said something to Rooney, then began to work through the crowd toward Morton. She was obviously frightened. Eyes flitting. Trying to camoflage herself amongst the revelers.

Another day the counselor might have met her half way. No longer.

He remained nonplused as she approached. But when he lifted his chin to face her his eyes popped in disbelief. She was in one of the lick your chops erotic stage gowns. And nothing else! It halted at her pubic hair where a two inch boundary of cowgirl fringe took over. The thing was without buttons, and hung wide open in front. She made no effort to conceal herself. It was a déjà vu of the early locking box times when he'd been so staggered by her measurements. Morton and Muriel looked hard at her.

"I know you think I'm a slut," she said right off. "Joseph's been making me dance all night. He won't even let me tie this sash. If I do—" She clammed up. "If I have to dance one more time, I swear I'll hire somebody to blow my brains out."

Morton said, "I thought you were going to your parents' place in Pasadena."

"I guess I lied. I do that sometimes. I'm sorry, Morton. I felt safe enough. I didn't really believe Joseph would..." She trailed off.

"It's all right, Annise. I'm here now. You won't have to dance anymore."

She looked at him like he was stone cold crazy. She said, "I haven't been home since yesterday morning. Did you try to call?"

"Yes," said the counselor.

"Joseph's lost it, Morton. He forced me to leave the Fraction House with him the other day. Then he went to my place and did God knows what inside. He made me wait in the car. I heard crashing sounds. Anyway, Sassafras hasn't been fed for two days. I really need to get back to the apartment."

"Then go back," said Morton.

"It's not so easy."

She pushed up her sleeve. Deep bruises were clustered over her biceps and shoulders.

"Joseph sent me to show you this," she said.

Annise glanced toward Rooney, who was still at the bar, and the group of partiers around him. Morton came to his feet. She lifted her leg and laid it cantilevered across the stool. The Catholic was exposed to the barroom in a way she'd never offered him in her bed.

"Look at this," said Annise.

She pointed to slash marks cross-hatched on her inner thigh. Apparently from a razor blade, or razor knife perhaps. Morton's head began to throb. The combination of the vulgar and the stimulating twisted his thoughts like a pit of recently severed snake heads.

"He told me if I don't agree to the abortion he's going to finish the job later tonight," she said.

"What job?"

"The butcher job. I can't abort our Toni. He's going to get a coat hanger and untwist it except for the hook and tear the baby out of me. He will, too. I know he will. I do everything he says, Morton. Why does he treat me this way?"

Roxanne appeared. She leaned over the bar and examined Annise's wounds. Morton could see the sadness in her eyes, and he thought of how much of her life had been wasted around this sort of thing. Was Annise too, about to squander away her youth?

"I don't know what I could do. I'll try to help if you want," whispered the barmaid.

Morton said, "You've got surgery tomorrow, Annise. I'm driving you, remember?"

"Surgery?" she squeaked.

The blonde was dumbfounded. She held out her arms. "This is ludicrous," she said. "Can't you see I'm a prisoner? Don't you understand what's happening here? Why the hell do you think I'm dressed like this? Before you came Joseph made me dance in front of all these people. Do you think I want to go around with this robe hanging open? I'm not going to any stupid surgery. I'll be lucky to get out of here alive." A second passed. "And so will you," she added icily.

"I'll explain it to the Gestapo," clarified Morton. "I mean, to Mad Dog. I intend to lay it out in a way he'll understand."

Morton turned from her. "Bring me a draft, Roxanne," he said. "And bring Muriel one too."

He checked his wallet. There was a single twenty, but that was all. He checked the secret compartments. Nothing.

"Relax," he said to the blonde. "You're free to say a prayer if you want, but I doubt it'll do much good in a place like this."

"I doubt it too," she muttered beginning to move away.

~~~

Joseph's whiskey-sharded voice chimed in close behind them.

"Why you little heathen! Haven't got the guts even to pray, have you?" chastised the Gestapo. Morton heard the telltale lisp. Such a peculiar anomaly for a brutish womanizer.

Joseph slapped Annise's naked butt. Not playfully, but hard, like someone doling out a punishment. At the sound of the crack a number of patrons whipped their heads excitedly.

"They're on me," declared the Gestapo when the beers arrived. "And bring us all a round of Snakebites for old time's sake, Roxanne. Pour one for yourself too."

Joseph pulled out a cigarette. He was carrying a large manila envelope under his arm. He squeezed it awkwardly while he fumbled with a tattered, double-wide match pack and began a bizarre ritual of ripping off matches, missing the strike, and tossing them onto the bar beside the glasses of beer and the small tumblers of Snakebites.

Rooney idled up. Physically, he was a small person, and with a smart-alecky contrivance, like a man who might be carrying a weapon, he placed his motorcycle helmet on the counter using both hands.

Joseph was guiding Annise—manhandling might have been a better word—to make her to belly up to the bar for her drink. He seemed to have mentally lynched her. She wore high heels, like the other dancers, and she twisted her ankle as the Gestapo shoved her against the rail. She made the tiniest of squeals at the pain. Obediently she hunched over her Snakebite.

Positioned as she was, Morton could make out the red hand print glowing on her behind.

Pain. Tears. They could be hot, she'd said. They could be perfectly bad, in a fiery do-or-die way which offered a twisted, screwball pleasure. But this of course wasn't true. Bad was bad, no matter how you cut it. She sure wasn't grinning now.

"Unbelievable, the evil in that man," Morton said to Muriel. And he didn't particularly care if he was overheard.

* * *

Chapter 87

At last the Gestapo had his sleek black cigarette going. He puffed it like a steam engine, put his lips on Annise's ear and exhaled the thick white smoke along the side of her face.

"Drink up," Morton saw him mouth out.

The counselor shook his head at Muriel in disgust. She, however, was stretching a glance to Joseph implying something like admiration. Was she actually winking at the guy? Couldn't be.

Muriel picked up her Snakebite, slid off the stool and maneuvered between Joseph and Rooney. The Gestapo shoved his pile of bent matches off to the side. He turned his attentions to Muriel.

"I got your message on my answering machine, babe," he said going soft. "You don't know how happy it makes me, you wanting to come back to us and all."

"Message? You left Joseph a message?" said Morton to Muriel.

The Gestapo slung his arm around her shoulder. She put her lips to his ear and whispered something. Joseph's eyebrows rose. A black gleam of sexual appetite flashed behind his pupils. He was nodding 'yes,' and Muriel wasn't objecting.

Morton's mouth went cold and cottony, like dry ice.

Muriel downed her drink in one giant swig and snapped the glass onto the bar. Very strange.

"God, that's good," she breathed. "Buy me another one, Joseph?"

"Roxanne! Another round of Snakebites!" called the Gestapo, thrilled.

Morton moved up behind Muriel. "What the hell's the matter with you?" he whispered.

"Stay out of this, Allison," intervened Joseph. "I've got her all warmed up to sign these papers. I'm on a roll, or couldn't you tell?"

Buck Buchanan

"A roll straight to hell," said the counselor.

Joseph opened the envelope. He spread copies of the forms from Marshmont, Peterson & Liam, the corrupt videotape attorneys, across the bar top.

Muriel swayed, picked up one of the nearby mugs of beer and drank half of it. Even Annise appeared surprised at Muriel's gusto for the party.

"You should have heard her cutting loose on my answering machine, Allison. It was quite a sexy earful. Your girl here made *very* flattering remarks about the new Director." Joseph puffed his chest.

"You haven't heard?" he continued. "She's coming back to me. To Dar/Neese, I mean. When is it you said we'd getting in the tub again?" he asked Muriel. "Monday, isn't it? Goddamn, that's tomorrow! My how time flies!"

"In the tub! What are you talking about?" cried Morton. "What's he talking about, Muriel?"

Rooney uncapped his pen and handed it to Joseph. Joseph made a manipulative mini bow and passed it to Muriel.

"Sign on the dotted line, sweetheart, and it's all sewed up," said the Gestapo.

Morton snatched the pen. "She's not signing anything," he said.

"Correct me if I'm wrong, Allison. But thanks to your Teenage Pregnancy Campaign she's now her own Guardian. She's free to sign whatever she wants," returned Joseph. "Now give her back the pen."

Morton found himself lost. And when he got lost he invariably reverted to what Harvey had taught him. 'When torn with doubt, do nothing,' suggested the Freudian. 'Close your mouth. Even close your heart, if need be. Step back. Reassess. Then, if you've got the guts, release the hammer thong on your six-shooter and prepare to draw.'

Poor Harvey. By the time he'd mustered the guts it was too late.

Morton and Muriel met eyes, but he was unable to gain a clear meaning. He handed her back the pen.

Roxanne brought the Snakebites. In passing one to Morton she leaned close and whispered, "Joseph's way out of himself. By this time of night he's capable of anything. I know him. All hell's about to break loose."

Muriel gulped down the rest of the beer. Morton was astonished as she set her hand to the paper. But suddenly she wobbled. Her eyes rolled upward in their sockets. She grabbed the Gestapo, not Morton, for support.

"Jesus fucking Christ, she's drunk!" exclaimed Joseph, steadying her. "How long you been feeding her alcohol today, Allison?"

"I want to sign. I want to get in the tub, Joey," slurred Muriel, her hand making loose circles in the air.

Her knees began to buckle. The Gestapo jerked her upright. He forced her fingers onto the document. Morton and Annise looked on in disbelief.

"You're coercing her, Schopen!" exclaimed the counselor. "There's plenty of witnesses here. If she signs all blown out from Snakebites that form won't mean a thing."

For an instant Morton picked out a curious lucidity in Muriel's eye. A magical heart beam running between them, like fire on the edge of a glacier. Trust?

She said to Joseph, "I want it legal. I don't want nothing unlegal about it."

Joseph's temples were a map of tortuous, pressure-packed veins. "Sign it, bitch," he hissed.

"But if I do, it might be annulled. Couldn't annulled happen? We'd never get to—" She halted and smiled lewdly at the Gestapo.

"Annulled? Where'd you learn that?" queried Joseph.

"Morton taught me. He said if somebody tried to kidnap a person to Venezuela and marry me up he could have it annulled. He said it'd be like it never happened. We don't want a backfire on Dar/Neese. I mean, on an important thing like my signature. Do we, Joseph?"

The Gestapo tore the pen from Muriel's hand, wheeled and flung it violently across the bar. Aimed or not, it struck Roxanne hard in the back of the neck, drawing a crooked twig of blood.

Morton's fists clenched. He lurched toward Joseph, but somehow Muriel aligned herself between them and deflected him sidelong into the crowd.

Pushing. Shoving. Slapping women around. It was all par for The Green Room course.

Frantically Joseph fetched another match pack from his pocket and started slashing the weak cardboard matches across the strike zone.

"Roxanne!" he called.

She moped over. She was holding a damp rag against her neck.

"Roxanne, baby. I'm sorry. I really am," moaned the Mad Dog.

"You've had a lot to drink. Go on home, Joseph. It'd be the best thing for everybody," she said.

Muriel leaned to Morton. "I think we better get out of here," she whispered.

"I said I'm sorry for Christsake," persisted the Gestapo. "Can't we make up? Here, have a cigarette."

Roxanne was wary. Joseph looped his middle finger into her leotard top and dragged her to him. He stuffed one of his cigarettes in her mouth. Ominously, he said, "Now hold still while I light it."

The Gestapo ripped off one of the matches, but instead of lighting Roxanne's cigarette, he pushed up her lip, and in the deformity where her teeth grew outward from high in her gums he jammed the match.

"Don't move," he warned.

With your deviant's theatrical sense of calculation he stripped off another match and wedged it between the next protruding tooth. He lifted the other side of her lip and twisted in two more matches.

The Gestapo pointed and began to count. "Two! Three! Four! Four match sticks! What talents you have."

He quickly downed a Snakebite. "Hold still, Roxanne. Rooney, where's my camera when I need it? I should have a picture of this."

The counselor couldn't take it any longer. Inside him a rage the size of Harvey Mueller himself had taken shape. His stomach did not lift into his throat. He was not bristling with venom as he'd expected. Instead he was as clear as a carving knife of severed glass. Muriel, however, was attuned to his fast burning fuse.

"Don't look at them, Morton," she said, drawing him aside.

Out of nowhere really, Muriel kissed the counselor. A long, deep kiss right there at the bar. Had Joseph seen them? Morton could feel the veracity of her passion. The disturbance with Roxanne kept intruding from beyond, but for a few hang-fire moments he was able to block the upcoming onslaught of trauma.

"I think I'm going crazy," muttered Morton. "Is a person crazy if they feel like killing a man?"

"Probably," returned Muriel. "I'm crazy, and I felt like killing him every day for the last two years."

Morton said, "So why were you sucking up to him over there? And what was all that about your phone message?"

"Please don't be mad, Morton. I wasn't really kissing up to Joseph," said Muriel.

She was sober as a judge. Remarkable.

"I was trying to take the heat off Annise by putting it on me instead. You understand, don't you? And about the phone message, I want you to know—"

Joseph bellowed, "You're not laughing, Annise. Don't you think Roxanne looks funny?"

Annise jerked her head away.

"You're not drinking either. In this part of town holding back on the juice is an insult."

He pushed her Snakebite closer.

Annise stared straight ahead, like a zombie. For once she did not bat her eyelashes.

"I can't drink that, Joseph," she said.

The Gestapo laughed. "Because of the baby? You're protecting her health?"

Annise lowered her head.

"Little Toni is long gone history," he said. "Drink up. It'll help do her in. Chase it with this," he added handing her a full mug of beer.

Joseph wrapped his forearm around Annise's head, lifted the shot glass and began dumping the mixture of schnapps and whiskey between her quivering lips. With the maniac's spur of the moment change of mind, he suddenly tried to drive the dud matches between Annise's pearl white teeth.

He pushed Roxanne away to concentrate on his newest victim. Just his style. Annise went rigid with fear. Her teeth however were too well formed for the trick, so the Gestapo squeezed her lips together with his thumb and forefinger, stuffing in the matches until her face looked like the grill of an antique car.

"Now give us a kiss, you dirty cunt," he said.

Joseph laid his mouth over Annise's, wilted match sticks and all. It was such a savage display even the biker drug dealer seemed surprised.

Morton moved to intervene, but Muriel pulled him back by his shirttail. In the split second he glanced away there came a sickening cracking sound, which meant human injury.

Annise was holding the side of her head. Her glass, swan-shaped earring had been smashed to powder. Pieces of it lay scattered in the folds of her satin robe. There were tiny oozing cuts along her neck. She reached for a napkin. Many people had seen what happened, yet there was no change in the music or dancers' mannerisms.

'L.A. 2000:' Sex Asylum

The Gestapo's hand had taken a nick. He stared insanely at the little wedge of blood. Morton had held himself back as long as he could.

"Let me go," barked the counselor yanking free of Muriel's grasp.

"All right. But first put this under your arm," she whispered. "Joseph won't know what it is. It might be enough to scare him."

Secretly she undid a button of his shirt and wedged her empty beer mug under his arm.

"Look here what you did to me, woman," whined the Gestapo squeezing the pinpricks of blood off his fingers. "I ain't through with you yet. I ain't through by a long shot."

Using the backs of both hands, like a swimmer, Morton pried Joseph and the blonde apart. Muriel cringed. Confronting the Gestapo on his home turf simply wasn't done.

Annise was stiff with fright. A few of the match sticks remained in her mouth. One by one the counselor began removing and dropping them conspicuously onto the floor. He made a point of looking beyond Joseph to meet Rooney's eyes, showing them both he meant business. Rooney, the candy man, as drug dealers on the Strip were called, seemed nervous and kind of stupefied. He worked his beer mug back and forth in front of his motorcycle helmet.

All became quiet. Eyes lined the bar. More looked on from the tables.

"He... He didn't mean anything by it," stammered Annise.

The Gestapo stared violently at Morton.

"Of course he meant something. He meant to call you ugly names. He meant to degrade you," said the counselor.

Annise shied away.

"I heard the whole thing. I was sitting right there," continued Morton. "He called you a dirty cunt, didn't he?"

She was frozen.

"You don't have to stand still for his abuse. No one should ever stand for that kind of crap."

He looked at the Mad Dog. Morton lifted Joseph's empty beer mug and handed it to Annise. She cradled it with both hands, confused.

"That man hit you. If you want to even things up smash him in the face with this beer mug," he said.

Annise was shaking badly. Blood trickled down the side of her long, flawless neck.

"You don't have to be afraid," said the counselor. "Just take the mug and smash that bastard in the face with it. I can personally guarantee your safety."

Joseph eyed him up and down, street-fighter style. He started to grin, but the smile was cold lard and failed to materialize. One of his black cigarettes smoldered in the nearby ash try. Morton picked it up.

"The best thing would be to take a few puffs off this cigarette, which I know is his," he said. "Then shatter that mug across the bastard's face. As I say, Annise, you have nothing to be afraid of. I'm guaranteeing your protection in whatever you choose to do. But if it were me, I would never allow anyone to get away with that."

Morton held the burning cigarette at his side. Long moments passed. Their eyes shot from person to person. Annise stretched out her arm and carefully placed the mug back on the bar top.

"Come on, Joseph. Let's get out of here," said Rooney reaching for his helmet. He drained his glass. Rooney—the candy man who could never be too cautious, lest the authorities be waved in. He nudged Joseph's shoulder and turned to leave.

The Gestapo hesitated. Then, without a word, he about-faced and took steps toward the door.

Rooney found his way outside. Recall the Bonnie and Clyde flash point change of focus, the counselor warned himself. Sure enough, the Gestapo pivoted with a quick, tight rotation. A bluff charge?

Annise had come to her feet, teetering though, what with the spike high heels. At Joseph's advance she recoiled into one of the stools, tripped and tumbled to the filthy, cigarette butt covered floor, her hair splayed out like a platinum halo. As in the battle in Annise's bedroom Morton had another fear of a possible miscarriage.

The counselor cemented his ground. The Gestapo's jaw worked as if he were chewing worms. His shoulders began to square off. The air liquefied with adrenaline. Joseph was about to attack, it was clear, when his experienced criminal eye alighted on the bulge inside Morton's shirt.

The counselor took a moment to look around at Muriel. He was still holding Joseph's black cigarette. He set it in the ash tray and laid his hand gingerly down on the bar top, like a gunslinger.

They could hear the Jaguar starting up outside. The horn sounded. Joseph whipped his head at the noise.

Muriel was helping the blonde off the floor.

"Annise is coming with me," said Morton looking directly at Joseph. "Roxanne," he called. "If there are any more problems with this fellow, I want you to phone me right away. Night or day, it doesn't matter. Do you understand?"

No answer. Everything cold and vicious.

Joseph inched closer, blinking his eyelids, grinding his jaw.

Morton set one leg slightly in front of the other.

"I'm going to give you my address too, Roxanne. In case there's something you might want to say to me in person. It's 330 Somerset Drive, #5," he began. He looked over at her. "You're not writing."

Muriel got a pen from her purse and passed it to the barmaid.

"Do you hear?" he repeated without breaking eye contact with the Gestapo.

"I hear," said Roxanne.

The Jaguar horn began to blow again.

"You're a killer, Joseph," said Morton. "You've killed twice. It's not going to happen again." The Gestapo scrutinized the bulge under Morton's arm.

"You'd better wake up, Allison. I might kill a third time," returned Joseph. He reached slowly behind his back.

The counselor's shirt was unbuttoned two down from the neck. He eased his hand to his chest and let it rest there, like he'd seen in those pictures of Napoleon.

"So you finally admit it," said Morton. "A man like Harvey doesn't go down easy. I figured sooner or later you'd have to brag about it."

Joseph turned toward the enormous vanity behind the bar and nodded to one of the dancers, apparently the second in charge after Roxanne. Morton recognized her as the one in the tiger-striped miniskirt from time he'd happened into The Green Room on his mental health day. At any rate, she and Joseph had some sort of connection, for a sudden blast of music obliterated the brittle air of the standoff. As if on cue, dancers stormed the stage and began to strip down.

The last thing Morton saw conclusively was the Gestapo's thumbs down signal to the stage girl. The lights dimmed to near blackness.

Joseph's hand lanced out from behind his back. Through the shadows came a macabre glint of steel. A knife?

The counselor had only a micro-second to render judgment. Joseph was lunging at him! Or was it the unruly crowd making for the turmoil? The Gestapo's hand seemed at Morton's temple. A death click trembled in his ear.

In a motion which felt practiced for months, Morton drew the empty beer mug from his shirt and slashed it through the darkened air. A crunching sound of glass meeting bone as the heavy mug shattered across the side of Joseph's head.

The Gestapo went down, bleeding out quickly from above the eye. Other lacerations, deep ones, checkered the side of his face. Morton called for assistance, but the lights remained low. Had no one noticed? Had the counselor attacked without cause? He looked frantically around, but saw no knife.

Rooney was there, hooking the Gestapo under the arms and dragging him toward the door. Worried, Morton pressed behind them through the crowd. Near the entrance Joseph's appendages began to move. He hadn't been killed, thank God!

The Gestapo was quickly returning to himself. He found a handkerchief and pressed it to his wounds. He looked demonically around the place, as if he'd lost something dear to him. He was going to live. Yes, the Gestapo was going to live after all.

A moment later they disappeared through the double doors.

* * *

Chapter 88

Morton returned for the girls.

Gradually the room came back into focus, the rough wooden posts, the old-timey pictures on the walls.

Roxanne brought a glass of water for him. As he went to drink he heard the ice rattling. His arm had begun to shake.

Muriel snatched him by the shirtfront. "Look," she said. She lifted her foot. Under it was Annise's pearl-handled derringer. "Joseph dropped this when you hit him."

"I guess he was really going to shoot," said Morton.

Annise was observing them. "It's my gun," she said. "I want it back."

"What for?" said Morton.

"You know what for. In case I have to— Shit, forget it."

She reached for it. Morton held her away, for this was the very weapon she claimed she'd kill herself with if she ever got pregnant. No, if she ever got *raped*—that was the word she used. Which, depending on the moment to moment whimsy of her interpretation, could have been what Joseph had done.

Morton scooped the weapon from the edges of the shadows and slipped it into his pocket.

Roxanne came and thrust a plastic bag into Annise's arms. "Here are your things, honey. Now you all go. Run as fast as you can."

Morton took each girl by the hand and started a push and pull drive toward the exit. The threesome made it to the doorway, but thinking better of it, Morton tugged them toward the enormous mirrored window looking out to the parking lot.

Rooney's bike was on the sidewalk, not ten feet away through the glass. The window was tinted, but Morton could easily see Joseph attempting to kick start the Harley under the streetlamp. Blood was draining eerily down his face. How come everything seemed so topsy-turvy with your evil doers?

Always swapping vehicles, switching sexuality from bi to straight to— Well, best not think of this right now.

The motorcycle roared to life. Joseph wasn't astride it yet. Odd? No, probably too loaded, mulled the counselor. And now he was unscrewing the cap on the gas tank, dipping in the bloody handkerchief and letting it dangle over the edge of the tank. The Gestapo fished for his matches.

Morton grasped the scenario. Joseph was concocting a giant Molatov cocktail! The counselor watched in shock as the Gestapo struck the handkerchief aflame.

The headlight beamed on, blindingly bright. Morton heard a clack, which was the gearbox shifting into first, though Joseph was still to the side of the bike. The cycle revved so loud in another second the engine would have blown. Then the grating sound of the clutch releasing.

The riderless cycle lifted like a rearing stallion and charged toward the plate glass window. Morton dove right and crashed to the floor, dragging the girls down with him. The bulk of the motorcycle followed after them in an enormous firebomb through the window. A blur of burning chrome and a million splintering mirrors as the great slab of glass disintegrated.

Everyone scrambling for safety. People's hands at their faces in terror. The bike on its side spinning erratic ellipses due to the rear wheel remaining engaged. Catching ankles and legs of people and hurling bodies to the floor, where the gasoline ignited with a deep bass *whomp*.

Heat and smoke enveloped the room.

On his hands and knees Morton clawed his way toward the double doors, desperately encircling Annise and Muriel with his flailing arms. Raw gasoline had spilled across the old unvarnished flooring. He could feel where it dampened the cuffs of his pants. Like a hundred mini Satans darting to life from the sprayed-out fuel flames began to dance wildly through the alleyways between the tables. The motorcycle was crashing from table to table and gyrating around, the back tire billowing a black acrid smoke into the flames.

People were hurt and screaming.

Morton went woozy. A strange crop of fire, like windblown wheat, was brewing hauntingly alongside him on the floor. He tried his best to crawl through the flames. At any moment the place might ignite in a big way.

He felt a hand on the back of his shirt weakly pulling him to his feet. It was Muriel. Her other hand was in Annise's cape of hair. She was attempting to haul them both to safety.

Suddenly the overhead sprinkling system activated. A frying pan sizzle as the water boiled up into steam, and a new mass of heavy gray smoke fogged the barroom.

Morton struggled to his feet. In an awkward, hunched over ball, the three of them staggered to the door.

Outside, a melee of people, hurt to various degrees, were rushing in all directions. Alarms were sounding. Sirens in the distance became louder. Vehicles were screeching away. The Jaguar was long gone.

At last Morton was able to breathe. He hustled the girls to his truck.

Inside The Green Room the sprinklers seemed to be doing their job. A lot of smoke and hysterical patrons continued to pour from the building.

Roxanne emerged. She was rounding up her dancers and trying to help the injured to safety. Morton started to get out of the truck to give her a hand, but she waved him off and came to the window. A deformed pause interrupted the drama, like during an eclipse when all the birds stop chirping.

"You all get out of here," she said. "It's possible Mad Dog might try to frame you for this. He's done that sort of thing before."

Morton hesitated.

"I'll deal with the police," said Roxanne. "This has got to look like an accident. Like somebody fell off the bike and it just came through the window. Otherwise we'll be shut down in a heartbeat."

The barmaid blended back into the crowd.

Annise said, "Wait, Morton. There's my plastic bag. It's got my clothes and the shopping I did for little Toni. Can we get it?"

Dressed in only the charred blue robe, her high heels long lost in the chaos, Annise leapt from the truck and pushed people aside until she was able to snatch the bag from the pavement. Quite a force she could be when she wanted to.

Morton fired up the truck and wheeled hard left.

Muriel shoved open the door, then slid across the seat to make room.

Annise hopped in with the package, and the pickup pealed rubber into the smoke-streaked florescence of Hollywood Boulevard. Soon they were lost among the streetwalkers and the slow automobile traffic of the lonely johns.

* * *

Chapter 89

Morton telephoned Trina Lopez. He told her what happened in The Green Room.

"Is Joseph following you?" she asked nervously.

"No. He's hurt. He'll have to lick his wounds a while."

"Joseph found out I tested Harvey's drugs, Morton. And yours too. I told you he had me fired. He's out for blood." She was terrified.

"We need a safe place, Trina. Vera could probably help, but if Joseph doesn't know where you live—"

"You come here, amigo. All three. Let me tell you the way."

~~~

The freeway ride to Trina's was like a frozen pond with three hot marbles melting their own separate holes through the surface of the ice. It was always evident when two people had made love. Especially the two least expected. An indefinable smell? A secret which was no secret at all, but a loud scream of independence.

Annise's silence told the story. She leaned around Muriel and said, "Christ, Morton, I hardly know what's happening anymore. Why do you pull this shit? We could have all been killed back there."

Jealousy? Grateful exhaustion mixed with the inexhaustible bad girl mentality? Well, never underestimate an L.A. blonde, particularly one scorned in sex, the counselor reminded himself.

~~~

Trina Lopez eyed Annise with great suspicion. The blonde hadn't changed clothes. She still wore the flimsy Green Room robe, and it was well known that the conservative in the RN's heart rebelled at any nudity outside the shower curtain.

Morton noticed bruises on Trina's neck. He leaned her head sideways.

"Joseph came to my other apartment," she explained. "He tried to beat me. He was drunk on something and I got away. I am so frightened, Morton."

"Don't worry, Trina. I'm here now. You'll be safe. I promise."

Protect Trina? Protect Annise Chastain? Protect Muriel? And what about Gordon? For that matter, what about himself? Hell, he'd have to guard the whole City of Angels from the madman. But how? Buy a rifle? Write a letter to the Arbitrators? Give testimony with only paranoids and schizophrenics to back you up?

Although Annise wore the troubling outfit, and certainly could use a cleaning up, Trina, the dedicated nurse took over. She spotted the second degree burns on Muriel's legs and forearms and hustled her into the bathroom. "We'll be a few minutes," she said.

Annise started to put her hands on her hips, then didn't. People said beauty was only skin deep, and in the case of the blonde Morton worried they might be right.

"I know about the videotapes," said the counselor when they were alone. "Joseph sent a copy to Muriel to blackmail her into going back to the Fraction House."

Annise shrugged complacently.

"I was just starting my job, Morton. I thought she was her own Guardian. Joseph told me she was."

"Rape is rape whether she's her own Guardian or not."

Silence.

"I saw the tape, Annise. I know you had sex with her," pressed the counselor.

"Big deal," she returned. "So did you."

They eyed each other harshly.

Annise said, "And anyway, I didn't know she was so stoned."

"Bullshit. It was blatant in the tape."

"I was high as a kite myself. He gave *me* drugs too. Or didn't you notice? I hardly knew we were doing it."

Morton gave one head lowering nod. There was no use going on with this.

"You don't have anything to bitch about," added Annise. "You found your soul mate. It's her, isn't it?" She lifted her nose in the direction of the bathroom.

Annise pulled tight her robe. She paced around the room.

"I've got to get back to my apartment, Morton," she said. "I need my things for tomorrow. All my best makeup's there. And Sassafras will be famished."

This was true. She would need her clothes, the health insurance forms... But Sassafras? Well, maybe Annise had a nurturing instinct after all, thought Morton. He was always being so judgmental. Ease off, why don't you?

"Your apartment will be the first place Joseph goes looking," he said. "Make a list. I'll run by tonight and get your stuff."

Annise stepped into Trina's kitchen for a piece of paper.

"Are you through with me? I have to make a call," she said lifting the wall phone.

"Who to?"

She whipped her head. "To Wanda Novice. Not that it's any of your business."

～～

Trina and Muriel came out of the bathroom. Muriel's arms were wrapped in thick layers of gauze. Surprisingly, she had makeup on, though applied somewhat haphazardly. She must have used Trina's. The blonde wrinkled her nose from the kitchen.

"Love you too, Wanda," said Annise hanging up the phone.

She entered the living room with the list for Morton.

"Wanda's stuck at the Fraction House," Annise informed them. "I guess Joseph had enough sense to make her be in charge over there. Somebody's gotta do it. Anyway, she can't take me to surgery tomorrow."

"I thought I was taking you," said Morton. "I came back from the mountains so I could—"

"You are."

Words. What a lot of mumbo jumbo they amounted to. What, really, did they have to do with communication?

Annise grabbed her plastic bag and went into the bathroom.

"I'll brew us some tea," said Trina heading into the kitchen.

~~~

Muriel came up close to Morton. "I'm glad for what you did tonight. With Joseph, I mean. It's like you were a he-man in one of those muscle magazines. You're so strong. Only I'm worried you'll be hurt."

"Maybe it's better than hurting Joseph," said the counselor. "And anyway, I don't feel very strong."

"Not to yourself. But when I touch you— Whew!" She stroked his biceps. "It's like you're God, only with broad shoulders and blue eyes. It's why I love you so much. You always stand up for what's right."

"I know you weren't drunk in the bar," said Morton. "I saw the Gestapo's eyes light up when you whispered in his ear."

Muriel looked down. "Doesn't a girl have to do a little wrong sometimes to get a little good in return?"

"No. Wrong ain't right, Muriel, no matter how you cut it," said the counselor shaking his head.

"Do you think what I did was wrong?" she asked.

"I'm not sure. What did you do?"

"Well, I had kind of a plan. I thought it up as soon as I knew Joseph killed Harvey."

"A plan?"

"I called Joseph's machine and told him I wanted to come back to the Fraction House."

"You shouldn't have, Muriel."

"Tonight in The Green Room I realized I could still go through with it. I offered him something he could never pass up in a million years."

"What was that?"

"To meet him tomorrow and go in the tub. I told him real sexy too."

"You what!"

"I told him I wanted to take drugs. I told him I wanted to be like Annise and get molested real dirty like. You've been protecting us too long, Morton. Now it's my turn to protect you. I'm going to use my plan and take care of him."

"What plan?"

"I'm going to let him get on me in the tub like he always did. He's got these silver handcuffs, and I'm—"

"Annise's handcuffs?" exclaimed Morton.

"I don't know whose they are. He keeps them in the desk drawer. I'm going to say I want them for something special. He'll like that. So I get out of the tub and throw the lamp in and he'll be killed. I can still do it, Morton."

"A lamp?"

"Lamps kill people on TV."

"*Electrocution* is what kills people. It's too dangerous. You might kill yourself instead."

"I know," agreed Muriel. "The last time they gave me electrocution shocks I nearly died."

"Electric shock *therapy*," corrected the counselor. "You had electric shock therapy."

Muriel frumped her lips.

Well, she'd be needing more mainstreaming, more normalization as far as murder plots went.

"We're not trying to kill the guy, Muriel," countered Morton. "But I like your idea about setting him up. We've got to do something big, or else the sky really will fall in on us."

"Yes. Let's set him up. He's set everybody else up. It's our turn."

"I was thinking," mulled the counselor. "We could rent a camcorder easy enough. You get him to take his clothes off and climb in the tub. Let him put the handcuffs on you. That shows duress and imprisonment. He'll look like the Marquis de Sade. I'll open the door and film him in the act. We'll use his own tricks. We'll get videotape evidence."

"Won't it look setup though?" wondered Muriel.

"What difference does it make? He does what he does. He's a therapist. He's the Dar/Neese Director. People with those titles don't use handcuffs and strip down naked with their patients. Or at least they're not supposed to."

Muriel pursed her lips in thought. "He locks the Therapy Room door, Morton. You won't be able to get inside with the camcorder."

"Yes, I will. His OCD kicks in every six minutes. He has to check the hallway. When he peeks out I'll barge in and tape him naked, with you handcuffed behind him. If we do it right he'll convict himself."

"Do you think it would work?"

"I think so," replied the counselor. "Where would the keys to the handcuffs be? You'll have to unlock yourself while I'm filming so we can make our getaway."

"They'll be on the table by the tub. That's where he always leaves them."

"Can you unlock yourself?"

"Probably."

"Then you'll have to run into Harvey's office and call the police. All right?"

"All right."

"With this kind of proof any court would put the screws to him," said Morton. "And the Arbitrators will too. He'll be run out of L.A. for good."

"I'll do it," said Muriel.

"Wait a minute," said Morton. "What if he catches on to what we're doing? You won't have any way to protect yourself."

"I'll think of something. I can use my shampoo to squirt in his eyes. I've done it before."

"One problem though. We have to get those porno tapes of you and Annise out of Harvey's safe. We have to make sure his office door is open."

"The safe is always locked, Morton."

"We'll have to take the entire thing. It's heavy though. We'll need help," considered the counselor.

"What about Gordon? He's always saying how videotape is so phony. And a videotape full of lies is even phonier. He'd be happy to help, I'm sure of it."

Morton nodded cautiously.

Muriel said, "But isn't it stealing if we take Harvey's safe? The police might come after us. And even if we steal it, how are we going to break it open?"

The counselor pondered a moment. "I believe I know someone. He's a friend of Annise's."

"Friend?" Muriel lifted her nose suspiciously toward the bathroom.

"Lance Stonesipher," said Morton. "Rodney Stonesipher used to be her boyfriend. You met him in Venice, remember? Lance is his brother. He's a safecracker by profession. I've heard a lot about him."

Muriel looked concerned. "Won't I still be my own Guardian though? If I am it'll be legal for Joseph to assault me."

"Get this through your head once and for all, Muriel. Rape is *never* legal."

"Are you sure? Annise always told me a *little* rape was better than none at all."

"Some counseling," muttered Morton.

"I know what we'll do," said Muriel. "Joseph wants me to sign all those forms. The ones giving my Guardianship back to Dar/Neese. I'd have to do it in his office."

"In Harvey's office," said Morton.

"Right. I'll start signing. I'll do it real slow. Before we finish I'll say I'm feeling hot and dirty and want to go in the tub right away. He gets excited easy. We won't be able to finish the signing."

Morton raised his eyebrows. "Damn, you're steamy," he said.

"It's thanks to you," she returned smiling.

"So you'll hustle him into the Therapy Room?" said Morton.

"Uh huh. I'll squeeze his hand and pull him down the hall. He won't even think of locking Harvey's door."

Their heads moved close in deep consultation as they discussed the details. Of the two urges Harvey said we all had: the want to be wanted and the urge to communicate, which were really the same urge when you got down to it—well, Morton felt them both galloping through him like a herd of unruly kittens. The war was still raging, and the reality of the mines were everywhere, yet he was fulfilled in his heart. It was such a beautiful and awkward sensation he kept shaking his head in disbelief, which Muriel mistook for disagreement.

"Don't pay any attention to me. I'm nuts," he whispered to her.

"Nuts?" she said looking distressed.

"Nuts about you, Muriel. Don't worry, it's a good kind of neurosis."

Muriel grinned ear to ear. This was what he'd always sought in those years he worked with her. Funny how things turned out. They had to become lovers to unlock the mystery. So what? It was right as rain, and nobody was going to tell him any different, by God!

~~~

Annise emerged from the bathroom. She was wearing her Victoria's Secret shorts and her Frederick's of Hollywood turtleneck top with the chest area cut out to show off her cleavage.

Spontaneously Morton said, "You were wearing *that* with Joseph? No wonder he—"

Muriel put her fingers over his lips and shushed him before he could finish.

Annise dumped the *JC Pennys* bag onto the carpet. It was full of baby clothes, rattles, shoes the size of a person's thumb. She began toying insanely with the items.

"Just a few things for baby," she said. "No sense procrastinating till the last minute, is there?"

Morton knew he had to get out of there. He guided Trina aside. He whispered to her about Annise's surgery the next morning. About the Gestapo breaking up her apartment.

"You should be aware, Trina, Joseph killed her beagle. That's how far he's gone. I'll have to go over there and do something with the carcass. Annise doesn't know yet."

Trina gritted her teeth. "I understand."

Morton kissed her on the forehead. Trina turned beet red.

"You're a hell of a friend," he said.

"I, uh, am soon finished the tea," stammered the RN, struggling to gain her composure. "We girls will have it."

She hurried into the kitchen.

* * *

Chapter 90

By the time Morton got to Annise's apartment he realized how drained he felt. He climbed the stairwell and let himself in. He stepped quickly past the kitchen, refusing to acknowledge the stiff hind legs of Sassafras extending across the linoleum.

The apartment was busted up, as Wanda said. The stereo had been knocked over, the leather bound volumes of the Maccabees scooped off the bookshelves. It appeared worse than it was. Except for one thing: Sassafras was truly dead. There was none of her humble padding around, no more soft bark to say hi when you were down.

Morton went to the bedroom. The praying hands were still praying. There was a new plaster Madonna suckling the baby Jesus. And in the rim of the mirror—how could he have missed it these weeks?—was a snapshot of Wanda Novice.

The way it had all gone he expected to feel an isolation in there, a sorrow, or a bitterness maybe. Instead the place glowed with a warm, smoky ease. Finally, alone with himself, he recognized it had been them *together* who'd generated the chill. A couple not meant to be a couple was like a giant zero, like a ghost walking in and out of rooms. No one could see them. No one could hear them, except when they argued of course. And whatever emptiness existed in the world or in other people became enlarged and intensified, not relieved or comforted by their forced togetherness.

He moved to the calendar. He needed to verify little Toni's conception date. Annise *was* strict with some things, and the notations were easy to figure out. The 6th of June had been the big day. And yes, alongside his own M.A., the initials J.S. were clearly marked. She wasn't referring to any Joel Sincowitz either.

Her locking box was open on the bed, its contents spilled across the unmade covers. Not so different from other times he'd been there, really.

At the foot of the mattress was a mound of shredded paper. Morton examined the debris. He could make out the slitted stocks and bonds, the numerous tests for sexually transmitted diseases, the pregnancy confirmation, her negative HIV titer. He even recognized *My Confessions*, which by this time had thickened into a booklet. It too had been sliced into tiny strips. The work of Joseph's razor knife, surely. The Gestapo could do things out of pure meanness, but Morton suspected he'd been after some damaging evidence. Annise's style was to lay down who did what in a meticulous fashion, and more importantly, when. So he destroyed her Confessions hoping to obliterate any record of his involvement with her.

Morton had a sudden thought. *My Confessions* would be on the Imagineer 3000. He pulled the machine from the top drawer and booted up. But nothing. No files. No data. Everything on the hard drive had been deleted.

Morton recalled the cuts on Annise's thigh in The Green Room. She'd been telling the truth. The Gestapo had sunk to torture.

The counselor began stuffing the confettied papers back into the box. Perhaps they could be salvaged, pasted together or something.

As he worked he felt the pistol tapping against his ribs through his jacket pocket. He'd forgotten to remove it after the incident at the Green Room, and like an amputated leg envisioned it staring up at him, causing pain. The .38 caliber *Smith & Wesson* she never for the first instant intended to use on the rapist, right?

"I could never shoot anybody," she'd told him with such sincerity. "The Bible tells you to turn the other cheek."

He'd given a snicker at her use of the word cheek, what with its double meaning. At the time he hadn't known she was actually turning it over in the forbidden brothel style ways he feared. Still, it was no joke.

What they'd undertaken hadn't been rape though, had it? *Their* sinning had been done willingly, he felt. Honestly, so to speak.

Morton recalled the conversation with Muriel long ago about whether Annise wanted to be drawn out. No, he decided, what she wanted was to draw people in. Bring them *toward* her. The Rodneys. The Joels. The Wanda Novices. Even the Joseph Schopens. Impale herself with humanity, or at least the semblance of humanity, so she'd be safe and warm against her death, or her purgatory, or whatever she was trying to protect against. It was as if she were on a quest to become full. Not the fed kind, but rather the sated till you were sick to your soul kind.

Morton scratched his head. The heart to heart with Annise was way past due.

Wasn't this the truth of it? The outside was one thing. Better yet, if you were a magnificent blonde and had the guts for it, simply put the cast of characters inside yourself. Own them in your screwy way. Keep yourself surrounded, insulated from the inside out as it were. If you swallowed a constant diet of hot irons that never left the fire you could really get heated up proper. Now he knew what she meant when she talked about having two hearts. Only she'd been speaking of Joseph Schopen's heart she'd become one with. Because it had been Joseph's little Toni right from the start. And she'd known it all along.

On the other hand, maybe the Pope really was about to take his high-flying royal dump and like a sewage line suck away those ignorant scabs of Catholic emotion. Yes, he would casually rise from the throne, look, then flush the nasty business down the special pipeline which led straight to magnificent Pasadena blondes. That Annise Chastain—locked in a world of her own with the Devil sharpening his claws on the plywood back door. Who'd think it to look at that beautiful, sculpted face? And, sad to say, her Devil was mere reality.

He kept thinking of the derringer. After all, she had tried to get the gun back in The Green Room. What was she planning to do with it? Who could tell, maybe she believed God himself was so desperate for a tight piece of Pasadena evil only a good solid suicide would settle his craving.

Morton could just picture it. She'd limp home from the hospital, recuperate for a few days while she got it all straight in her head. Then, late one night, she would sit calmly at the vanity. Cigarette going. Wine glass half full. All decked out in her church clothes for the first time since the surgery, only with that weird little pistol freed from the box and waiting there under the soft red lights. She would think over and over about all those hells inside her that could never be made good, until she'd driven herself half crazy with guilt.

Finally, she'd take the gun into her hands. Profoundly. Religiously, even. Yet with all the wild-eyed desire rolling round in her heart that she knew only a strong man could penetrate. Or, he wondered glancing up at the photo of Wanda, a strong woman?

The counselor began to straighten the room, make the bed. If you saw no facts, and spoke no facts, were there no facts? When a tree fell in the forest was there no sound without an ear to capture it? Well, no one stayed as blind as the ones who refused to see. Beware of those who went around with their eyes slitted like dimes, for they faked blindness and could hear better than radar on bats.

For the first time he smelled a stench, which he knew was Sassafras decaying.

～～

Morton went into the kitchen and pulled several trash bags from under sink. He moved quickly, hoping to shorten the misery, until he saw the pills.

Around Sassafras's bowl were a handful of light green capsules. No, not capsules, but the halves of capsules. They'd been opened and the powder dumped into the beagle's favorite dish, eggdrop soup and hamburger, the treat Morton always kept handy in the refrigerator.

He checked closer. These were the old Librium pills, which he knew were filled with Dilaudid. From the looks of it Sassafras had passed out before she could even finish her dish. Poor girl. Her dose had been immense, more than enough to kill her.

Morton dumped the food. The capsules that weren't empty he flushed down the toilet. Why hadn't he gotten rid of this crap when he first thought of it?

Were there more pills in the bedroom? He became alarmed for Annise. If she was suicidal she'd find a way to get her hands on them.

He checked the locking box. No, the pills were gone now. At least that stage of the drama was over.

Nevertheless, Morton felt guilty. How many of these deaths could have been prevented if he'd been more alert? What was more, could he allow Muriel to place herself in such jeopardy while he floundered around trying to log the Gestapo's sins on videotape? Could he really risk Muriel's life in the name of justice when he knew damn well Joseph Schopen would run the dagger through whoever's heart got in his way?

Such torment he was experiencing. He ought to be grateful, for it was nothing compared to the pressures Muriel must have felt. Or Annise. Or even Sassafras. On the other hand, self torment was an act of perception, wasn't it? Not real, except inside your brain. It was said a person could remain serene in the midst of turmoil if his mind was fittingly composed. Enraged? Tranquil? Didn't you have to embrace them both if you intended to waste a man?

He felt the lifelessness of Sassafras as he struggled to fit the corpse into the layers of plastic bags.

He thought again of Muriel. Of her rape. She demanded justice.

He thought of Sally Featherman.

Then he thought of Harvey Mueller, the gentle caretaker he'd been schooled under. Harvey's bleeding ashes were crying out from the negative ionic dirt beneath the Organic Therapy Garden rose bushes. His very urn begged for the hangman's knot to be cinched around Joseph Schopen's barbaric neck.

Easier said than done. A quarter inch thick beer mug splitting across the Gestapo's forehead had only made the guy mad. Muriel was right. They would need help.

* * *

Chapter 91

It was 1:00 a.m. Morton checked to see if the phone was working, then dialed the Fraction House. Wanda answered.

"Hi, Wanda."

"Hi, Morton," she said recognizing his voice.

"I'm over at Annise's. She's not here. Don't worry, she's safe for now." The counselor hemmed and hawed, dodging the Sassafras issue, which Wanda seemed to understand. Finally he said, "I'd like to talk to Gordon, if you wouldn't mind."

"He's not allowed to receive calls. Joseph's had him on restriction to the Fraction House grounds," said Wanda.

"Why?" asked Morton.

"Well, that's the problem. He really didn't do anything. He's the next one up to become his own Guardian you know."

"I know," said Morton.

"I think Joseph's pulling the same deal with Gordon he tried with Muriel. He's desperate for his funding. So he filled out a bunch of forms saying Gordon's regressed lately."

"Has he regressed?" asked the counselor.

"No. Actually, a lot of us think he's been doing better. But then this blow up with Annise happened. And Gordon knows more than anybody about Joseph chasing after Muriel."

Morton's eyes narrowed. "I realize Gordon knows. But how do *you* know?"

"Joseph's completely out of touch, Morton. I guess when Harvey was here they kept each other's personalities in bounds a little. But now that Joseph's got the Directorship he's really gone over the edge. He's become pretty transparent."

Wanda took a deep breath.

"He practically dragged Annise out of here by the hair the other day," she said. "But the whole time he was talking about Muriel. Obscene crap came out of his mouth, Morton. It was hard for us to believe."

"Believe it," said the counselor.

"What I'm saying though, is when Joseph left Gordon told me he was going over to Muriel's. He said Joseph was about to murder her and he had to protect her."

"Gordon has courage."

"I couldn't stop him. He said it was something he had to do. He just left."

"I'm proud of him," said Morton.

"But don't you understand? He violated Joseph's restriction to the Fraction House. Do you know what this means, Morton? It means Roselawn has open season on him. All Priscilla has to do is find him roaming around Culver City and handcuff him into her ugly white van. He'll be put back in that hellhole forever."

"Didn't he come back from Muriel's?" asked the counselor.

"Sure, he came back. But he wanders in and out as he pleases. He doesn't have any faith in me. And Joseph's never around. Anyway, he'll be quick down the tubes if Priscilla sees him two feet off Dar/Neese property. We really can't afford that, can we? Losing Gordon and all, I mean?"

Morton said, "Is Gordon there now, Wanda?"

She gave a long sigh.

"It's Annise's life we're talking about," he pressed. "It's Muriel's life too."

"And yours," admitted Wanda.

Morton was quiet.

"All right. I'll put him on," she said at last. "It'll take me a few minutes to run him down."

~~~

The counselor waited. His body hummed he was so exhausted.

"Morton, is that you?" asked Gordon skeptically.

"It's me," he returned.

"I've been so worried. I was over at Muriel's. She wasn't home. The place looks all emptied out. Did Joseph strip it?"

"Muriel is safe. I took her up to the mountains camping. Don't tell anybody, but she's at Trina Lopez's now."

"Joseph about killed your poor synthetic blonde," said Gordon. "I mean, you know, Annise Chastain. He abducted her right from the cafeteria. Probably fifty people saw it."

"Really?"

"Yep. But nobody did anything to stop it. Not even the staff."

"Why not?" exclaimed Morton.

"It's hard to say. She had on this boob busting outfit. A lot of us thought she was working her next move on him. Using her dumb reverse psychology to make him take a bigger interest. She's like that, you know."

"I know," said Morton.

"She makes me nervous," volunteered the paranoid.

"Gordon, I'd like to ask a favor. Besides Muriel, you're my only real friend. I need your help in a big way."

"Anything," said Gordon.

"It's very dangerous. Joseph's got these sick porno tapes of him and Muriel. Only he phonied it up to look like it was me and Muriel. Anyway, what I have to ask is—"

The counselor went on to describe the details. Gordon was an intelligent man. His interest peaked when Morton mentioned how the videotape, already synthetic in Gordon's mind, had been tampered with by Joseph, which made it phonier than phony.

"This sort of caper deserves your attention," suggested the counselor.

Morton explained how they'd have to use Muriel for a decoy in the tub in order to film the Gestapo as the ugly predator he was.

"Now comes the important part," he continued. "Somehow you'll have to get that monster safe out of Joseph's office."

"Harvey's office, you mean?" said Gordon.

"Right. The tapes are inside. I think you'll be able to slide it—"

Morton thought hard. Sliding the safe might be possible, but it would require two people. And the noise and scraping of getting the bulky chunk of metal to the end of the hallway...

Gordon said, "Harvey's safe uses two keys, doesn't it?"

"Yeah," said Morton.

"You once told me when the keys were ready the lock would appear. I'll always remember that. It was one of the best pieces of therapy I've ever heard."

"It was?"

"Yep. Why don't you try those two keys in your briefcase?"

"Very optimistic, Gordon," praised the counselor. "But this isn't your Friends of Psychics Network. Reality is a lot tougher nut to crack."

Morton had an abrupt awakening. Or recollection, call it. Because— Yes, those keys in his briefcase were the ones he'd slipped from Harvey's shirt pocket the day he died. Minutes earlier the Freudian had been into his safe for a new bottle of nitro. Damn if the paranoid wasn't right on the money. These *were* the missing keys Annise alluded to that day on the freeway! She'd been right after all in her accusations. What was it about your *slightly* mentally ill, your *not* so idiot savants like Gordon Theodoricus that they could put a Rubik's Cube together when half the puzzle had fallen out in the aisle?

"Did anybody ever tell you what a rare jewel you are, Gordon?"

"I believe you might have said it once. I'm not sure though. I've been having trouble with my memory lately."

"We won't have to push the safe down the hallway after all. You'll open it with the keys. It's tricky, but I'm sure you can handle it."

"I'll do my best," Gordon assured him. "I'm psyched for this. Really psyched."

Morton sat on the rug and took his time refining the details with his friend. It was critical for every step in the process to be synchronized. Joseph's OCD would come in handy. His habit of checking the Therapy Room door every six minutes—and he was always punctilious to the split second on his gold Rolex watch—this would make it easier to pull off.

"I want to help Muriel," said Gordon. "I want to help Annise too. They're both batty in the belfry, but that's the way we like our women, isn't it, Morton?"

"I guess so," agreed the counselor reluctantly. "I guess we do, Gordon."

They hung up.

~~~

Morton checked the list and gathered the items Annise asked for. Her makeup case. Her sexy, white silk dress to wear home from the hospital. Her blow dryer. Everything a traveling blonde would need.

He had an urge to telephone Muriel with the revelation of the missing keys and how Gordon was coming in with them on the plot. This however he did not do, for Sassafras lingered luridly in the kitchen.

He turned to his task.

At last he had her triple bagged with Heftys and four metal ties twisted around the top where he'd spun closed the plastic.

He hoisted the rigid body, cradling it lovingly. He blinked back tears as he started down the steps. It was hard labor. Why was death so heavy to bear compared to the tail wagging lightness of the living? He hunched into the burden as he descended.

At the awkward turn in the stairwell Sassafras's legs caught in the weakened seams of the bags. Her toenails shot through, and both feet popped out like switchblades, nearly cutting Morton's face.

The counselor retied the bags, then proceeded down the stairs.

The body thumped loud in the truck bed. A number of the neighborhood lights clicked on, as if they'd been waiting expectantly for Annise Chastain to meet such an end. Here at last was their proof. Well, neighbors too were predictable. They'd also seen Joseph Schopen and his repugnant gold Jaguar lurking in the alleyways.

Regarding Sassafras, what was Morton going to tell Annise? That she'd run away? Been stolen?

He couldn't lie. He'd just go ahead and drive the body to the vet right now. Not the vet. To one of those all night animal hospitals. They'd handle the remains. He'd pay for what he had to.

As for informing Annise—this was no longer part of his duties. Better for the husband, er, the significant other rather, to break the news.

Yes, he'd find the animal hospital and call Wanda from there. She could deal with the rest.

Morton drove away.

* * *

Chapter 92

Morton left the Santa Monica All Night Animal Hospital at 4:00 a.m. On the drive back to Trina's he dragged his briefcase from beneath the seat. The two keys—the ones to Harvey's safe—were zipped into the inner pocket. Sweet.

At Trina's he tapped softly on the door. Muriel let him in, then returned to the sofa where she'd been sleeping.

"Where's Annise?" he asked nervously.

"In Trina's room. She only has one bed."

Annise and *Trina*, speculated the counselor briefly?

Morton told Muriel about the wonderful discovery of the safe keys in his briefcase.

"This means we don't have to steal the thing in thirty seconds and have a big bloody mess in the hallway."

"Bloody?" she said. "You're not going to stab him or something, are you?"

Jesus, how you had to watch your wording, reflected Morton.

Muriel said, "My date with Joseph is for three o'clock. I whispered it to him in The Green Room."

"Good. You better call him first. Or ring his beeper if he's not in his office. Get a cab to the Fraction House. Make sure Joseph is in the Therapy Room at four. That's when it's going down. Annise should be finished with her surgery way before then. Here, take these."

Muriel closed her fist around the two brass keys like a guerrilla fighter celebrating victory.

"Give them to Gordon when you get there," instructed the counselor. "I called him from Annise's. He's in this with us, Muriel."

"OK," she said.

"All he'll have to do is swipe the cassettes, wait for my all clear signal and bolt down the hallway. He's going to go burn them."

"How's he going to burn them?"

"He'll toss them in the giant drier in the laundry room. They'll melt in a few seconds. We already talked about it."

Muriel said, "But, Morton, if you open the Therapy Room door with a camera in your hand you know Joseph is going to fight. It'll be a huge face down."

"He'll probably be naked. We'll catch him helpless. We'll all get out of there as fast as possible."

"Joseph's never helpless," replied Muriel.

"We have no choice," said Morton. "As soon as I shoot the film you run into Harvey's office and call the police. They're used to coming to the Fraction House. They'll arrive in two minutes."

"Try thirty minutes," she said.

The counselor was tired to the bone. His eyes began to drift shut under the stress.

Muriel extended her arms and beckoned him to her. They hugged. How fine she felt. In one way her body formed up petite and soft against him, while in another she was the size of all the life he'd lived up till that moment.

They kissed. He was weary beyond himself, yet somehow the kiss worked into passion. They sunk into each other's arms like two glasses of cool water poured across a burning timber.

Romantic? Sexy? Dirty? Absolutely yes it was! Every bit of this, and more! Why did the human heart insist on boiling so much hotter when risk was involved? Careful though, for Trina and Annise were already tossing and turning in the next room, he could feel the vibes right through the walls.

Timing. It was everything in this life, wasn't it? Well, there'd be a future for these things, decided Morton settling in beside her on the sofa. An unfolding of hope and realistic dreams, where they'd carve out a sun-drenched existence in the Virgin Islands, sailing yachts by day and dancing flamenco fashion at night... So tired he was... So very tired and sleepy...

* * *

Chapter 93

It was daylight when he awakened to Annise's voice in the kitchen. No problem. He was dressed. Nothing inappropriate had occurred.

"We've got to be at the Surgery Center at nine," she called to him. "You better start pulling yourself together. We should eat somewhere first."

They went to Vera's. Part way there Morton thought he heard an odd sound, like a whimper. He turned, but she was the same as before, elbow out the window, smoking.

"Everyone who has ever lived has had to do this thing. I'm no different, I guess," she muttered.

She pushed back her hair.

"Even... Even Jesus of Nazareth had to do it, Morton. And he was almost God."

"Do what, Annise?"

She sagged her head far down. "Die," she whispered heavily.

Morton pushed her shoulder playfully. "Life is always better after a depression," he joked optimistically. She did not smile.

~~~

In the parking lot she waited for him to come around and open the door. She dove into his arms.

"I'm so afraid," she breathed.

Her muscles were hard and tight. He massaged them.

"It'll be OK, baby," he said.

Annise drew back. "Listen, I've been sick of the *baby* bullshit for a long time now. Can we please dispense with it?"

~~~

Annise ordered sausage and eggs.

"I didn't think patients were allowed food before surgery," said Morton.

"I told you, I'm going under a local. I'll be awake the whole time. And anyway, I'm supposed to eat for two now."

"They know you're pregnant, right?"

Annise frumped her lips. "Cut me some slack for Christsake. Everything is fine, Morton."

It was early, but already Vera's lunch special was being prepared. All day long the smells of turkey roasting in the oven would sift like fine Thanksgiving memories through the restaurant. A homespun wave of nostalgia passed through him for the couple they might have been. Honestly, though, nothing had changed. But then everything was always changing. Loose ends were everywhere. They both were aware of that, and by degrees a sourness crept into the air.

Annise was in the trendy white silk dress. She usually wore it with a sash tied tight at the waist, but today it hung loose, maternity style, although he knew she couldn't be showing yet. She reached over and touched his hand.

"You know, Morton, I can be so attracted to you sometimes. Especially like this morning when you're kind of wild looking and didn't comb your hair."

The counselor gathered up his courage. He leaned back in the hard wooden booth.

"There's something we need to discuss, Annise. It's about little Toni."

"Can't this wait?" she returned. "Can't we try to feel halfway pleasant with each other for once?"

He swallowed hard. "I have to say this before I get sidetracked. I'm not her father," he blurted.

Annise dug into her purse. She placed her compact on the table, her lighter. Next came the booklet she'd been studying, something put out by one of Wanda's Harmonic Convergence friends called, *You Can Take It With You.*

"Did you hear what I said? I'm trying to tell you—" he started.

'L.A. 2000:' Sex Asylum

"Do you know what pride is, Morton?" interrupted Annise.

He thought it over. "Isn't it when you want something someone else has, but you're too afraid to steal the thing?" he asked.

She shook her head very far from side to side. "Nooo," she sang. "It's when somebody acts like they like you when they actually don't like you at all."

"I've told you right from the start how I felt, Annise. I wanted you. I really did."

She pursed her lips. "I'm not talking about you and me. I'm talking about you and Muriel," she clarified.

She peeled the cellophane off a breadstick and took a loud bite.

"What about her?" asked the counselor.

Annise leaned forward. "I know you've been seeing her. And I know how naïve you are about these things, Morton. Christ, look at the way you've been with me."

He carefully stirred his coffee.

"Sometimes I think we're like candy to each other," said Annise. "Only the kind with a sickening cherry in the middle. You know, the ones that make you want to spit them out the second you chomp down?"

Morton gulped the rest of his coffee and pushed the cup to the edge of the table for a refill. Vera quickly appeared with the pot.

"I've got my pride too," she continued when they were alone again. "I don't want you going around thinking you got away with something. Because you didn't. All you got was a little drug-blasted schizophrenic, and everybody knows it too."

Morton's eyes rose with a haunting sense of reality. People were eating and drinking. The warm vibration of rational conversation was all around them. Annise stroked his wrist, and for a fleeting moment his mind flashed over their twisted history. Broiled lobster hot? Ice water cold? Pre-destined? Or as random and misguided as a meteor blazing out over the roof of The Amazon Bar and Grill, over The Shamrock, over the slobs and the prostitutes in The Green Room? Through it all, reflected the counselor, one thing had remained the same. Which was her cunning. Which was the magnificent blonde baring another lightning bolt of the old ultra-femininity to the boys at the bar. How much of their maladjustment had been Morton spreading his colorful peacock tail and hoping for the best result?

Vera arrived with Annise's eggs. She dug immediately in. The counselor had no appetite. He stuck with coffee.

"Have you ever thought of marrying Joseph?" he asked her.

Annise stiffened. "Why is there this thing inside me that always wants to tell you to fuck off?" she replied.

"Answer about Joseph," he pressed.

She shook her head.

"Because he's not the father?"

"Yes," she said. "I mean, no. Not only that."

Annise's eyes opened wide. She turned her head toward the table beside them and stared at the people there.

"Joseph's no father," she said. "He's too macho. I'm sure his sperm's fine though. You're the father type, Morton. Look at how you've rebonded with Muriel and made a woman of her. You'll do the same for little Toni. I know you will."

"Uh, Annise—"

"Why are you saying all this, Morton?" she asked. "It seems to me you ought to be facing up to your own obligations, not other people's."

Morton leaned onto the table. "I want to be honest with you, Annise. I think I should tell you I had a good look at your calendar last night."

"Oh?" she said.

He proceeded to outline how he'd identified the J.S.'s marked across the important week. Across the whole damn summer in fact. But particularly, *particularly* on the 6th of June. He told her how he'd been racking his brain to figure it all out. He tried to lay it down as humanely as possible.

"I'm not out to hurt you," he explained. "I'm just saying I've finally put it all together, and I know I'm not the father."

"Yes, you are," she countered.

"Think back for a minute. It was the day you told me to make you do it, remember? You kept saying, 'Make me. Make me.'"

She tilted her head.

"And right afterwards you ran over to the calendar and started writing things on it."

"Well, what of it?"

"That's the only night it could have been, isn't it? June 6th. It's marked to high heaven."

"That's it," agreed Annise. "I timed it perfectly."

"And you planned it way in advance, didn't you? That's what your horseplay in Venice was about—I mean, waiting till Thursday for the T-back date. You knew you were going to ovulate."

Annise picked up her napkin and blotted the grease off the top of one of her sausage patties. It was as if she wanted to speak but had lost the clues to the puzzle.

"You were trying to trap me," said Morton.

"Not to trap you. To collect what's good about you," she suddenly admitted.

"Only it wasn't me you collected. I started coughing. I got a tickle in my throat like I do a lot of times. You know how I hack when I get overheated. I was holding my chest and coughing, remember? I know you think I— Well, finished off, I guess you'd call it. But I didn't, Annise. I was just wheezing and trying to hack up phlegm. Honestly, that's all it was."

She glared angrily at him.

"I'm telling the truth. You can wait till she's born and have the tests. But I can guarantee you right now I am not the father of the little Toni you're carrying. Plus, I know you were with Joseph earlier that day."

Annise looked dazed. "What are you trying to say?"

Morton leaned close. "I'm saying, Annise, that I didn't—" He glanced around. "Ejaculate," he whispered. "And if I didn't, and you're pregnant, then someone else did."

"You don't know what you're saying," she mumbled.

"I admit I never figured out what aroused you," said Morton. "It seems like the only time you were very happy was when you were bad, or being punished. I don't know. It's too deep for me."

"I *was* bad. Do you think— Do you think if I sinned the day little Toni got made she'll turn out wicked? It could happen you know. Evil spirits are everywhere these days."

"She'll be all right," waved the counselor.

"Even if she was conceived in a den of iniquity like the back of The Green Room?"

"The Green Room!"

"Don't you understand, Morton? I wanted you to be the father, not some demon-possessed rapist like Joseph. I can't help what excites me. I've been shoveling coal in Hades since day one. But little Toni shouldn't have to suffer for my bad deeds, should she?"

"Are you telling me Joseph raped you in The Green Room?"

Annise nodded dismally. "You're making a big deal out of this. But why is it so different from the night *you* made me? You know I never wanted to do it in the first place."

Morton sighed and rubbed his temples.

"I wanted to believe it was you who got me pregnant. Anybody would have done the same thing if they were in my shoes. I'd have been good at it too, Morton. We'd have gotten married. I could have fooled us both for twenty years."

"Is that all we'd have been married? Twenty years? What would happen then? Divorce?"

"Of course not. Catholics aren't allowed to get divorces. But by then you'd probably be irritated with me and separate or something. Maybe leave me and Toni to fend for ourselves like a lot of Catholic husbands do."

"Leave you? Why?"

"Well—" She stalled. Meekly she said, "For still seeing Wanda. I know you'd be hopping mad about something like that."

"Wanda! Jesus Christ, this is insane, Annise."

"Are you calling love insane?" she countered. "Because just between me and my maker, Morton, Wanda loves me to the bottom of her heart."

She glared harshly at him, exposing a thin hard line of teeth. She pushed her plate away, rose and walked out.

* * *

Chapter 94

Morton took care of the bill.

It seldom rained in L.A., and full months could pass without a shower, but today a smoky patchwork fog hung over the street lamps. A light drizzle had begun to fall.

Annise was waiting at the truck. Strands of her hair were matted web-like across her forehead. All those times with her, he kept thinking as he unlocked the door. All the fire they'd generated. Whether good or bad, it made no difference now.

At the Surgery Center they emerged from the truck and walked to the entrance. For a fog soaked moment they lingered under an awning of each other for all the old times, for the way their quest for happiness was so much the same even if their heads wouldn't allow them together.

A gust of wind rustled against Morton's back. It nudged him forward. Annise too drifted a degree, and suddenly their lips met. He could hear the spit of rain tapping against their clothes for those seconds, then it was over. They hung there, staring forlornly at one another.

She opened the door to the Surgery Center. Her face glowed purplish as the fog mixed with the interior light. Tiny rivulets glistened across the tops of her breasts. Then came the weird staring into each other's eyes, which meant both everything and nothing.

"There is a hero in all this, Morton," she said. "But I want you to know it's not you. I don't want you ever thinking it's you. Do you understand?"

There was a cold, vibrating pause.

"I'll tell you who the hero is," said Annise. "It's Wanda Novice. She's the one who perseveres the way a decent person is supposed to."

"I understand," he said.

"Wanda's the one who deserves the real credit. In fact I'm going to give her a call. I'm going to ring her up right now. What do you think of that?"

"Well, if you feel it's wise—"

"It might not seem wise to you, but that's because you have no idea what sort of a woman Wanda is inside."

"What kind is she?" wondered the counselor.

Annise put her hands on her hips. "I can tell you this much. She's not the kind who gets in bed with a person just to cough a bunch of goddamn phlegm all over them."

"What exactly does she do in bed with them?" he asked her.

At that Annise spun on her heels and stepped toward the Nursing Station. The door closed slowly behind her, leaving Morton outside in the thickening rain.

He took a moment then to cup his hands to the glass and watch as the heads in the waiting room rotated one by one in reverence to her beauty. He was used to this by now. Yes, she was still the magnificent blonde. Silk bodice over torso like lake water lapping the hull of a boat, designer dress eddying lazily around her ankles, face dazzling each of them.

The picture seemed so unlikely. She was *too* blonde, *too* exquisite. For a moment he fantasized at what she might become in the next ten years. But the thought flitted away in the next gust of breeze. He took his hands from the window. Love. The truth of the matter was that if in the end you didn't achieve it you left the person alone, you had to.

Morton returned to his truck.

* * *

Chapter 95

The counselor hardly had time to mourn his parting with Annise. Foremost now was acquiring the video camera.

He drove to Rip's Rentals on Wilshire and used his credit card to lease a Sharp Viewcam. This was the type Joseph used, and Morton was familiar with its operation. More importantly, it was the kind you aimed from the chest, glancing downward into the viewfinder rather than holding it to your eye like the others. Should a punch be thrown, he reasoned, best to have the machine low on the body, and a lanyard, like this one had, securing it around your neck.

As he left the store the counselor paused to check his watch. A week of living might have passed, yet it was still only 10:00 a.m. While every aspect of his life would be hanging out to dry a few hours in the future, now, for the first time in months, he had nowhere to go. He felt like a fly in a giant web of asphalt. Well, yes, he did have one final errand. The Dar/Neese Credit Union held his last $100. Fortunately he could get that from any ATM. How he would pay off the credit card for the Viewcam rental was anybody's guess.

Morton crossed the street to the pay phone. Whatever their differences, he couldn't bring himself to leave Annise alone in her time of need. He dialed the Surgery Center.

The secretary wasn't very agreeable. Perhaps Annise had mentioned something about keeping him away. The counselor jutted his jaw.

"Look, this is Dr. Morton Chastain. I'm her husband. I have a right to know when she'll be going home."

"Oh! Dr. Chastain! I'm so sorry. We're running a little late. Your wife will be in Recovery after lunch. She won't need you until then. My apologies, sir. I'm sure you're a busy man."

"Thanks," he said. "I am."

Morton hung up the receiver. A group of sexy looking office workers happened to be strolling by. Was it his ego, or were they actually eyeballing him? They were sporting those chic L.A. ultra-miniskirts, the red high heels.

What section of town was this anyway, he wondered? Could these by any chance be high-life call girls working the brunch shift? Or were they *real* high-lifes dolled up to look like call girls? Joseph, in his boob bar wisdom, called this the Barbie doll syndrome, so universal was the modern woman's desire to be perceived as a curvaceous Eve in erotic fishnet stockings. Well, the Gestapo wasn't wrong about everything.

A wave of disorientation passed through Morton, like when you're lost, and though you're pretty sure you know the way back you still feel a terror you might forget. That you might *never* get back.

Snap out of it, Allison. Space out on the curves and you'll run into the ditch for sure. The Barbie Doll Syndrome? More like the Chastain Stimulus/Response Syndrome. After all, she exhibited the behavior and he'd given the hormonal response at every intersection. They all gave the response. Vera had her frowns. Joseph raged with control fetishes. Wanda shot from the hip, so to speak, but in the end simply wanted a companion.

None of this would have been unusual, except Annise sucked it up like ice cream into a Dirt Devil vacuum. Then she carried the pureed results around in a gold embroidered pouch and called it her personality. Her people were like her handbags. One day she might carry a suede Morton Allison instead of a silk Wanda Novice. Either would do, it seemed, and no one was going to criticize your top of the line runway blonde for either choice. Not in this day and age.

~~~

Morton started the drive back across the city to the Surgery Center. He didn't have to go by way of the Strip, but he decided to anyway. No need to hurry.

At the intersections he stared wanly off toward the mountains. They were brown, phony looking humps way in the distance. Although he had been there only yesterday, he could scarcely recall the smell of the pines, the goose-bump glisten of the lake water under the high winds.

How playful Muriel had been around their campsite. Sweet little Muriel Gonska, the schizophrenic, who had never found her place in the big city. Trying, yes. She was always trying her hardest to make a go of it, yet inevitably finding she didn't quite fit the mold. Why was that, when she seemed so sane and rounded to Morton?

He drove on. Idling. Accelerating. Making his way with the others through the smog and the shallow wheezes of exhaust.

He remembered more of their late night talk. Muriel had been explaining about the itches. The hundred million she said were always swarming over you.

"The only thing you have to decide— And *you* have to decide, Morton, is where you need to scratch."

In the end, that was what it amounted to, of course. The itch and where you chose to scratch. He'd wedged onto an elbow. The last coals flickered out. Her face had begun to drift in the moonlight from the way the trees kept crossing above them.

That Muriel. She was a person you had to admire. As he was finding with this Joseph mess, she was someone to contend with in a real life way. After all, she'd miraculously weaseled herself out of Roselawn. She'd become the prize pupil at the Fraction House. She'd even found her way to freedom and raised the dinky Culver City apartment to levels of high art. Who could predict what she was capable of in the big picture? For all Morton knew she might be married to him and beginning to live happily ever after in another week or two. Never underestimate the power of a person they called crazy.

As he drove he kept thinking how in the tent she'd been so serene, so unified with nature in all its incomprehensible forms, from pickup truck to lakeside fishing. Emblazoned on his mind was how accurate she'd been in their joining. It was as if she'd slipped supernaturally free of herself, and became something entirely different. Which was... What? *Him*, he wondered? A metamorphosis into some as yet untrodden part of his soul?

Was this what sex amounted to when you truly cared about someone? That your security blankets were interchangeable? That your warmth and allegiance to a person boiled down to the small silk fringes of courtesy?

～～～

The truck chugged on. Soon he found himself passing The Green Room. The doors were propped open, as usual, only this time due to the hammer and nail renovations going on inside.

What was it Joseph told him when he first started with Dar/Neese? Yes, he'd said it the drunken night bar hopping as they stared together at the naked dancers.

"Hell might be other people, Allison. But it's also yourself. Never forget that," grunted the Gestapo over his Snakebite.

At the time, Morton hadn't been sure which of them Joseph was referring to. Now though, he understood when a person said a thing, particularly if it was about hell, it had mostly to do with themselves.

～～～

The counselor parked in the Cedars-Sinai lot, across the street from the Surgery Center. There was still time to kill. He decided to window-shop the few nearby stores. Soot and oddball pieces of litter blew across the sidewalks as he began to walk. Sirens were roaring in from all directions, though no one seemed to notice.

He wandered up the road until he came to an outdoor magazine stand. He paused on the sidewalk to page through the periodicals. It was a spooky, hollowed out time. Annise back there under the knife. The asphalt going dark, then turning bright and sparkling again as the dark rain clouds rushed by.

On the front of one of the tabloids Morton noticed a photograph of a blonde who looked like Annise. There was her black sequined dress, her patented platinum hair cascading all down the front. He opened the paper and found the article. A starlet, yes, she was, but not Annise.

Another picture caught his eye. He picked up the magazine. This one definitely had the eyes, those sharp green emeralds beneath the sky blue mascara. But no, no, not the right cheek bones.

Morton glanced across the shelf. My God, if they weren't *all* Annises! Each with the perfect nipple-skin lips, the pearly teeth, their hips cocked seductively into the sunlight the way Annise was always cocking hers.

The counselor found it difficult to take his eyes off the photos. Would he ever wake up to the great synthetic sham of the makeup artist? Would he ever quit skipping like a dopey tin man down the Yellow Brick Road? Maybe you had to stick your fingers in your ears to avoid being led astray by some tickle-your-nuts Marilyn Monroe voice.

Morton moved farther down the road. He noticed a card shop, and realized these were establishments catering to the surrounding Medical Complex. Through the window he could see joke books along the back wall. That's what Muriel needs, he thought excitedly. A book of jokes. A good laugh after a few rotten, death defying days. That's exactly what she needs!

He went inside and started going through the selections. None however offered the relaxed, giggly sort of humor he was looking for.

He took his time, until at last he found one. It was a small silver booklet called, *The Laidman's Gospel*. At least it had a funny, irreverent theme, which she might get a kick out of. When he peered inside the jokes were so dirty and sacrilegious the counselor had a second thought. In the end though nothing else intrigued him.

At the front desk, as the lady cashier was nervously bagging the booklet, Morton glimpsed a gold Jaguar passing by. Joseph's? The committee inside the counselor's head began to worry. But doctors drove Jaguars too. Joseph wouldn't risk going after her in the Recovery Room, would he? Besides, the hospital had their own security guards. Still, better get back there, just in case. She'd be coming out of the Operating Room any minute.

~~~

Outside the glass Surgery Center doors was a girl selling flowers from a small cart. She was a teenager, and wearing sexy shorts to stimulate business. Her eyes were wide and beautiful, but when Morton began to speak he saw her squinting in an attempt to read his lips. She was no more than sixteen years old, and a deaf mute according to the laminated nametag around her neck.

"I need your prettiest flowers. Which ones here are best?" he asked, meticulously mouthing the words.

She pointed to the elegant, long-stemmed roses. Lovingly she fanned the petals, picked up a small black slate and wrote, "These are nicest. Expensive though."

"How much?"

She wrote: "$30."

Hmmm. Incredibly overpriced. But nothing could stand up to dollar by dollar scrutiny when the person was in true need. Overpriced? Yes, but for the right reason, obviously. He said, "They're for someone very special. I'll take a dozen of those white carnations too."

Annise would be thrilled. Of all the flower types, she always said carnations were the purest.

The child was overjoyed at the size of the sale. She placed the carnations in a complementary vase, then wrapped the roses with white tissue and an outer stabilizer of green foil. God, what extraordinary communication!

Morton paid and turned to go. From behind he heard a childish groaning through the wind. The girl trotted over. On her slate she wrote, "You forgot your roses." She ran back to the stainless steel counter for the package.

"I didn't forget. Those are for you," replied the counselor holding up his hand.

She squinted at him in disbelief. Suddenly, overwhelmed with gratitude it seemed, she said, "Thank you. Thank you so very much! You wouldn't believe the shitheads around here. They're so hostile and ugly. Especially the doctors. You must be the nicest man ever lived."

Morton grinned at the compliment and began to walk away. After a few steps it hit him. She'd talked! Jesus H. Christ! He'd been duped yet again. She wasn't a deaf mute any more than Annise Chastain was a virgin!

"You spoke. You spoke right out loud. You can understand everything I'm saying, can't you?" exclaimed Morton.

The girl dipped her eyes, and in your classic Annise Chastain style gave a shy, I'm-not-as-innocent-as-you-think nod from under her bangs.

Morton was stunned at the weirdo right and wrong balance going on here. Well, at least the girl had looks. That was something, wasn't it? Normally he'd hang around and analyze an event this bizarre. But for now, like a dog just out of the drink, he'd have to shake it off and get on down the road. Duped? Yes. Yet he was an over-sensitive type, and couldn't ask for his money back if he wanted to remain the nicest man in the world.

Much like he'd done with Harmonic Convergence he backpedaled a short distance, then turned and headed into the hospital.

* * *

Chapter 96

An orderly showed the counselor to the gymnasium-sized Recovery Room. Many cubicles were partitioned off for privacy with white canvas.

As he entered Annise's area Morton found the curtains undulating, though there was no wind. It was as if ghosts had recently slipped away from among the pleats. Instinctively he checked behind him. No one.

A large black nurse appeared. Pathology, she said, had taken the tumor over to the Cedars-Sinai lab for assessment. They'd completed what she called, "a frozen section," to test for cancer. Early tests of the cells, as expected, proved benign. There was no malignancy.

"She'll be all right?" asked Morton.

"Of course. Not a thing to worry about."

"Wonderful," said the counselor.

"She had a local, as you know," said the nurse. "She was awfully tense so we gave her a shot of Valium. But I don't need to tell you all this, Dr. Chastain. You're familiar with the routine."

"Valium? Is that safe, with her pregnant and all?"

"Pregnant?" The nurse became alarmed. "She's not pregnant. She signed a waiver—"

Morton recognized what had happened. As if in confidence he said quietly, "Don't worry. I know what she was thinking. She's been wanting to make me a father for a long while. Sometimes her fantasies—"

The nurse held up her hand in sympathy. "Say no more. I need to see to the monitors." She disappeared through the cloth barrier.

～～

Annise had on one of those tie-in-the-back smocks. An arm was crooked up under her cheek. She was resting on her stomach, and the gown had worked conspicuously open around her buttocks. Her legs were splayed apart. A funky instant of eroticism magnified the tiny room. Morton's spirit of nostalgia lifted. Under the worst of circumstances she was still an incredible beauty.

He put the flowers on the bedside table with her purse. In the process the vase tipped, spilling a curl of water. He noticed an odd looking towel hanging on the coat rack against the wall. Hurriedly he lifted it off. But this was no towel. It was... Could it be? Yes, it was a wig! Not a wig, a fall, rather. A hair thickener made to blend with her real hair. Jesus, this was too much. Where would the shock and the lies end?

The counselor set the hairpiece back on the hook. He would liked to have been angry, but instead he welled with a sympathy for how deep her contradictions went.

"Where have you been?" said Annise. Morton jumped.

"Christ! You scared me," he gasped.

"I can be on my side. Jus' not on my back," she muttered sleepily.

Morton reached up and pulled the curtain shut. He got a Kleenex and dabbed at a string of saliva drifting over her lips.

"I have to stay here an hour. Observation or something. The doctor said it'll take three weeks to heal."

Annise rolled sideways. As she did this she discovered how exposed she'd been.

"You— You weren't looking up my smock before, were you?" she asked tugging it down.

Morton hesitated. "No, not really."

"Not really? What do you mean? I want to know. Were you staring at me when I was passed out?" Her forehead rumpled. She seemed very disturbed.

"Well, to be honest, Annise, it was hard not to. In fact, you got me a little excited." He smiled.

"Then you really *did* do it!"

"You looked good," he defended. "Why shouldn't I pay attention to your—"

"Jesus Christ in heaven!" she cried squeezing the sheets.

Her bandage had shaken loose. She winced. Many seconds went by. Had she drifted off? He found a washcloth and wiped at her brow.

"It doesn't really matter who sees what anymore. It's all been killed anyway," she said lifting her head.

"I wish you wouldn't say those things, Annise. You're still woozy, you know. You might be misunderstood."

"Oh? How?"

"Well, it seems like you're trying to hurt me sometimes. I know you don't really mean to."

"Don't you get what's happening, Morton?" she said. "God is doing a number on me He's punishing me. He hates me. He's always hated me. And now—" She clenched her teeth. "Now look what you've done."

"What have I done?"

"I'm deformed. You can't deny that," she said blandly.

"Not badly deformed."

"But I'm the one who's had to pay. It all comes straight down to the soul. Everything in this rotten world comes right down to how dirty your soul is." Her eyelids closed, then bolted open again. "Sometimes the only way you can see these things is when you're on drugs," she added.

So true, he thought. On the other hand, it didn't seem mere Valium could have gotten her this high.

"Please stop, Annise. Can't you see you're making a fool of yourself?"

"Are you calling me a fool?"

Her eyes were wide and discerning. Something had clicked.

"I said, are you calling me a fool?"

"I guess I am," he said.

In a lightning bolt of motion her hand shot out to slap him. Morton caught it. After a moment she quit struggling.

"That's why I'm here," she mumbled.

"What?"

"I said, this is why I'm cut open and practically have cancer when I'm only twenty-three years old."

"What's the reason again?"

She puffed her cheeks. "Christ you're a shithead. Sin, Morton. *That's* the goddamn reason," she fumed.

"What about the other sick people, Annise? What about people around the world in hospitals? Are they all sick because of sin?"

"They're sick because of somebody you're on terribly intimate terms with. I suppose you know who I mean," she replied.

"Joseph?" he asked.

"*Lucifer*," she whispered hotly. Her voice was like gravel under the wheel of a truck.

Maybe she was right, he reflected. Maybe she could weasel enough credit to build a mansion on the fault line and have the Madonna keep it safe. Drink down her quart of wine each evening for the next thirty years and call the hangover hormones. Plenty of people lived that way, didn't they? Perhaps not in Oregon, but in west L.A. they sure did.

The counselor checked his watch. It was 2:10 p.m.

"I'm quite aware, thank you, how ugly and bad I am," she went on. "At first I wanted you to be nice to me. And damnit, you *were* nice. I couldn't believe it. Only it made me mad, Morton. Because people who are evil don't deserve being nice to. Frankly, that's why I get along with Joseph. Don't get me wrong. Some days I know I'm good and pretty. On them I deserve being nice to, but it hardly counts because of how bad I've been before, and I end up wasting the day in utter misery."

The counselor stroked her shoulder. "It's OK," he soothed, but he could feel her shudders.

"I ought to shoot myself," said Annise. "One pull of the trigger and put this stupid nightclub scene to sleep. None of the drinks are made right anyway."

Morton gripped the metal rail. For so long he'd tried to deny his hurt, but now it was flying at him full force.

"I've thought about it, you know," continued Annise. "Do you honestly believe my pistol was for that abortion nonsense?"

"You mean you lied about all that?"

"Ouch!" she exclaimed. She'd been moving too much. The wound was hurting her. Red blots appeared in the covers.

"Ever since the first day I met you I've been scared sick straight through myself. I mean like in horror movies when you're frightened half to death. Please, I'd rather you left now. I'll find a way home."

She whipped her head away. In so doing she happened to notice the flowers on the table. Morton slid them toward her.

"No," she muttered. "Get rid of them. Go ahead. Drop them in the trash can."

"Won't you smell them, Annise? I know they're your favorites." He held the vase toward her.

"Carnations?"

"Uh huh."

"This is a perfect example of our problem, Morton," she informed him. "What I *like* is totally irrelevant. What I *need* is a dozen super expensive *roses*. Champagne is better than brandy anytime, even if you hate champagne. I wish you'd get these ideas through your head."

She sighed heavily.

"I want you to disappear from my life," she said. "I've wanted that right from the beginning."

Morton happened to notice the bulge in his back pocket. He was visited by one of his dubious grayscale ideas, similar to the fitful Teenage Pregnancy Campaign, where his motives tended to run off the page. For once he decided to indulge it.

"All right, Annise. I'll leave," he said. "Only I'd like you to know, I took a long walk when you were in surgery, kind of sorting this out. I had a chance to pick up something special for you."

She looked hesitantly over her shoulder. "Really? Something besides the flowers?"

"Yes. I'd like to give it to you, if you'll have it. It might help cheer you up."

Her eyes opened big and girlish, like when he'd first met her. "Well, OK," she said.

Morton brought the small silver booklet from his back pocket.

"I didn't have a chance to wrap it," he said.

Annise gave a crooked smile and opened the cover. She began to flip through the book. Graphic photos were on every third page. They were in brilliant surrealistic color. The see-through angel and devil costumes bloomed vividly to life. He grinned over at her.

Annise's bosom began to heave. She shot bolt upright on the bed, her hindquarters taking all the pressure.

"What is this?" she asked, holding it between her red, quivering fingernails. "*The... The Laidman's Gospel?*"

She gazed dumbfounded at the booklet. Her eyes streaked to his, and for a split second a strange and pure truth ran between them.

"You're... You're trying to fuck with me," she sputtered.

She held the booklet far out in front of her. Her weight had fallen directly on the incision, but she didn't seem to notice.

"You're trying to twist my mind, aren't you?"

She said this so straightforwardly he went ahead and answered her.

"Well, yes. I guess I am," said Morton.

By weird terrified degrees her eyes lifted toward him. "Oh my God! You really *are* evil!" she moaned.

She dropped the booklet and thrust her hands to her face in disgust. With a sudden flash of venom she rose to her knees and swept the vase off the table. It shattered against the wall. The white heads of the carnations tore away from the stems and rebounded Helter Skelter across the tiling.

Many seconds went by. She was blinking and eyeballing everything except him. Morton observed her across a distance that seemed like a million miles. A sadness was there. And maybe she was right about this too. Maybe it had been there from the start.

The bandage was cockeyed and bright red. It was a crude sight. Gradually their gaze fell to the sheets. Together they ogled the wet, grapefruit sized blots of blood. Still more was throbbing out.

Annise went wobbly and lightheaded. She clutched the side rail to keep her balance. Morton was able to catch her by the shoulders as she lost consciousness and collapsed onto the mattress.

Something was very wrong. He lifted her gown. The dressing had worked completely off. The wound lay open like a torn orange rind, jagged and peeled up from the meat below. He sponged at the blood with a sheet end. He could see that the stitches were properly knotted at the ends, yes, but they weren't holding the wound together. He looked closely. They had been snipped through in the middle, or sliced maybe, reopening the incision.

Morton pressed the sopping bandage into place. In the folds of the covers he noticed several small green capsules. How did *they* get there?

He fished quickly through the sheets. He discovered four pills, altogether. Librium? Of course not. Dilaudid! A sudden intuition presented itself. The Jaguar! And as for the severed stitches, Joseph's razor knife had apparently found more action.

The counselor hit the red emergency call button. "Nurse!" he cried.

"What's the matter?" said someone from behind.

Morton spun. It was Wanda.

That's right, Joseph would have taken over at the Fraction House by now, planning for his encounter with Muriel.

At the Social Worker's unusual sounding pitch Annise began to come around.

"Is that you Gary?" she said wearily.

Wanda looked hurt. "Gary?" echoed the Social Worker.

"I think she's talking about the Assistant Priest over at St. Dunstan's," explained Morton. "From what I understand his voice is a little like yours. Try to forgive her. She's a bit out of it."

Wanda noticed the bloody mattress. While she was diverted, Morton slipped *The Laidman's Gospel* out of the covers and into his back pocket.

"Why is her dressing off? What have you done to her, Morton?" said Wanda.

The black nurse scurried in. Morton pointed to the zigzag of sutures. "They've come undone," he said. "See there."

The nurse jerked open a drawer and started applying gauze and elastic tape to stanch the bleeding. Wanda found a pair of scissors and tried to help.

Annise was exceedingly groggy. Morton leaned to her ear. "Someone cut your stitches, Annise. Tell me, was Joseph here?"

For an instant her eyes went clear as ice. "Yes," she said. "How did you know?"

"Did he make you take pills? Stay awake now." He shook her slightly. "Look." He opened his palm and showed her the capsules. "Did you take any of these?"

"Uh huh," she said.

"How many?"

"Two or three is all. They're pain killers, Morton. He doesn't want me to suffer."

"No pain in the hereafter, my friend," he countered. "Those pills are pure Dilaudid, Annise. I'm sure of it. They're what he gave you to give me instead of the Librium you thought it was."

"You're such a goddamn know it all," she fired. "Joseph came to make sure they did a good job of the surgery. He's not mad at me anymore. He's not like you. He wants us to be friends."

"He just tried to murder you and the baby, Annise."

"With drugs?"

"With drugs and his razor knife. He cut the stitches so you'd bleed out. Dilaudid and a big loss of blood and you'd be a goner for sure."

Annise squinted at him with her childlike confusion.

"Do you think the pills will hurt little Toni?" she asked.

"I don't know. Are you positive you only took two?"

"He tried to thumb a bunch of them into my mouth. I only swallowed two though. Somebody was coming so he said he had to run."

"He had to run, all right," muttered the counselor.

A male nurse in a white lab coat entered the room. He and the black woman conferred in secret. Morton could tell they knew the incision had been tampered with. They eyed him skeptically. Once again Joseph had set him up and gotten away with it. Why did doing the right thing always seem to incriminate a person?

Annise's eyelids twitched with the growing effects of the narcotic. Her pupils rolled upward into her skull. Suddenly she threw up, the debris spewing like quarters out of a slot machine over Morton's forearm.

"There's not supposed to be anything in her stomach! She had the instructions. Nothing by mouth after midnight!" cried the male nurse.

In a panic he tilted Annise's fine blonde head to the side.

Morton's eyebrows did not rise. Her lies had become so thick he'd come to expect full reversals by now. Eating before the surgery? Swallowing dangerous pills? Was she attempting suicide perhaps? And therefore attempting to murder her child to boot? Or was this simply stupidity combined with a hyper Catholic cover-up of her guilts? Was she really capable of caring for a little Toni, he worried?

Wanda had a sponge and was clearing the half chewed eggs from Annise's lips. Well, maybe the Social Worker knew how to raise a child, hoped the counselor. On the up side, he wouldn't have to mention the pills Annise had taken, since the residue had just been expelled with her breakfast.

The black nurse left the room. In a minute she returned with several other staff members. They hung tensely outside the cubicle. Morton realized he was under suspicion.

He checked his watch. It was almost three. He had to get out of there.

All at once he had a vision of Muriel naked in the Therapy Room tub. He shivered, and remembered she was going to need something to cover up with when the action started.

With a confident air of authority the counselor threw back his shoulders and strode to the wall hook which held Annise's wig and her bag of street clothes. Included was yesterday's blue satin robe, the one from The Green Room. Morton formed the fabric into a ball and shoved it in his pocket.

In the corridor he set his jaw and said, "Nurse, I want those sheets changed immediately. Get someone to clean up the broken glass and the mess on the floor. I don't know which of you is responsible for the broken sutures, but you can damn well bet I'm going to find out."

He hurled them one of Annise's slit-eyed looks, which said, 'Better cover your rosy red backsides, if you know what's good for you.' Then he walked briskly into the distance.

It was said that people got out of the way for a man who knew where he was going. It worked the same for a man who *pretended* he knew, didn't it? Doors opened fastest for the ones who raised the biggest stink. Right or wrong, this was The American Way.

* * *

Chapter 97

Morton parked at Vera's and walked up the hill to the Fraction House. The camcorder was already loaded with videotape and strapped diagonally across his chest.

According to the plan, Joseph should be well occupied by this time.

The counselor had Muriel's key to get in through the front doors. As he jogged the steps he caught sight of someone climbing the exterior fire escape leading to Harvey's window. He moved to the side of the building. It was Gordon. Already the blueprints were changing.

Every few seconds the paranoid glanced shakily behind, as was his habit. He wore a black beanie hat and a dark blue sweater, cat burglar style. He noticed Morton and gave a short wave.

Sunlight slanted sharply across the aging aluminum siding, placing the rickety iron stairs in a deep concealing shadow. Hmmm, not such a bad idea, reflected the counselor as Gordon disappeared through the window.

Morton looked up and down the street. He too scaled the fire escape. At the top Gordon helped him inside and snapped shut the window. The counselor's heart pounded in his ears. Harvey's wall clock read 3:45. So far, so good.

Gordon whispered, "Muriel said she could throw the latch on the window. She felt it'd be safer than Joseph maybe catching me in the hallway."

"Good thinking," agreed Morton.

The Custody Reinstatement papers were on Harvey's desk. Morton shuffled through them. Muriel had signed about half the stack, just as she said she would.

Gordon produced the two safe keys.

"You know what to do," said Morton.

Gordon nodded.

Buck Buchanan

"When you get hold of the tapes, go *back* down the fire escape. Then go in the front lobby and down to the laundry room. Don't risk running through the hallway," said Morton.

"All right," said Gordon.

The paranoid hiked up his pants and began to crawl under Harvey's—now Joseph's—giant mahogany desk.

Once again Morton confirmed the time. It was 3:51. Three minutes were left before the Gestapo would have to inspect the hallway to comply with his nutty six minute Obsessive/Compulsive checking intervals.

Morton stepped out of Harvey's office into the bright florescence of the hallway. He edged along the wall to the door of the Therapy Room. There was no point trying to listen in, what with it being soundproof to protect the super-secret goings on inside. He rotated the filming lens to face directly forward.

The huge elementary school wall clock clicked over to 3:53. Morton sucked his breath. One more minute and *all* their futures would be up for grabs. He half expected Stacy or maybe some weak-willed Perry Barwick to come pussyfooting up the stairway and around the corner. But he knew better. Joseph wouldn't be sloppy this time. Especially with Muriel caving in to his desires. Joseph would have sealed the place off with the Russian army to guard his petty ego.

The Gestapo was in there molesting Muriel. Going through his ritual Therapy Session paces, his despicable games of male and female dancing in a field of flaming carbuncles. Hell in the here and now, the kind of gimmicks which stoked the coals of your Annise Chastains maybe, but not of your wiser Muriel Gonskas.

What was it Muriel had told him? A person wasn't safe if they weren't protecting themselves? The world could do bad things. You had to at least put a forearm in front of your face to block the blows.

The counselor tapped at his pants pocket and felt the strange question-mark outline of steel riding against his thigh. This was Annise's derringer, which he'd stashed away in The Green Room.

'L.A. 2000:' Sex Asylum

A mouse like noise was emitted from the other side of the door. The scratching and hissing of the vampire, as shallow and ominous as the lit fuse on a bundle of dynamite.

Morton didn't know much about religion but he did have a grateful streak, for how else could you predict a criminal's exact behavior at the moment of truth without the psychic wonder of his crazed obsessions? Joseph *had* to open the door precisely thirty-six inches—his age this year—and also at precisely 3:54 p.m. Once a man had bought into his fetish, from dominatrix to snuffer films, the rest of the world became a figment to him, unreal, insubstantial, giving way to the sole maniacal vision that was his insanity.

A checking compulsion had more to do with checking than finding. The counselor watched as the long brass handle traveled to the open position.

The door creaked inward. Morton pivoted flush to the entrance. Although the camera was self-focusing he could not afford to look up lest the lens veer from its target. Capture the scene at all costs, that's what he was here for.

~~~

Morton looked downward to the tiny three inch screen of the viewfinder and pushed the red record button. Joseph was stark naked. A vile, hairy sight, the dark sausage unconcealed between his legs. Next came the Gestapo's glazed over shock of misapprehension Morton had hoped for.

The counselor thumbed the zoom to focus on the tub. Through the viewfinder a nude Muriel was standing in a few inches of water. Her wrists were locked together by Annise's silver handcuffs; her arms still wrapped in Trina's white gauze, only now water-soaked with spots of red beginning to leak through.

Right away Muriel struggled to reach for the key on the table. Her contortions caused Morton to cringe. It was all as she said it would be. This was real life. Harsh naked was plain harsh naked, far removed from the glitter-cloud illusions and drug addled gold-digging of The Green Room.

At the first flush of confrontation the Gestapo fell prey to his stylized jerks and gyrations. He shook it off quick though, and lunged for his pants.

To the counselor's surprise a scattering of the green Librium pills, which were Dilaudid, were laid out on the table, along with his cigarettes, lighter, razor knife, etc. Perfect! More incriminating evidence! Morton panned across the paraphernalia. He was getting valuable footage.

From behind came a noise. Morton turned to see Gordon pushing Harvey's ancient safe down the hallway. No longer was the floor kept super slippery like in the old days, and the metal base kicked up a nerve grating squeal as it cut into the linoleum.

The counselor bolted into the corridor. "Gordon, what the hell are you doing?" he cried.

"The keys wouldn't work, Morton. It was too heavy to take down the fire escape," he panted.

The paranoid's shoulder was pinned against the huge square of steel. Like a locomotive he continued to maneuver the safe toward the stairs.

"Did you turn the dial?" gasped Morton.

"What dial?"

"You've got to turn the dial to zero and throw the lever. I thought you knew that. Quick, Gordon, give me the keys."

The paranoid didn't seem to hear. With incredible strength he just kept driving the safe down the hallway.

Morton started to follow, but fearing for Muriel's safety he about-faced toward the Therapy Room.

Joseph Schopen's distorted face ballooned in front of him. So close the counselor could see blood encrusted sutures from where the beer mug had hit.

The Gestapo's razor knife swept through the air. Morton lunged backwards. The blade narrowly missed his midsection, making a metallic clatter as it crossed the body of the camcorder.

The counselor seized Joseph's forearm. But the Gestapo was stronger, and grasping Morton's hand he slowly coiled it around, bearing the knife tip down toward Morton's chest. The two hovered there in mid-struggle.

At the last instant the counselor whipped his elbow upward onto the heel of Joseph's palm. The knife twisted sideways, slashing through the nylon lanyard of the camcorder. The machine crashed to the floor and Morton had a flash the film would be ruined. But no, this was videotape. Even with the camera broken the evidence would still be there.

The Gestapo slammed his boot against the camcorder, like kicking a football. It rebounded wall to wall in the direction of Harvey's office.

Joseph gripped the knife so hard his knuckles went white. Morton was about to be run through, he knew it. He reached into his pocket. In the next instant his arm extended, aiming the *Smith & Wesson* point black at the Gestapo's forehead.

"Drop the knife, Schopen," said Morton.

The Gestapo looked where the video camera had come to rest near Harvey's office. Then he looked left to the other end of the hallway where Gordon was frantically spinning the safe dial and trying to simultaneously turn the keys.

Beyond Joseph, Morton could see Muriel inside the Therapy Room battling to free herself from the handcuffs. She still wasn't dressed.

"Drop it, Joseph," repeated the counselor. "I'm protecting my two best friends. I'll kill you if I have to."

Joseph was in his skin tight designer jeans. No shirt. His physique trim and impressive. Even the angular gash on his forehead appeared important, like an actor made up for exactly this role. The Gestapo hesitated a moment under the threat, as any full-blooded criminal would. He choked the handle of the knife.

Morton drew back the hammer on the pistol. The loud series of clicks awakened Joseph to how heavy this incident was.

Surprisingly, the Gestapo opened his fingers and let the knife fall away. He turned and started down the hall toward Gordon.

"Hold it, Joseph!"

Morton aimed the gun. Joseph ignored him.

The Gestapo said, "I know you, Allison. You'd never shoot an unarmed man. There's not a document in your alligator briefcase could get you out of that jam."

He proceeded toward Gordon.

Morton tore into the Therapy Room. The handcuffs proved too tight on Muriel's wrists for her to insert the key without help. They hadn't accounted for this. Morton quickly snapped them open, knocking over like dominoes the bottles of shampoo and perfumy creme rinses lining the tub. One was the high priced *Cloister Creme Rinse*, Annise's special brand. What was it doing *here*? In his heart though, he knew.

He pulled Annise's balled up robe from his pocket.

"Wear this," he said. "I got him on tape, Muriel. The camcorder's in front of Harvey's office. Run get it, then call the police."

Morton raced back into the hallway. He was met with the sight of Joseph's fist striking Gordon's head in a series of heart-sinking thuds. The awful sound reverberated across the cold wall tiling. Time after time the Gestapo slammed mercilessly into the paranoid's face, like in a street fight. He jerked at Gordon's balled palm for the safe keys, attempting to pry them from his fingers.

Morton ran so fast his vision went blurry. Joseph realized he was about to be tackled, and with a vicious spin landed a final savage punch on Gordon's jaw.

Suddenly the Gestapo had the keys. His last blow sent the paranoid tumbling down the steps, gripping helplessly at the banister, falling head over heels toward the long floor length window. A river of blood streamed around Gordon's eyes and cheeks as he collapsed on the landing.

Joseph was right. The counselor was not a cold blooded killer. In fact, he hardly remembered that the pistol was still in his hand as he closed on the Gestapo.

Joseph had tasted blood. He was in the chest beating flow of the fight, and he had a lot to protect. He was a weight trainer of sorts, but nothing prepared Morton for his sudden clean and jerk power lift of Harvey's safe. It rose as if levitated, then came hurtling toward him, a square of blackness which obliterated the gun and the counselor's great charge.

The safe struck him hard in the chest. Morton crunched to the floor. He sucked helplessly for breath. Was his lung punctured? The left side of his abdomen seemed caved in. Were his ribs snapped in two from the impact of the steel?

The pistol had sprung free. The Gestapo calmly stooped and picked it up, letting the muzzle dangle over Morton's head as he decided what to do next.

How much time had passed? A minute maybe? Twenty seconds? Where was Muriel?

The counselor clutched his side and craned his neck toward the far end of the hallway. The Sharp Viewcam was still on the floor. Joseph walked over and got it. He tied together the cut nylon strap and hung it over his neck. He saw the razor knife and picked that up too.

Morton gasped for air. He made an effort to stand, but found he could only grovel snail-like across the linoleum. He expected Joseph to turn into the Therapy Room for Muriel, but instead the Gestapo waltzed back to the safe and inserted the keys. Morton watched in agony as he spun the dial and dragged open the door. Calmly Joseph removed the tapes and put them in his back pocket.

It couldn't have gone any worse. The Gestapo was now in possession of every shred of evidence. Like it or not, he was home free.

"You're a murderer, Schopen," groaned Morton. "You might not pay today. But sooner or later you *are* going to pay."

"Nobody saw any murder," returned Joseph. "There's no evidence of murder."

"Saw? I *know*," said Morton.

Out of nowhere came one of the Gestapo's self-styled martial arts moves. The leather heel of his boot smashed into the bridge of Morton's nose. Blood spewed from his nostrils. The counselor blacked out for an instant, instinctively reaching toward the safe for support.

"You're a thief, Allison. You're robbing this place. You came in here armed." Joseph opened his hand and showed the pistol. "I've finally got the right to finish you off," said the Gestapo.

Slowly Joseph bent and wrapped his arms around the body of the safe.

On the landing below Morton could see Gordon starting to inch up the steps on his hands and knees. His lip was split. His eyes were bloody and puffy with cuts.

Morton pulled shallow breaths through his mouth to fight off the impulse to blackout. He pushed up to his elbow. Along the skewed angle of the flooring he saw Muriel edge out of the Therapy Room.

Joseph had the safe pressed chest high. The camcorder dangled around his neck.

"No!" cried Muriel flying down the corridor. Something was in her hand.

The rising safe cast a dark rectangle of shadow over the counselor's hunched torso. In another second his skull would be crushed. Muriel roared headlong toward the Gestapo.

"Stop, Muriel!" grunted Morton.

The counselor executed an erratic body roll, a veritable whirlwind of gut fortitude considering his busted ribs and the faucet of red running out his nose. Let the safe land where it may, he decided. And with the full force of his pain and rancor he whipped his legs into the Gestapo's ankles.

Joseph wavered, but did not fall. The safe teetered as he continued to drive it over his head. He split his legs to gain stability, to make certain the blow would be effective. The florescent overhead lighting, which came on automatically in the late afternoon, went dim as the Gestapo's inky form powered over the counselor like an eclipse.

A curious wetness traveled over Morton's trousers. He feared he had accidentally urinated. He could taste blood in his mouth. Desperately he struggled to remain conscious.

Urinated? No. This liquid was a slick, silica-like foam spreading out over the linoleum. Muriel was squeezing a plastic bottle of creme rinse, the super luxurious *Cloister* brand, under the Gestapo's slick-soled jodhpur boots. *Cloister Creme Rinse*—what a weapon!

Morton hugged his side to splint the pain. His eyes flooded with adrenaline. Here was his chance.

Muriel was squatting and squirting the creme rinse for all she was worth. The slimy mass lubricated the top floor landing like a coat of oil and dribbled over onto the first few steps. Morton could hear the plastic bottle squeaking and sputtering as more and more jetted out of the nozzle.

Once again the counselor gathered his courage. He hurled himself at the Gestapo's feet, rolling and lashing with his legs. Joseph's stance was wide apart. This time Morton connected with an ankle.

But that was enough. Muriel shot upward from her crouch and drove her shoulder into Joseph's hip. She was risking the giant safe collapsing on her. Joseph still had the pistol. He had his razor knife. She was gambling everything.

Then it happened. The safe door swung open as Joseph gyrated on the lubricated surface of the flooring. His feet skated from under him. Morton's kick and Muriel's shoulder lunge propelled the Gestapo backwards with an irretrievable momentum. Insanely, he did not let go of the safe. It was odd to see the ultra-cool ladies' man flailing like a clown for those seconds, his balance betraying him, his great Directorship reduced to a micro moment of terror and loathing for his enemies.

Morton could see hatred lasering from his eye. But hatred had always been in his eye, probably aimed at himself as much as at the rest of them.

Joseph's feet failed him. He stumbled on the top step. The two hundred pound pressure of the safe catapulted him head over heels down the stairs.

Gordon clutched the banister as the Gestapo and the clattering safe blew by. Muriel dove to Morton's side and held him tight around the shoulders.

Joseph's fall was doubled in speed by the weight of the steel safe. Strange what the mind will seize on in a crisis, for in the desperate tumble Morton kept seeing the iron door flopping open and shut in a kind of erotic slow motion. The Gestapo was like the picture of the atom with camcorder and metal box circling his cascading body in radical ellipses.

Like two shocked cats, Morton and Muriel lifted their heads. Joseph was going to hit the window. Had it ever been renovated to the shatterproof Plexiglas Morton had pushed for?

The safe separated from the Gestapo's hands. It plunged into the glass barrier with the sound of a lightning crack. The window buckled outward, leaving a huge gaping hole. Triangles of thick diamond-sharp glass forked in a weird kaleidoscope symmetry around the circle.

Unable to slow his fate, the Gestapo dive-bombed face first through the jagged mouth of glass. Morton and Muriel watched in disbelief as the bottom knives of crystal slit Joseph's gut diagonally from the liver to the top of the thigh. He was dissected before their very eyes, deep and bloody, like a long scalpel cut in an autopsy.

Joseph's bloodcurdling scream splintered the cool Los Angeles twilight as he plummeted down two and a half stories of thin air.

A milli-instant passed, followed by the gruesome sound of the Gestapo landing splat on the courtyard pavement.

And then—an echo chamber of silence! A vacuum of tile and Dura-lubed linoleum in the closed cylinder of the stairwell.

No safe. No camcorder. No wicked little derringer. All that remained was an eerie Halloween quiet, the likes of which had never been heard around the Fraction House.

Morton and Muriel owl-necked one another. Funny, there seemed no emotion in them at the very time when all the big emotion was coming down. The counselor recognized this phenomenon as Harvey's psycho-sensitive FUD factor: Fear! Uncertainty! Doubt! And all three stonewalling in your gut in order to come to terms with the gory details.

~~~

Muriel helped Morton down the stairs to the landing, her white forearm bandages unwinding behind them like lace off the long train of a wedding dress.

Gordon hobbled over, and together the three of them gazed dumbfounded through the shattered plate glass window. What they saw was repulsive beyond belief. Morton looked quickly to the paranoid. Gordon looked back as if to say, 'Any witnesses?'

"Look," said Muriel, her hair tossed about by gusts of late July wind streaming through the blown out serrations of the window. She pointed across the quadrangle.

"It's Annise over there by E-Wing," she said. "And I think that's Wanda beside her."

She was right. The stocky Social Worker and the svelte, aching-heart Catholic were clinging to each other outside the E-Wing doors. Apparently the blonde's surgery, together with Joseph's butcher job on the sutures hadn't left her as bad off as Morton first thought. Their mouths dangled open like people in pictures of when Jesus was on the cross—awestruck, and without an Antichrist Joseph Schopen to backlight their tumble-down world.

* * *

Chapter 98

There was no time to lose.
"Are you hurt bad, Gordon?" said the counselor.
"I'm all right. I'll go get the tapes. I'll do what we said with them."
He turned and jogged down the stairs.
For the first time since Morton had known him, Gordon did not look behind. He hardly seemed paranoid. Suddenly the counselor realized that it was Joseph who had been Gordon's paranoia problem all along. Who wouldn't be worried with a man like the Gestapo forever sneaking up behind him?
"We have to get downstairs," said Morton to Muriel.
She steadied him. They made their way to the first floor.
The counselor used the phone in the Staff Lounge to summon an ambulance. Then he and Muriel hobbled through the laundry room and out to the courtyard.
There was a U-shaped crush mark on Joseph's chest, like a horse's hoof. Somehow he must have somersaulted the safe in mid-air, for the metal edge had crashed into his sternum, doubling his injuries. He lay there filleted to the organs like a giant salmon, bleeding out in bushels over the cold cement. All just a few feet, reflected Morton, from where Harvey's ashes had recently been scattered.
A moment of everything hovering still as a number of the clients—Sam, Odette, Sally, and others—began to assemble behind the glass-encased hallway leading from C-Wing to the cafeteria. Their faces pressed distortedly against the windows. Insane looking people, yes, but once you got to know them not so insane. Their emotions? This was easy to interpret. Relief!
Gordon wasn't finicky. The more death entering the world was, according to his synthetic doctrine, a movie review on how backwards life traveled to begin with. Nothing to be frightened of there.

The paranoid walked directly to the pile of blood and guts that was Joseph slowly dying. The tapes, along with the pistol, the razor knife, and miscellaneous inner safe stuff had spilled in a parachute circle around the Gestapo. The camcorder lay a slight distance away. The housing was cracked, the lenses broken.

Morton and Muriel stepped over to the smashed Viewcam. The counselor removed the videotape and placed it in the pocket of his purple blazer.

As he did this he noticed several Polaroid photographs on the concrete. He bent down to look one over. It was a picture of Sally Featherman naked in the tub. A man's hand, Joseph's hand, was holding her still for the next installment of molestation. Perverts liked to see their handiwork objectified, recalled Morton. Well, it was more proof of the Gestapo's dirty deeds. The counselor gathered the scattered photos and slipped them in his pocket. They might be needed if Joseph survived his injuries, for Morton could see his chest still rising the slightest degree.

Gordon picked up the porn cassettes. "I'll dispose of these. I'll do it now," he said loud enough for Joseph to hear.

Like eyes in a severed head, the Gestapo glared blankly upward at the paranoid.

Gordon pried out the brown videotape with his fingernails and began ripping it from the plastic casing. The strand got longer and longer until it coiled over the pavement and snaked into Joseph's expanding stain of blood. Gordon did the same to the second cassette, the copy. Then he ground them both to bits with his feet, a macabre little dance of death around the human campfire.

Stacy Lung burst through the E-Wing doors. She bumped Wanda aside and rushed toward Joseph.

"Oh, my God!" she exclaimed, kneeling over him.

She reached to embrace him, but the Gestapo's condition was such a train wreck she couldn't find a safe place to touch.

"I called for an ambulance," said Morton. "It should be here any minute." The counselor heard a muffle in his voice. His nose had stopped bleeding, but red stains were veined down the front of his shirt and jacket.

Stacy backed slowly toward the center of the courtyard, all the while flitting severe eye contact between Morton and Joseph's zombie body. The counselor knew Stacy too well. In her eyes hung a sign which said, 'I really liked him, only now I don't have a date. And it's all due to you.'

Woodenly, Stacy said, "The ambulance should have been here by now. I'm going to call again." She scurried away.

Wanda and Annise edged up to Joseph's side, Annise limping noticeably. She should have been home in bed.

Morton and Muriel stood opposite them, shoulder to shoulder, staring down at the nauseating spectacle. Which was all anyone could do. It was like in a war where irretrievable damage left the healthy inept to offer aid and placed them on the extreme outside of the dying man's system of souls.

Wanda and Annise seemed dazed. They looked up to the jagged holed window on the second floor. Strange how no one commented on the specifics of what had happened. Not even Stacy. It was as if it *must* have occurred in exactly this way, and no one questioned it.

"I thought you were confined to bedrest, Annise," said Morton.

"She is," interjected Wanda. "She insisted on riding over here. She wants to come clean with Joseph."

"Come clean?" echoed Morton.

"Annise decided to confront him," said Wanda. "It's his baby. She's going after everything he's got. Legally, she's entitled to a hell of a lot. Maybe even Wojeck's fifty thousand."

Joseph's eyes were clouded from blood loss. He was immobile, but it was obvious he'd heard.

Annise held her belly. She looked down at the Gestapo.

"I'm going after your car," she said hard. "I'm going to take your bank account. I'm even going after your drug money."

Joseph began to jerk violently. He was in his death throes. It was looking like the two women would be raising little Toni.

But there was something awkward telegraphing between them. Did Annise and Wanda really want to be together? Or was this your post modern union of convenience, L.A. style, much like Morton's had been with Stacy? He detected not the warm, 'Hey, now we're together' look; but rather the, 'Hey, *now what*!' expression.

At last the counselor and the schizophrenic were arm in arm in public, a bona-fide couple anointed with the sacrificial blood of the enemy. Annise and Wanda looked them up and down, mystified to the core.

Finally they heard the sirens.

Annise and Wanda started walking away. No prayers this time. No swell clichés about some incomprehensible Harmonic Convergence up in the heavens.

Joseph's eyes moved minutely as they left, then rotated vacantly back to Morton and Muriel.

He gave a classic inward gasp for wind, exhaled, and died.

* * *

Chapter 99

There was only one thing in the world a person did on their own. And that was die. All else involved others. Morton breathed nervously. Being born, he knew, and every aspect of life thereafter, was social. But when you met your end you were the only individual ever who was *you*, and who in the next instant would no longer be you. It was a unique event, a disappearing act so effective only the most creative mythology could finagle a way to smuggle someone back. No matter who you were or how bad or good the time between had been, only one solitary event would be forever yours and yours alone. Your death. Think about it. Christ, it gave you cause to search for love.

These were the counselor's thoughts as he and Muriel moved slowly away from the dead man.

~~~

The ambulance arrived. A team of three paramedics hustled toward the body. They were obliged to apply resuscitative measures, but Morton knew it was too late.

Priscilla Daddio waltzed in, kid leather briefcase and all. What was she doing here?

That's right, remembered Morton, Priscilla monitored the police scanner round the clock, hoping against hope for this very scenario. At heart, she was an opportunist. She strode directly to the Gestapo and made her clinical assessment.

"Joseph Schopen is dead," declared Priscilla, the wheels under her widow's peak turning fast and furious.

Morton kept waiting for the one-two punch of threats and accusation. He was almost used to it. But not even Priscilla bothered to ask for the details.

She went to Wanda. "Legally, the state takes charge in emergencies such as these," said Priscilla. "Joseph's

Directorship falls immediately to Roselawn's senior Clinical Supervisor."

Wanda crossed her arms defensively.

"And Priscilla is this person," said Priscilla.

"You don't have a mandate unless a judge gives it to you," objected Wanda. "I'm next in charge here under Joseph. That means *I'm* the acting Director."

The two jawed on. A lot of hands on hips. Much frumping of the lips.

Gordon had bowed out. He now reappeared and tugged Morton aside.

"Here's Muriel's mail," he said. "I picked it up Saturday when I was at her apartment."

"Thanks," said Morton. He shuffled through it. "Hmmm. There's a letter from Wojeck. That's odd."

"You two need to beat the feet out of here," said the paranoid. "The police'll have to comb through this for hours. And they might still enforce that injunction."

"Morton's not leaving," interrupted Priscilla over her shoulder. "The authorities are going to need a full explanation."

"I witnessed the whole thing from right over there," said Wanda nodding toward E-Wing. "Can't you see Morton's hurt? He needs to go to the hospital."

"I saw it too," said Annise. "Joseph was trying to kill Morton. The lights had just come on upstairs." She pointed to the blown out hole in the Gestapo's peeping Tom window. "He's a murderer. He killed Harvey. It'll all come out soon enough."

True or not, Priscilla wasn't buying it. She'd insist on investigations, judicial committees, the whole ball of wax.

Annise and Wanda joined hands. Priscilla didn't raise an eyebrow. Who knew, maybe she went their way too.

Gordon whispered to Morton. "I'll distract Daddio while you all get away. She wants to do to me what Joseph did to Muriel."

"She wants to rape you?" said the counselor.

Gordon giggled. "I'm talking about my funding, Morton. I'm close to my own Guardianship. I've been acting out, I guess.

Priscilla wants me back at Roselawn. But if she gets Wanda's Directorship she'll want me here. We've got lots to talk about."

Priscilla interjected, "Why in the world is Muriel dressed this way, may Priscilla ask?"

For the first time Morton realized Muriel was still wearing Annise's skimpy robe from The Green Room, the one with cowgirl fringes just south of the border.

He was reminded of the night which had kicked off this crazy business. He'd come back from the mountains, alone and exhausted. The paramedics swarming over Muriel. The stains of blood on his carpet, on her dress. Annise confused and aimless, hanging limply around the periphery. And Priscilla Daddio trying to horn in for the big bucks, as usual.

Gordon stepped over and boldly tucked a curl of Priscilla's hair back around her ear. He began talking quietly to her. The paranoid possessed a charm so phony bigwigs were invariably convinced of his honesty and disarmed by it. In seconds he had Priscilla wrapped around his little finger. The counselor could practically see her ears perking up as Gordon articulated the tricky ins and outs of his funding block.

Morton saw his opportunity. He nudged Muriel. She gave a nod, took him by the hand and together they rambled through the laundry room and down the long corridor past the cafeteria.

All of a sudden his ribs didn't seem so urgent. Maybe they hadn't cracked in half after all.

A feeling of freedom wider than the state of Oregon swept around him like clean mountain air. They pushed through the grand double doors in the lobby, and fairly danced down the concrete steps to his truck.

* * *

Chapter 100

Whatever the extent of his injuries, Morton found he was able to drive. They were riding high above the ground. The engine sounded strong and solid.

No, be honest, the engine was backfiring and sputtering. It was weak as water, if he looked at it clearly. Quite a difference in interpretation there, decided the counselor as he turned onto La Brea and headed north toward the freeway.

Morton was under the pink umbrella of an exhilarating new perspective. Something like—well, like seeing reality. Like if you could experience the miracle of a single flower with perfect clarity your world would suddenly enlarge. It finally dawned on him how close to the junkyard his truck really was. Well, truth was truth. Accept it and move on.

Muriel scooted across the seat and hugged him around the neck. She nuzzled into his shoulder. He rested his hand on her knee. They hit a bump and it bounced to her thigh. A *bare* thigh, for Godsake, since she was still clad in the provocative Green Room robe. For many minutes they rode close like that.

"We're not running away," said Morton. "We'll have to deal with the police. Give statements or something."

"I know you wouldn't run," said Muriel.

"We might take a short vacation though. Kind of clear our heads before we get into another shoot out."

"A vacation? You mean like to Oregon? Somewhere like, I don't know, to Oregon maybe?"

"There's nothing to force you back to the Fraction House, Muriel. I've got the Sharp video I shot of Joseph right here if we have to prove anything." He tapped his jacket pocket. "We're not in jeopardy."

"I signed a bunch of papers in Joseph's office," countered Muriel.

"I saw them. We're safe there too. You'd have to have signed every last one to make it legal. You only got through about half."

They were quiet a moment.

Morton said, "The camcorder's ruined. It'll costs nine hundred dollars to replace. I'll have to find a way to pay Rip's."

"I'll be able to get a job now. I'll help you pay for it," said Muriel.

The counselor smiled. "Thanks. But I'm afraid there's work left for me at the Fraction House. Gordon is almost free, you know. And now with this big blow up Priscilla's going to try to steal his Guardianship. I can't let that happen."

"You're such a good man," said Muriel.

"You really think so?"

"I really think so."

They looked each other in the eyes. Only a fool wouldn't have felt the large and startling heat running between them. At last it was all feeling right. Yes, right and pure and truly good. And yet someone had died. Was the world at a loss because of it? Or was the world a *better* place because of it? This was your yardstick. Joseph's death? No matter how he analyzed it, the counselor couldn't find the tragedy.

~~~

At Beverly Boulevard Muriel noticed a sign pointing west toward Cedars-Sinai.

"We better run down to the Emergency Room," she said. "You're alive, Morton. And I'm going to keep you alive if it's the last thing I ever do."

There was one final piece of important business on the agenda. Morton bypassed the turn. He'd see to it now. Dried blood was encrusted in his beard. Muriel tried to dust it off.

"I must look a sight," said the counselor.

She reached around his mid-section to support the damaged ribs. She was no nurse, and Morton winced with pain.

"I'm sorry," she said. As she eased away she noticed the bulge in his back pocket.

"What's this?" she asked pulling out the sexy silver booklet he'd purchased back at the card shop. "*The Laidman's Gospel*?"

She turned through a few pages. Her eyes opened wide and crisp, shining it on with those magnetic aquamarine glaciers. Offended, worried Morton?

Miraculously, she grinned and turned another page.

She likes it, he realized! She actually likes it! What an incredible woman, he thought, as he watched her beginning to snicker at the jokes. And not a flimsy piece of one either, but the entire thing top to bottom, just like she'd told him.

"This is filthy," said Muriel looking over.

"I know. That's why I bought it for you," agreed Morton.

She flipped on through the pictures. She grinned mischievously, leaned and kissed him on the cheek.

"Thank you, Morton. I'll study it very hard. There's an awful lot about beautiful dirty lovemaking I don't know yet."

~~~

The counselor zoomed up the ramp of Hollywood Freeway and powered north. Muriel began leafing through the packet of mail Gordon had given them. She opened Wojeck's envelope.

"I wonder what Dad has to say," she muttered furrowing her brow.

Nervously, she peeked inside. Something startled her. Her palm shot to her chest as if to stop the flutters.

"Look at this. I think— I think it's fifty thousand dollars."

"It's what?"

"Fifty thousand dollars. It's the yearly check my father gives the Fraction House. Only it's not in Joseph's name. Or Harvey's either."

"Who's name is it in?" asked the counselor.

She held up what Morton recognized as an Insured Cashier's Check.

"He wrote a message. It's to you, Morton," said Muriel. "It says, '*I'm sorry for what I did in the old days. My daughter is her own free Guardian now. I love her. I know you're the only one big enough to take care of her, Morton. Best wishes, W.G.*'"

The counselor examined the check as they rumbled up the freeway.

"This is very weird, Muriel," he said at last. "Did you see? It's made out in the names of Morton Allison and Muriel Allison. It's actually typed in like that."

"What does it mean?" she said.

"It means we can't cash it unless we both sign the way it's written."

"So it's no good?"

"Not as long as our names are different. We'd have to both be Allisons. We'd have to show valid identification. You know, rubber stamps and notary seals, stuff like that."

Muriel looked over at him. "But we're not both Allisons," she said.

Her lips formed a sweet, unpresumptuous pout Morton was recognizing as unchained sensuality. That Muriel. She was a naïve puppy, maybe, but not *this* naïve.

All at once life seemed so natural. So... Well, *real*. He wasn't simply having a new look at his truck, this was a new look at *all* trucks, at everything on wheels, particularly womanhood. It was nothing like the ladies' polo match galloping around The Green Room. It was nothing like Annise Chastain either, the archetypal femme fatale, supposedly.

Morton exited the freeway.

"Is this the way to the hospital?" asked Muriel.

"It's important we straighten out any funky, leftover documents. Like your father's check, for instance. Like us being mistaken as counselor and client, for instance. My briefcase with all your fancy forms is right under the seat. The powers that be do not like it when names and titles and certain certificates don't come into line with the rest of their paperwork. We've got to change that."

"Conform?" she cried spontaneously.

"Why not, as long as it's a labor of love? I mean, you know, being pure and honest inside yourself regarding who you want to live with for the rest of your life. Absolutely yes, conform. That's what I say."

As if by divine intervention a great stone edifice appeared ahead. Morton pulled along the curb. Although she'd been here numerous times before, Muriel stared in awe at the giant building.

"Morton, this isn't the hospital! It's the Courthouse!"

He nodded.

"You weren't even planning on going to the hospital, were you?"

"I'll go. But first I need to marry you up. I don't want anybody else having claims on you. Only me. Only your husband." With dignity he added, "If you'll have me."

"If I'll have you? Only a certified nut would say no to an offer like that!"

Muriel leapt into Morton's arms. They hugged for a long time. Then they kissed.

THE END

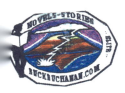

~ ABOUT THE AUTHOR ~

Buck Buchanan and his wife, Sandy St. Pierre, spent 7 years between south Florida and the Bahamas aboard their Morgan OutIsland sailboat, ***Gravity's Rainbow***. They relocated to a log cabin in the Appalachian Mountains of Southwest Virginia where Buchanan completed his novel, ***'L.A. 2000:' Sex Asylum***, and began assembling a collection of his published short stories entitled, ***'Imperative Orgy:' The Sweetwater of Suburbia***.

Buchanan has published in numerous literary magazines, professionally written and edited nonfiction texts, books of poetry, and novels. He supervised Group Homes for Autistic Children in San Francisco, and for Retarded Citizens in the Experimental Community of Columbia, Maryland. ***'L.A. 2000:' Sex Asylum*** won the Virginia Highlands Literary Contest in the novel category.

Buck Buchanan's writing resonates with a fast-paced narrative style turned with a voice that is at once polished and hardcore. As his titles indicate, these works present a notably unconventional approach to progressive, thought-provoking literature, highlighting the glossy sparkle of tomorrow's bizarre unreality.

Buchanan and his wife are currently aboard their Winnebago Motor Home where he is at work on his new novel, ***'The Mad Beach:' Follies & Fornications***. He holds a Master of Arts Degree in Literature from the University of South Florida.

'Imperative Orgy:' The Sweetwater of Suburbia, is now previewable on his website at BUCKBUCHANAN.COM.

* * *

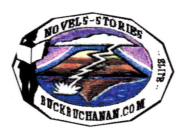